MW00345742

Copyright © 2021 by Sam Thomason -All rights reserved.

No part of this publication may be reproduced, distributed, or transmitted in any form or by any means, including photocopying, recording, or other electronic or mechanical methods, without the prior written permission of the publisher, except in the case of brief quotations embodied in reviews and certain other non-commercial uses permitted by copyright law.

This Book is provided with the sole purpose of providing relevant information on a specific topic for which every reasonable effort has been made to ensure that it is both accurate and reasonable. Nevertheless, by purchasing this Book you consent to the fact that the author, as well as the publisher, are in no way experts on the topics contained herein, regardless of any claims as such that may be made within. It is recommended that you always consult a professional prior to undertaking any of the advice or techniques discussed within.This is a legally binding declaration that is considered both valid and fair by both the Committee of Publishers Association and the American Bar Association and should be considered as legally binding within the United States.

CONTENTS

VEGETARIAN & VEGAN RECIPES

Creamy Gnocchi With Peas

INGREDIENTS for Servings: 2

1 pack gnocchi	1 tbsp butter
½ thinly sliced sweet onion	½ cup frozen peas
	¼ cup heavy cream
Salt and black pepper to taste	½ cup grated Pecorino Romano cheese

DIRECTIONS and Cooking Time: 1 Hour 50 Minutes
Prepare a water bath and place the Sous Vide in it. Set to 183 F. Place the gnocchi in a vacuum-sealable bag. Release air by the water displacement method, seal and submerge the bag in the water bath. Cook for 1 hour and 30 minutes. Once the timer has stopped, remove the bag and set aside. Heat a skillet over medium heat with butter and sauté the onion for 3 minutes. Add the frozen peas and cream and cook. Combine the gnocchi with the cream sauce, season with pepper and salt and serve in a plate.

Sweet Red Beet Dish

INGREDIENTS for Servings: 4

1 pound red beets, peeled and quartered	Salt and black pepper to taste
2 tbsp butter	6 oz baby romaine leaves
2 peeled oranges, chopped	½ cup pistachios, chopped
1 tbsp honey	½ cup Pecorino Romano cheese
3 tbsp balsamic vinegar	
4 tbsp olive oil	

DIRECTIONS and Cooking Time: 1 Hour 45 Minutes
Prepare a water bath and place the Sous Vide in it. Set to 182 F. Place the red beets in a vacuum-sealable bag. Add the butter Release air by the water displacement method, seal and submerge the bag in the water bath. Cook for 90 minutes. Once the timer has stopped, remove the bag and discard the cooking juices. Combine the honey, oil and vinegar. Season with salt and pepper. Throw the romaine leaves, orange, beets, and vinaigrette. Garnish with pistachio and Pecorino Romano cheese.

Curry Pears & Coconut Cream

INGREDIENTS for Servings: 4

2 pears, cored, peeled and sliced	1 tbsp curry powder
	2 tbsp coconut cream

DIRECTIONS and Cooking Time: 1 Hour 10 Minutes
Prepare a water bath and place the Sous Vide in it. Set to 186 F. Combine all the ingredients and place in a vacuum-sealable bag. Release air by the water displacement method, seal and submerge the bag in the water bath. Cook for 60 minutes. Once the timer has stopped, remove the bag and transfer to a large bowl. Divide in serving plates and serve.

Delightful Tofu With Sriracha Sauce

INGREDIENTS for Servings: 10

1 cup vegetable broth	1 tbsp rice wine
2 tbsp tomato paste	1 tbsp agave nectar
1 tbsp grated ginger	2 tsp Sriracha sauce
1 tbsp ground nutmeg	3 minced garlic cloves
1 tbsp rice wine vinegar	2 boxes cubed tofu

DIRECTIONS and Cooking Time: 1 Hour 10 Minutes
Prepare a water bath and place the Sous Vide in it. Set to 186 F. Combine well all the ingredients, except for the tofu. Place the tofu with the mixture in a vacuum-sealable bag. Release air by the water displacement method, seal and submerge the bag in the water bath. Cook for 60 minutes. Once the timer has stopped, remove the bag and transfer into a bowl.

Mushroom Soup

INGREDIENTS for Servings: 3

1 lb mixed mushrooms	2 tbsp thyme powder
2 onions, diced	2 tbsp olive oil
3 cloves garlic	2 cups cream
2 sprigs parsley leaves, chopped	2 cups vegetable stock

DIRECTIONS and Cooking Time: 50 Minutes
Make a water bath, place Sous Vide in it, and set to 185 F. Place the mushrooms, onion, and celery in a vacuum-sealable bag. Release air by the water displacement method, seal and submerge the bag in the water bath. Set the timer for 30 minutes. Once the timer has stopped, remove and unseal the bag. Blend the ingredients from the bag in a blender. Put a pan over medium heat, add olive oil. Once it starts to heat, add in pureed mushrooms and the remaining ingredients, except for the cream. Cook for 10 minutes. Turn off heat and add cream. Stir well and serve.

Grape Vegetable Mix

INGREDIENTS for Servings: 9

8 sweet potatoes, sliced	1 tsp minced garlic
2 red onions, sliced	Salt and black pepper

4 ounces tomato, pureed	to taste 1 tsp grape juice

DIRECTIONS and Cooking Time: 105 Minutes
Prepare a water bath and place Sous Vide in it. Set to 183 F. Place all the ingredients with ¼ cup water in a vacumm-sealable bag.Release air by the water displacement method, seal and submerge the bag in water bath. Set the timer for 90 minutes. Once the timer has stopped, remove the bag. Serve warm.

Green Pea Cream With Nutmeg

INGREDIENTS for Servings: 8

1 pound fresh green peas 1 cup whipping cream ¼ cup butter 1 tbsp cornstarch	¼ tsp ground nutmeg 4 cloves 2 bay leaves Black pepper to taste

DIRECTIONS and Cooking Time: 1 Hour 10 Minutes
Prepare a water bath and place the Sous Vide in it. Set to 184 F. Combine the cornstarch, nutmeg and cream into a bowl. Whisk until the cornstarch soften. Place the mixture in a vacuum-sealable bag. Release air by the water displacement method, seal and submerge the bag in the water bath. Cook for 1 hour. Once the timer has stopped, extract the bag and remove the bay leaf. Serve.

Effortless Pickled Fennel With Lemon

INGREDIENTS for Servings: 8

1 cup apple cider vinegar 2 tbsp sugar Juice and zest from 1 lemon	Salt to taste 2 bulb fennels, sliced ½ tsp fennel seeds, crushed

DIRECTIONS and Cooking Time: 40 Minutes
Prepare a water bath and place the Sous Vide in it. Set to 182 F. Combine well the vinegar, sugar, lemon juice, salt, lemon zest and fennel seeds. Place the mixture in a vacuum-sealable bag. Release air by the water displacement method, seal and submerge the bag in the water bath. Cook for 30 minutes. Once the timer has stopped, remove the bag and transfer to an ice-water bath. Allow cooling.

Allspice Miso Corn With Sesame & Honey

INGREDIENTS for Servings: 4

4 ears of corn 6 tbsp butter	1 tbsp canola oil 1 scallion, thinly sliced

3 tbsp red miso paste 1 tsp honey 1 tsp allspice	1 tsp toasted sesame seeds

DIRECTIONS and Cooking Time: 45 Minutes
Prepare a water bath and place the Sous Vide in it. Set to 183 F. Clean the corn and cut the ears. Cover each corn with 2 tbsp of butter. Place in a vacuum-sealable bag. Release air by the water displacement method, seal and submerge the bag in the water bath. Cook for 30 minutes. Meanwhile, combine 4 tbsp of butter, 2 tbsp of miso paste, honey, canola oil, and allspice in a bowl. Stir well. Set aside. Once the timer has stopped, remove the bag and sear the corn. Spread the miso mixture on top. Garnish with sesame oil and scallions.

Buttered Peas With Mint

INGREDIENTS for Servings: 2

1 tbsp butter 1 tbsp mint leaves, chopped	½ cup snow peas A pinch salt Sugar to taste

DIRECTIONS and Cooking Time: 25 Minutes
Make a water bath, place Sous Vide in it, and set to 183 F. Place all the ingredients in a vacuum-sealable bag. Release air by the water displacement method, seal and submerge in the bath. Cook for 15 minutes. Once the timer has stopped, remove and unseal the bag. Transfer the ingredients to a serving plate. Serve as a condiment.

Lemon & Garlic Artichokes

INGREDIENTS for Servings: 4

4 tablespoons freshly squeezed lemon juice 12 pieces' baby artichokes 4 tablespoons vegan butter 2 fresh garlic cloves, minced	1 teaspoon fresh lemon zest Kosher salt, and black pepper, to taste Chopped up fresh parsley for garnishing

DIRECTIONS and Cooking Time: 90 Minutes
Prepare the Sous Vide water bath using your immersion circulator and raise the temperature to 180-degrees Fahrenheit. Take a large bowl and add the cold water and 2 tablespoons of lemon juice. Peel and discard the outer tough layer of your artichoke and cut them into quarters. Transfer to a cold water bath and let it sit for a while. Take a large skillet and put it over medium high heat. Add in the butter to the skillet and allow the butter to melt. Add the garlic alongside 2 tablespoons of lemon juice and the zest. Remove from heat and season with a bit of pepper and salt. Allow it to cool for about 5 minutes. Then, drain the artichokes from the cold water and place them in a large resealable bag. Add in the butter

mixture as well. Seal it up using the immersion method and submerge underwater for about 1 and a ½ hour. Once cooked, transfer the artichokes to a bowl and serve with a garnish of parsley.

Nutrition Info: Per serving:Calories: 408 ;Carbohydrates: 49g ;Protein: 12g ;Fat: 20g ;Sugar: 5g ;Sodium: 549mg

Poached Tomatoes

INGREDIENTS for Servings: 3

4 cups cherry tomatoes 5 tbsp olive oil ½ tbsp fresh rosemary leaves, minced	½ tbsp fresh thyme leaves, minced Salt and black pepper to taste

DIRECTIONS and Cooking Time: 45 Minutes
Make a water bath, place Sous Vide in it, and set to 131 F. Divide the listed ingredients into 2 vacuum-sealable bags, season with salt and pepper. Release air by the water displacement method and seal the bags. Submerge them in the water bath and set the timer to cook for 30 minutes. Once the timer has stopped, remove the bags and unseal. Transfer the tomatoes with the juices into a bowl. Serve as a side dish.

Lovely Kidney Bean & Carrot Stew

INGREDIENTS for Servings: 8

1 cup dried kidney beans, soaked overnight 1 cup water ½ cup olive oil 1 carrot, chopped 1 celery stalk, chopped	1 quartered shallot 4 crushed garlic cloves 2 fresh rosemary sprigs 2 bay leaves Salt and black pepper, to taste

DIRECTIONS and Cooking Time: 3 Hours 15 Minutes
Prepare a water bath and place the Sous Vide in it. Set to 192 F. Strain the beans and wash them. Place in a vacuum-sealable bag with olive oil, celery, water, carrot, shallot, garlic, rosemary, and bay leaves. Season with salt and pepper. Release air by the water displacement method, seal and submerge the bag in the water bath. Cook for 180 minutes. Once the timer has stopped, remove the beans. Discard bay leaves and the rosemary.

Spicy Black Beans

INGREDIENTS for Servings: 6

1 cup dry black beans 3 cups water 1/3 cup lemon juice 2 tbsp lemon zest	Salt to taste 1 tsp cumin ½ tsp chipotle chili powder

DIRECTIONS and Cooking Time: 6 Hours 15 Minutes
Prepare a water bath and place Sous Vide in it. Set to 193 F. Place all the ingredients in a vacuum-sealable bag. Release air by the water displacement method, seal and submerge the bag in the water bath. Cook for 6 hours. Once the timer has stopped, remove the bag and transfer into a hot saucepan over medium heat and cook until reduced. Remove from the heat and serve.

Vegan Alfredo

INGREDIENTS for Servings: 6

4 cups chopped cauliflower 2 cups water 2/3 cup cashews ½ teaspoon dried oregano ½ teaspoon dried basil	2 garlic cloves ½ teaspoon dried rosemary 4 tablespoons nutritional yeast Salt, and pepper to taste

DIRECTIONS and Cooking Time: 90 Minutes
Prepare the Sous-vide water bath using your immersion circulator and increase the temperature to 170-degrees Fahrenheit. Take a heavy-duty resealable zip bag and add the cashews, cauliflower, oregano, water, garlic, rosemary, and basil. Seal using the immersion method. Submerge underwater and cook for 90 minutes. Transfer the cooked contents to a blender and puree. Use the Alfredo over your favorite pasta.

Nutrition Info: Per serving:Calories: 160 ;Carbohydrates: 10g ;Protein: 8g ;Fat: 11g ;Sugar: 1g ;Sodium: 282mg

Tofu Delight

INGREDIENTS for Servings: 8

2 tablespoons tomato paste 1 tablespoon grated ginger 1 tablespoon rice wine 1 tablespoon rice wine vinegar	1 cup vegetable broth 1 tablespoon agave nectar 2 teaspoons Sriracha sauce 3 minced garlic cloves 2 boxes cubed tofu

DIRECTIONS and Cooking Time: 60 Minutes
Prepare your Sous Vide water bath using your immersion circulator and raise the temperature to 185-degrees Fahrenheit. Take a medium bowl and add all the listed ingredients except the tofu. Mix well. Transfer the mixture to a heavy-duty resealable zipper bag and top with the tofu. Seal it up using the immersion method. Cook for 1 hour. Pour the contents into a serving bowl Serve!

Nutrition Info: Per serving:Calories:
186 ;Carbohydrates: 28g ;Protein: 10g ;Fat:
6g ;Sugar: 15g ;Sodium: 13mg

Rice & Leek Pilaf With Walnuts

INGREDIENTS for Servings: 4

1 tbsp olive oil	¼ cup currants
1 leek, thinly sliced	2 cups vegetable broth
1 minced garlic clove	¼ cup walnuts,
Salt to taste	toasted and chopped
1 cup rinsed wild rice	

DIRECTIONS and Cooking Time: 3 Hours 15 Minutes
Prepare a water bath and place the Sous Vide in it. Set
to 182 F.   Heat a saucepan over medium heat with oil.
Stir in garlic, leek and 1/2 tbsp of salt. Cook until the
leek is fragrant. Remove from the heat. Add in rice and
currants. Mix well. Place the mixture in a vacuum-
sealable bag. Release air by the water displacement
method, seal and submerge the bag in the water bath.
Cook for 3 hours.   Once the timer has stopped,
remove the bag and transfer to a bowl. Top with
walnuts.

Gnocchi Pillows And Caramelized Peas With Parmesan

INGREDIENTS for Servings: 2

1 pack, store-bought gnocchi	Fresh ground black pepper
1 tablespoon, unsalted butter	½ cup, frozen peas
½, thinly sliced sweet onion	¼ cup, heavy cream
	½ cup, grated Parmesan
Salt	

DIRECTIONS and Cooking Time: 30 Minutes
Prepare your Sous Vide water bath by dipping your
immersion cooker and raising the temperature to
183ºF Take a large zip bag and add gnocchi to the
bag   Seal using immersion method and cook for 1
and a ½ hours Take a cast iron skillet and place it
over medium heat   Add butter and allow the butter
to melt   Add onion and season with salt and Sauté for
3 minutes Add frozen peas, cream and simmer Stir
in gnocchi and stir well to coat with the sauce
Season with pepper and salt   Transfer to a platter
and serve!

Nutrition Info: Per serving:Calories 260,
Carbohydrates 5 g, Fats 20 g, Protein 15 g

Garlic Mushrooms With Truffle Oil

INGREDIENTS for Servings: 2

10 mediums to large button mushrooms	2 tbsp of truffle oil
2 cloves, garlic,	1 tbsp of fresh thyme,
minced	chopped
3 tbsp, olive oil	Salt/Pepper

DIRECTIONS and Cooking Time: 1 Hour
Prepare your Sous Vide water bath by attaching the
immersion circulator and setting the temperature to
185ºF.   Mix the olive oil with the truffle oil and the
rest of the ingredients. Add the mushrooms and make
sure that they are well coated with the oil mixture.
Place the mushrooms into a sealable plastic pouch and
seal using a vacuum sealer or the water displacement
method.   Place into the water bath and cook for 1
hour.   Once the mushrooms are cooked, remove
from the bag, drain and toss in a grilling pan to sear,
until golden brown.   Serve hot and garnish
optionally with some extra thyme on top.

Nutrition Info: Per serving:Calories 330,
Carbohydrates 4.4 g, Fats 34.1 g, Protein 1.5 g

Easy Vegetable Alfredo Dressing

INGREDIENTS for Servings: 6

4 cups chopped cauliflower	½ tsp dried basil
2 cups water	½ tsp dried rosemary
2/3 cup hazelnuts	4 tbsp nutritional yeast
2 cloves garlic	
½ tsp dried oregano	Salt and black pepper to taste

DIRECTIONS and Cooking Time: 1 Hour 45 Minutes
Prepare a water bath and place the Sous Vide in it. Set
to 172 F.   Place the hazelnuts, cauliflower, oregano,
water, garlic, rosemary, and basil in a vacuum-
sealable bag. Release air by the water displacement
method, seal and submerge the bag in the water bath.
Cook for 90 minutes.   Once the timer has stopped,
remove the contents and transfer into a blender and
blend until pureed. Serve with pasta.

Momofuku Brussels

INGREDIENTS for Servings: 2

2 pounds of Brussels sprouts with stems trimmed and slice up in half	1 tablespoon, rice vinegar
	1 and a ½ teaspoon, lime juice
2 ¼ tablespoon, extra virgin olive oil	12 pieces, thinly sliced Thai chills
¼ teaspoon of kosher salt	1 small sized minced garlic clove
¼ cup, fish sauce	Chopped up fresh mint
2 tablespoons, water	
1 and a ½ tablespoon, granulated sugar	Chopped up fresh cilantro

DIRECTIONS and Cooking Time: 40 Minutes
Prepare your Sous Vide water bath by dipping your
immersion cooker and raising the temperature to
183ºF Take a heavy-duty re-sealable bag and add

Brussels sprouts, salt, and olive oil   Seal it up using immersion method and cook underwater for 40 minutes   Take a small sized bowl and add fish sauce, sugar, water, rice vinegar, lime juice, garlic and chills to prepare the vinaigrette   Once the cooking is done, transfer the Brussels to an aluminum foil lined baking sheet   Heat up your broiler to high   Broil the Brussels in your broiler for about 5 minutes until they are just slightly charred   Transfer them to a medium-sized bowl and add the vinaigrette   Toss well   Sprinkle a bit of cilantro and mint   Serve!

Nutrition Info:Per serving:Calories 126, Carbohydrates 6 g, Fats 10 g, Protein 3 g

Cabbage & Pepper In Tomato Sauce

INGREDIENTS for Servings: 6

2 pounds cabbage, sliced	1 tbsp sugar
1 cup sliced bell pepper	Salt and black pepper to taste
1 cup tomato paste	1 tbsp cilantro
2 onions, sliced	1 tbsp olive oil

DIRECTIONS and Cooking Time: 4 Hours 45 Minutes
Prepare a water bath and place the Sous Vide in it. Set to 184 F.   Place the cabbage and onion in a vacumm-sealable bag and season with the spices. Add in tomato paste and stir to combine well. Release air by the water displacement method, seal and submerge the bag in water bath.Set the timer for 4 hours and 30 minutes. Once the timer has stopped, remove the bag.

Mustardy Lentil & Tomato Dish

INGREDIENTS for Servings: 8

2 cups lentils	1 tbsp butter
1 can chopped tomatoes, undrained	2 tbsp mustard
1 cup green peas	1 tsp red pepper flakes
3 cups veggie stock	
3 cups water	2 tbsp lime juice
1 onion, chopped	Salt and black pepper to taste
1 carrot, sliced	

DIRECTIONS and Cooking Time: 105 Minutes
Prepare a water bath and place Sous Vide in it. Set to 192 F. Place all the ingredients in a large vacumm-sealable bag. Release air by water displacement method, seal and submerge in bath. Cook for 90 minutes. Once the timer has stopped, remove the bag and transfer to a large bowl and stir before serving.

Tomato Soup

INGREDIENTS for Servings: 3

2 lb tomatoes, halved	3 tbsp olive oil
1 onion, diced	1 tbsp tomato puree
1 celery stick, chopped	A pinch sugar
	1 bay leaf

DIRECTIONS and Cooking Time: 60 Minutes
Make a water bath, place Sous Vide in it, and set to 185 F. Place all the listed ingredients except salt in bowl and toss. Put them in a vacuum-sealable bag. Release air by the water displacement method, seal and submerge the bag into the water bath. Set the timer for 40 minutes.   Once the timer has stopped, remove the bag and unseal. Puree the ingredients using a blender. Pour the blended tomato into a pot and set it over medium heat. Season with salt and cook for 10 minutes. Dish soup into bowls and cool. Serve warm with a side of low- carb bread.

Easy Two-bean Salad

INGREDIENTS for Servings: 6

4 oz dry black beans	Salt to taste
4 oz dry kidney beans	1 tsp sugar
4 cups water	1 tbsp champagne
1 minced shallot	3 tbsp olive oil

DIRECTIONS and Cooking Time: 7 Hours 10 Minutes
Prepare a water bath and place the Sous Vide in it. Set to 90 F. Combine the black beans, 3 cups of water and kidney beans in 4-6 mason jars. Seal and submerge the jars in the water bath. Cook for 2 hours.   Once the timer has stopped, remove the jars and top with shallots, kosher salt and sugar. Allow resting. Seal and immerse in the water bath again. Cook for 4 hours. Once the timer has stopped, remove the jars and allow chilling for 1 hour. Add olive oil and champagne and shake well. Transfer to a bowl and serve.

Cabbage Wedges

INGREDIENTS for Servings: 2

2 tablespoons, unsalted butter	1 medium-sized savoy cabbage cut up into wedges
½ teaspoon, kosher salt	

DIRECTIONS and Cooking Time: 4 Hours
Prepare your Sous Vide water bath by dipping your immersion cooker and raising the temperature to 183ºF   Take a large sized zip bag and add 1 tablespoon of butter, salt, and cabbages   Mix well and seal using immersion method   Cook for 4 hours and remove the cabbage, pat dry using kitchen towel   Take a tablespoon of butter and add to a medium-sized skillet over medium heat   Allow the butter to melt and add cabbages   Sear for 5-7 minutes until golden   Serve and enjoy!

Nutrition Info:Per serving:Calories 42,
Carbohydrates 4 g, Fats 2 g, Protein 2 g

Cauliflower Broccoli Soup

INGREDIENTS for Servings: 2

1 medium cauliflower, cut into small florets	1 onion, diced
½ lb broccoli, cut into small florets	1 tsp olive oil
	1 clove garlic, crushed
	½ cup vegetable stock
1 green bell pepper, chopped	½ cup skimmed milk

DIRECTIONS and Cooking Time: 70 Minutes
Make a water bath, place the Sous Vide in it, and set it to 185 F. Place the cauliflower, broccoli, bell pepper, and white onion in a vacuum-sealable bag and pour olive oil into it. Release air by the water displacement method and seal the bag. Submerge the bag in the water bath. Set the timer for 50 minutes and cook. Once the timer has stopped, remove the bag and unseal. Transfer the vegetables to a blender, add garlic and milk, and puree to smooth. Place a pan over medium heat, add the vegetable puree and vegetable stock and simmer for 3 minutes. Season with salt and pepper. Serve warm as a side dish.

Curry Ginger & Nectarine Chutney

INGREDIENTS for Servings: 3

½ cup granulated sugar	2 tsp curry powder
½ cup water	A pinch of red pepper flakes
¼ cup white wine vinegar	Salt and black pepper to taste
1 garlic clove, minced	Pepper flakes to taste
¼ cup white onion, finely chopped	4 large pieces nectarine, sliced into wedges
Juice of 1 lime	
2 tsp grated fresh ginger	¼ cup chopped up fresh basil

DIRECTIONS and Cooking Time: 60 Minutes
Prepare a water bath and place the Sous Vide in it. Set to 168 F. Heat a saucepan over medium heat and combine the water, sugar, white wine vinegar, and garlic. Moving until the sugar soften. Add lime juice, onion, curry powder, ginger, and red pepper flakes. Season with salt and black pepper. Stir well. Place the mixture in a vacuum-sealable bag. Release air by the water displacement method, seal and submerge the bag in the water bath. Cook for 40 minutes. Once the timer has stopped, remove the bag and place in ice bath. Transfer the food on a serving plate. Garnish with basil.

Shallot Cabbage With Raisins

INGREDIENTS for Servings: 4

1 ½ pounds red cabbage, sliced	2 sliced shallots
¼ cup raisins	1 tbsp apple balsamic vinegar
3 sliced garlic cloves	1 tbsp butter

DIRECTIONS and Cooking Time: 2 Hours 15 Minutes
Prepare a water bath and place Sous Vide in it. Set to 186 F. Place the cabbage in a vacuum-sealable bag. Add the reamaining ingredients. Release air by the water displacement method, seal and submerge the bag in the water bath. Cook for 2 hours. Once the timer has stopped, remove the bags and transfer into serving bowls. Season with salt and vinegar. Top with the cooking juices.

Sesame Zucchini Miso

INGREDIENTS for Servings: 2

1 zucchini, sliced	1 tsp sesame oil
¼ cup white miso	Salt to taste
2 tbsp Italian seasoning	2 tbsp sesame seeds, toasted
2 tbsp sake	2 tbsp scallions, thinly sliced
1 tbsp sugar	

DIRECTIONS and Cooking Time: 3 Hours 15 Minutes
Prepare a water bath and place the Sous Vide in it. Set to 186 F. Place the zucchini in a vacuum-sealable bag. Release air by the water displacement method, seal and submerge the bag in the water bath. Cook for 3 hours. Once the timer has stopped, remove the bag and transfer to a baking sheet. Discard the cooking juice. For the miso sauce, combine the miso, sake, sugar, Italian seasoning, and sesame oil in a small bowl. Whisk until smooth. Brush the zucchini with the sauce and caramelize for 3-5 minutes. Serve on a platter and top with sesame seeds.

Mushroom & Truffle Oil

INGREDIENTS for Servings: 2

10 large button mushrooms	1 tablespoon chopped fresh thyme
3 tablespoons truffle oil	1 clove thinly sliced garlic
3 tablespoons olive oil	Salt, and pepper to taste

DIRECTIONS and Cooking Time: 60 Minutes
Prepare the Sous-vide water bath using your immersion circulator and raise the temperature to 185-degrees Fahrenheit. Take a large bowl and add the truffle oil, mushrooms, olive oil, garlic, and thyme Season with some pepper and salt. Transfer the mushroom mixture to a large Sous-vide resealable zip bag and add the mixture to the bag. Seal it up using the immersion method. Submerge underwater and cook for 1 hour. Once cooked, drain the mushrooms and discard the cooking liquid. Take a large skillet

and put it over medium heat for 3 minutes. Add the mushrooms and sear for about 1 minute to brown it. Transfer the cooked mushroom to a serving plate and season with pepper and salt. Top it up with thyme. Serve!

Nutrition Info:Per serving:Calories: 440 ;Carbohydrates: 28g ;Protein: 19g ;Fat: 28g ;Sugar: 6g ;Sodium: 314mg

Minty Chickpea And Mushroom Bowl

INGREDIENTS for Servings: 8

9 ounces mushrooms	1 tsp paprika
3 cups veggie broth	1 tbsp mustard
1 pound chickpeas, soaked overnight and drained	2 tbsp tomato juice
	1 tsp salt
	¼ cup chopped mint
1 tsp butter	1 tbsp olive oil

DIRECTIONS and Cooking Time: 4 Hours 15 Minutes
Prepare a water bath and place the Sous Vide in it. Set to 195 F. Place broth and chickpeas in a vacumm-sealable bag. Release air by the water displacement method, seal and submerge the bag in water bath.Set the timer for 4 hours. Once the timer has stopped, remove the bag. Heat oil in a pan over medium heat. Add in mushrooms, tomato juice, paprika, salt, and mustard. Cook for 4 minutes. Drain the chickpeas and add them to the pan. Cook for another 4 minutes. Stir in butter and mint.

Sage Roasted Potato Mash

INGREDIENTS for Servings: 6

¼ cup butter	4 tsp salt
12 sweet potatoes, unpeeled	6 tbsp olive oil
	5 fresh sage sprigs
10 garlic cloves, chopped	1 tbsp paprika

DIRECTIONS and Cooking Time: 1 Hour 35 Minutes
Prepare a water bath and place the Sous Vide in it. Set to 192 F. Combine the potatoes, garlic, salt, olive oil and 2 or 3 thyme springs and place in a vacuum-sealable bag. Release air by the water displacement method, seal and submerge the bag in the water bath. Cook for 1 hour and 15 minutes. Preheat the oven to 450 F. Once the timer has stopped, remove the potatoes and transfer into a bowl. Separate the cooking juices. Combine well the potatoes with butter and the remaining sage springs. Transfer into a baking tray, previously lined with aluminium foil. Make a hole in the center of the potatoes and pour the cooking juices in. Bake the potatoes for 10 minutes, turning 5 minutes later. Discard the sage. Transfer to a plate and serve sprinkled with paprika.

Oregano White Beans

INGREDIENTS for Servings: 8

12 ounces white beans	1 cup chopped onions
	1 bell pepper, chopped
1 cup tomato paste	
8 ounces veggie stock	1 tbsp oregano
1 tbsp sugar	2 tsp paprika
3 tbsp butter	

DIRECTIONS and Cooking Time: 5 Hours 15 Minutes
Prepare a water bath and place the Sous Vide in it. Set to 185 F. Combine all the ingredients in a vacumm-sealable bag. Stir to combine. Release air by the water displacement method, seal and submerge the bag in water bath.Set the timer for 5 hours. Once the timer has stopped, remove the bag. Serve warm.

Cream Of Tomatoes With Cheese Sandwich

INGREDIENTS for Servings: 8

½ cup cream cheese	2 tbsp olive oil
2 pounds tomatoes, cut into wedges	⅛ tsp red pepper flakes
Salt and black pepper to taste	½ tsp white wine vinegar
2 garlic cloves, minced	2 tbsp butter
½ tsp chopped fresh sage	4 slices bread
	2 slices halloumi cheese

DIRECTIONS and Cooking Time: 55 Minutes
Prepare a water bath and place the Sous Vide in it. Set to 186 F. Put the tomatoes in a colander over a bowl and season with salt. Stir well. Allow to chill for 30 minutes. Discard the juices. Combine the olive oil, garlic, sage, black pepper, salt, and pepper flakes. Place in a vacuum-sealable bag. Release air by the water displacement method, seal and submerge the bag in the water bath. Cook for 40 minutes. Once the timer has stopped, remove the bag and transfer into a blender. Add in vinegar and cream cheese. Mix until smooth. Transfer to a plate and season with salt and pepper if needed. To make the cheese bars: heat a skillet over medium heat. Grease the bread slices with butter and put into the skillet. Lay cheese slices over the bread and place over another buttery bread. Toast for 1-2 minutes. Repeat with the remaining bread. Cut into cubes. Serve over the warm soup.

Broiled Onions With Sunflower Pesto

INGREDIENTS for Servings: 4

1 bunch large spring onions, trimmed and	2 cloves garlic, peeled
	3 cups loosely packed

halved	fresh basil leaves
½ cup plus 2 tbsp olive oil	3 tbsp grated Grana Padano cheese
Salt and black pepper to taste	1 tbsp freshly squeezed lemon juice
2 tbsp sunflower seeds	

DIRECTIONS and Cooking Time: 2 Hours 25 Minutes
Prepare a water bath and place the Sous Vide in it. Set to 183 F.   Place the onions in a vacuum-sealable bag. Season with salt, pepper and 2 tbsp of olive oil. Release air by the water displacement method, seal and submerge the bag in the water bath. Cook for 2 hours.   Meanwhile, for the pesto sauce, combine in a processor food the sunflower seeds, garlic, and basil, and blend until finely chopped. Carefully add the remaining oil. Add in lemon juice and stop. Season with salt and pepper. Set aside.   Once the timer has stopped, remove the bag and transfer the onions to a skillet and cook for 10 minutes. Serve and top with the pesto sauce.

Brussel Sprouts In White Wine

INGREDIENTS for Servings: 4

1 pound Brussels sprouts, trimmed	½ cup white wine
½ cup extra virgin olive oil	2 tbsp fresh parsley, finely chopped
Salt and black pepper to taste	2 garlic cloves, crushed

DIRECTIONS and Cooking Time: 35 Minutes
Place Brussels sprouts in a large vacuum-sealable bag with three tablespoons of olive oil. Cook in Sous Vide for 15 minutes at 180 F. Remove from the bag.   In a large, non-stick grill pan, heat up the remaining olive oil. Add Brussels sprouts, crushed garlic, salt, and pepper. Briefly grill, shaking the pan a couple of times until lightly charred on all sides. Add wine and bring it to a boil. Stir well and remove from the heat. Top with finely chopped parsley and serve.

Provolone Cheese Grits

INGREDIENTS for Servings: 4

1 cup grits	2 tbsp butter
1 cup cream	1 tbsp paprika
3 cups vegetable stock	Extra cheese for garnish
4 oz grated Provolone cheese	Salt and black pepper to taste

DIRECTIONS and Cooking Time: 3 Hours 20 Minutes
Prepare a water bath and place the Sous Vide in it. Set to 182 F. Combine the grits, cream and vegetable stock. Chop the butter and add to the mixture. Place the mix in a vacuum-sealable bag. Release air by the water

displacement method, seal and submerge the bag in the water bath. Cook for 3 hours.   Once the timer has stopped, remove the bag and transfer into a bowl. Stir the mixture with the cheese and season with salt and pepper. Garnish with extra cheese and paprika, if preferred.

Citrus Corn With Tomato Sauce

INGREDIENTS for Servings: 8

⅓ cup olive oil	3 tbsp lemon juice
4 ears yellow corn, husked	1 serrano pepper, seeded
Salt and black pepper to taste	4 scallions, green parts only, chopped
1 large tomato, chopped	½ bunch fresh cilantro leaves, chopped
2 garlic cloves, minced	

DIRECTIONS and Cooking Time: 55 Minutes
Prepare a water bath and place the Sous Vide in it. Set to 186 F. Whisk the corns with olive oil and season with salt and pepper. Place them in a vacuum-sealable bag. Release air by the water displacement method, seal and submerge the bag in the water bath. Cook for 45 minutes.   Meantime, combine well the tomato, lemon juice, garlic, serrano pepper, scallions, cilantro, and the remaining olive oil in a bowl. Preheat a grill over high heat.   Once the timer has stopped, remove the corns and transfer to the grill and cook for 2-3 minutes. Allow to cool. Cut the kernels from the cob and pour in tomato sauce. Serve with fish, salad or tortilla chips.

Quinoa & Celeriac Miso Dish

INGREDIENTS for Servings: 6

1 celeriac, chopped	Juice of ¼ a large lemon
1 tbsp miso paste	5 cherry tomatoes roughly cut
6 cloves garlic	
5 sprigs thyme	Chopped parsley
1 tsp onion powder	8 ounces vegan butter
3 tbsp ricotta cheese	8 ounce cooked quinoa
1 tbsp mustard seeds	

DIRECTIONS and Cooking Time: 2 Hours 25 Minutes
Prepare a water bath and place the Sous Vide in it. Set to 186 F.   Meanwhile, heat a skillet over medium heat and add the garlic, thyme, mustard seeds. Cook for about 2 minutes. Add butter and stirring until browned. Combine with onion powder and set aside. Allow to cool at room temperature. Place the celeriac in a vacuum-sealable bag. Release air by the water displacement method, seal and submerge the bag in the water bath. Cook for 2 hours.   Once the timer has stopped, remove the bag and transfer to a skillet and stirring until golden brown. Season with miso. Set aside. Heat a pan over medium heat, add tomatoes,

mustard and quinoa. Combine with lemon juice and parsley. Serve by mixing the celeriac and tomato mix.

Crispy Garlic Potato Purée

INGREDIENTS for Servings: 2

1 pound sweet potatoes	2 tbsp olive oil
5 cloves smashed garlic	Salt to taste
	1 tsp rosemary, chopped

DIRECTIONS and Cooking Time: 1 Hour 20 Minutes
Prepare a water bath and place the Sous Vide in it. Set to 192 F. Combine all the ingredients and place in a vacuum-sealable bag. Release air by the water displacement method, seal and submerge the bag in the water bath. Cook for 1 hour. Once the timer has stopped, remove the potatoes and transfer to a baking tray foil-lined. Cut the potatoes in rounds and sprinkle with garlic oil. Bake for 10 minutes in the oven at 380 F. Garnish with rosemary.

Vegan Steel Cut Oats

INGREDIENTS for Servings: 2

2 cups water	Cinnamon and maple syrup for topping
½ cup steel cut oats	
½ teaspoon salt	

DIRECTIONS and Cooking Time: 180 Minutes
Prepare the Sous Vide water bath by using your immersion circulator and raise the temperature to 180 degrees Fahrenheit. Take a heavy-duty resealable zipper bag and add all the listed ingredients except the cinnamon and maple syrup Seal the bag using the immersion method and submerge underwater. Cook for about 3 hours. Once cooked, remove it and transfer the oats to your serving bowl. Serve with a sprinkle of cinnamon and some maple syrup.

Nutrition Info: Per serving:Calories: 141 ;Carbohydrates: 19g ;Protein: 5g ;Fat: 6g ;Sugar: 6g ;Sodium: 87mg

Germany's Potato Salad

INGREDIENTS for Servings: 6

1 ½ pound, Yukon potatoes, sliced up into ¾ inch pieces	Salt
	Pepper
½ a cup of chicken stock	½ a cup, chopped onion
4-ounce, thick bacon cut up into ¼ inch thick strips	1/3 cup, apple cider vinegar
	4 thinly sliced scallions

DIRECTIONS and Cooking Time: 1 ½ Hours

Prepare your Sous Vide water bath by dipping your immersion cooker and raising the temperature to 185ºF Take a heavy-duty re-sealable bag and add potatoes alongside the stock Season with some salt and seal up the bag using immersion method Submerge the bag underwater and let it cook for 1 and a ½ hours Take a large sized non-stick skillet and place it over medium-high heat Add bacon and cook for about 5-7 minutes Transfer it to a paper towel-lined plate using a slotted spoon Make sure to keep reserved fat Return the skillet to medium-high heat and add onions Cook them for a 1 minute Once the cooking is done, remove the bag from the water and return the skillet to medium heat again Add the bacon and add vinegar Bring it to a simmer Add the contents of the bag to the skillet and stir well to combine and allow the liquid to come to a simmer Add scallions and toss well Season with some pepper and salt Serve warm!

Nutrition Info: Per serving:Calories 75, Carbohydrates 5 g, Fats 3 g, Protein 7 g

Potato & Date Salad

INGREDIENTS for Servings: 6

2 pounds potatoes, cubed	1 tbsp lemon juice
5 ounces dates, chopped	3 tbsp butter
	1 tsp cilantro
½ cup crumbled goat cheese	1 tsp salt
	1 tbsp chopped parsley
1 tsp oregano	¼ tsp garlic powder
1 tbsp olive oil	

DIRECTIONS and Cooking Time: 3 Hours 15 Minutes
Prepare a water bath and place the Sous Vide in it. Set to 190 F. Place the potatoes, butter, dates, oregano, cilantro, and salt in a vacumm-sealable bag. Release air by the water displacement method, seal and submerge the bag in water bath.Set the timer for 3 hours. Once the timer has stopped, remove the bag and transfer to a bowl. Whisk together the olive oil, lemon juice, parsley, and garlic powder and drizzle over the salad. If using cheese, sprinkle it over.

Rosemary Russet Potatoes Confit

INGREDIENTS for Servings: 4

1 pound brown russet potatoes, chopped	1 tsp chopped fresh rosemary
Salt to taste	2 tbsp whole butter
¼ tsp ground white pepper	1 tbsp corn oil

DIRECTIONS and Cooking Time: 1 Hour 15 Minutes
Prepare a water bath and place Sous Vide in it. Set to 192 F. Season potatoes with rosemary, salt and pepper. Combine the potatoes with butter and oil. Place in a vacuum-sealable bag. Release air by the

water displacement method, seal and submerge the bag in the water bath. Cook for 60 minutes. Once the timer has stopped, remove the bag and transfer into a large bowl. Garnish with butter and serve.

Honey Drizzled Carrots

INGREDIENTS for Servings: 4

1-pound baby carrots	3 tablespoons honey
4 tablespoons vegan butter	¼ teaspoon kosher salt
1 tablespoon agave nectar	¼ teaspoon ground cardamom

DIRECTIONS and Cooking Time: 75 Minutes
Prepare the Sous-vide water bath using your immersion circulator and increase the temperature to 185 degrees Fahrenheit   Add the carrots, honey, whole butter, kosher salt, and cardamom to a resealable bag   Seal using the immersion method. Cook for 75 minutes and once done, remove it from the water bath.   Strain the glaze by passing through a fine mesh.   Set it aside.   Take the carrots out from the bag and pour any excess glaze over them. Serve with a little bit of seasonings.

Nutrition Info: Per serving: Calories: 174 ; Carbohydrates: 42g ; Protein: 2g ; Fat: 1g ; Sugar: 31g ; Sodium: 180mg

Paprika Grits

INGREDIENTS for Servings: 4

10 ounces grits	10 ounces water
4 tbsp butter	½ tsp garlic salt
1 ½ tsp paprika	

DIRECTIONS and Cooking Time: 3 Hours 10 Minutes
Prepare a water bath and place the Sous Vide in it. Set to 180 F.   Place all the ingredients in a vacumm-sealable bag. Stir with spoon to combine well. Release air by the water displacement method, seal and submerge the bag in water bath. Set the timer for 3 hours. Once the timer has stopped, remove the bag. Divide between 4 serving bowls.

Thai Pumpkin Dish

INGREDIENTS for Servings: 6

1 medium pumpkin	Fresh cilantro for serving
2 tbsp vegan butter	Lime wedges for serving
2 tbsp Thai curry paste	
Salt to taste	

DIRECTIONS and Cooking Time: 2 Hours 20 Minutes
Prepare a water bath and place the Sous Vide in it. Set to 186 F.   Cut the pumpkin into wedges slices and take out the seeds. Reserve the seeds. Place the pumpkin wedges, curry paste, butter, and salt in a vacuum-sealable bag. Release air by the water displacement method, seal and submerge the bag in the water bath. Cook for 90 minutes.   Once the timer has stopped, remove the bag and squash until softened. If required, cook for 40 minutes more. Transfer to a serving plate and top with curry sauce. Garnish with cilantro and lime wedges.

Vegetable Caponata

INGREDIENTS for Servings: 4

4 canned plum tomatoes, crushed	6 garlic cloves, minced
2 bell peppers, sliced	2 tbsp olive oil
2 zucchinis, sliced	6 basil leaves
½ onion, sliced	Salt and black pepper to taste
2 eggplants, sliced	

DIRECTIONS and Cooking Time: 2 Hours 15 Minutes
Prepare a water bath and place the Sous Vide in it. Set to 185 F. Combine all of the ingredients in a vacumm-sealable bag. Release air by the water displacement method, seal and submerge the bag in water bath. Set the timer for 2 hours. Once the timer has stopped, transfer to a serving platter.

Herby Mashed Snow Peas

INGREDIENTS for Servings: 6

½ cup vegetable broth	Salt and black pepper to taste
1 pound fresh snow peas	2 tbsp chopped fresh chives
Zest of 1 lemon	
2 tbsp chopped fresh basil	2 tbsp chopped fresh parsley
1 tbsp olive oil	¾ tsp garlic powder

DIRECTIONS and Cooking Time: 55 Minutes
Prepare a water bath and place the Sous Vide in it. Set to 186 F.   Combine the peas, lemon zest, basil, olive oil, black pepper, chives, parsley, salt, and garlic powder and place them in a vacuum-sealable bag. Release air by the water displacement method, seal and submerge the bag in the water bath. Cook for 45 minutes. Once the timer has stopped, remove the bag and transfer into a blender and mix well.

Sous Vide Turmeric And Cumin Tofu

INGREDIENTS for Servings: 4

1 pack, firm tofu, drained and cut to ½ inch thick pieces	1 tsp, cumin
	2 tbsp, lime
	3 tablespoons olive oil
3 cloves, garlic,	Kosher salt/Pepper

minced	
1 tbsp, turmeric	

DIRECTIONS and Cooking Time: 2 Hours
Prepare your Sous Vide water bath by attaching the immersion circulator and setting the temperature to 180ºF. Arrange the tofu pieces on a flat surface (you can use a baking tray) and place on the fridge for 15 minutes. In a small bowl, combine all the rest of the ingredients to make a marinade. Take the tofu pieces out of the fridge and dip into the marinade, making sure all pieces are well coated. Transfer the marinated tofu on a sealable pouch (lying flat) and seal using a vacuum sealer or the water displacement method. Submerge into the water bath and let cook for 2 hours. Take out of the pouch carefully and serve as it is or with lettuce or Roca leaves as a garnish.

Nutrition Info:Per serving:Calories 220, Carbohydrates 5.4 g, Fats 16.9 g, Protein 11.7 g

Mixed Vegetable Soup

INGREDIENTS for Servings: 3

1 sweet onion, sliced	1 tsp red pepper
1 tsp garlic powder	flakes
2 cups zucchini, cut in	2 cups vegetable stock
small dices	1 sprig rosemary
3 oz Parmesan rind	Salt to taste
2 cups baby spinach	
2 tbsp olive oil	

DIRECTIONS and Cooking Time: 55 Minutes
Make a water bath, place Sous Vide in it, and set to 185 F. Toss all the ingredients with olive oil except the garlic and salt, and place them in a vacuum-sealable bag. Release air by water displacement method, seal and submerge the bag in the water bath. Set the timer for 30 minutes. Once the timer has stopped, remove and unseal the bag. Discard the rosemary. Pour the remaining ingredients into a pot and add salt and garlic powder. Put the pot over medium heat and simmer for 10 minutes. Serve as a light dish.

Easy Broccoli Puree

INGREDIENTS for Servings: 4

1 head broccoli	3 tbsp butter
1 cup vegetable stock	Salt to taste

DIRECTIONS and Cooking Time: 60 Minutes
Prepare a water bath and place the Sous Vide in it. Set to 186 F. Combine the broccoli, butter and vegetable stock. Place in a vacuum-sealable bag. Release air by the water displacement method, seal and submerge the bag in the water bath. Cook for 45 minutes. Once the timer has stopped, remove the bag and drain. Reserve the cooking juices. Put the broccoli into a blender and puree until smooth. Pour some cooking juices. Season with salt and pepper to serve.

Light Broccoli Sauté

INGREDIENTS for Servings: 4

1 pound fresh broccoli	Salt and black pepper
¼ cup butter, melted	to taste

DIRECTIONS and Cooking Time: 45 Minutes
Prepare a water bath and place the Sous Vide in it. Set to 183 F. Chunk the broccoli in quarters. Place them in a vacuum-sealable bag. Season with salt and pepper. Add in butter. Release air by the water displacement method, seal and submerge the bag in the water bath. Cook for 30 minutes. Once the timer has stopped, remove the bag. Serve

Delicious Chutney Of Dates & Mangoes

INGREDIENTS for Servings: 4

2 pounds mangoes,	¼ cup dates
chopped	1½ tsp yellow
1 small onion, diced	mustard seeds
½ cup light brown	1½ tsp coriander
sugar	seeds
2 tbsp apple cider	Salt to taste
vinegar	¼ tsp curry powder
2 tbsp freshly	¼ tsp dried turmeric
squeezed lemon juice	⅛ tsp cayenne

DIRECTIONS and Cooking Time: 1 Hour 45 Minutes
Prepare a water bath and place the Sous Vide in it. Set to 183 F. Combine all the ingredients. Place in a vacuum-sealable bag. Release air by the water displacement method, seal and submerge the bag in the water bath. Cook for 90 minutes. Once the timer has stopped, remove the bag and pour into a pot.

Tasty Spicy Tomatoes

INGREDIENTS for Servings: 4

4 pieces cored and	2 tbsp olive oil
diced tomatoes	1 tsp dried oregano
3 minced garlic cloves	1 tsp rosemary
	1 tsp fine sea salt

DIRECTIONS and Cooking Time: 60 Minutes
Prepare a water bath and place Sous Vide in it. Set to 146 F. Place all the ingredients in a vacuum-sealable bag. Release air by the water displacement method, seal and submerge in the bath. Cook for 45 minutes. Once the timer has stopped, remove the tomatoes and transfer to a plate. Serve with toast French bread slices.

Buttery Artichokes With Lemon & Garlic

INGREDIENTS for Servings: 4

4 tbsp lemon juice	Salt, to taste
12 baby artichokes	1 tsp dill
4 tbsp butter	Ground black pepper, to taste
2 minced fresh garlic cloves	Chopped up fresh parsley for serving
1 tsp fresh lemon zest	

DIRECTIONS and Cooking Time: 1 Hour 45 Minutes
Prepare a water bath and place the Sous Vide in it. Set to 182 F. Combine cold water with 2 tbsp of lemon juice. Peel the artichokes and chop thinly. Transfer to the water and allow resting. Heat the butter in a skillet over medium heat and cook the dill, garlic 2 tbsp of lemon juice and zest. Season with salt and pepper, allow cooling for 5 minutes. Drain the artichokes and place in a vacuum-sealable bag. Add in butter mixture. Release air by the water displacement method, seal and submerge the bag in the water bath. Cook for 1 hour and 30 minutes. Once the timer has stopped, remove the artichokes and serving in a bowl. Top with parsley.

Perfect Curried Squash

INGREDIENTS for Servings: 6

1 medium-sized winter squash	1 to 2 tablespoon, Thai curry paste
2 tablespoons, unsalted butter	½ teaspoon, kosher salt
Fresh cilantro	Lime wedges

DIRECTIONS and Cooking Time: 1 ½ Hours
Prepare your Sous Vide water bath by dipping your immersion cooker and raising the temperature to 185ºF   Slice the squash into half lengthwise and scoop out the seeds alongside inner membrane Keep the seeds for later use   Slice the squash into wedges of 1 and ½ inch thickness   Take a large sized zip bag and add squash wedges, curry paste, butter, salt and seal using immersion method   Submerge and cook for 1 and ½ hours   Remove the bag and slight squeeze it   If soft then take out, otherwise cook for 40 minutes more   Transfer to serving platter and drizzle a bit of curry butter sauce   Top with cilantro and enjoy!

Nutrition Info: Per serving:Calories 152, Carbohydrates 5 g, Fats 12 g, Protein 6 g

Braised Swiss Chard With Lime

INGREDIENTS for Servings: 2

4 tbsp of extra virgin olive oil	2 pounds Swiss chard
	1 whole lime, juiced
	2 tsps sea salt

2 garlic cloves, crushed	

DIRECTIONS and Cooking Time: 25 Minutes
Thoroughly rinse Swiss chard and drain in a colander. Using a sharp paring knife roughly chop and transfer to a large bowl. Stir in 4 tablespoons of olive oil, crushed garlic, lime juice, and sea salt. Transfer to a large vacuum-sealable bag and seal. Cook en sous vide for 10 minutes at 180 F.

Herby Balsamic Mushrooms With Garlic

INGREDIENTS for Servings: 4

1 pound Portobello mushrooms, sliced	1 minced garlic clove
1 tbsp olive oil	Salt to taste
1 tbsp apple balsamic vinegar	1 tsp black pepper
	1 tsp minced fresh thyme

DIRECTIONS and Cooking Time: 1 Hour 15 Minutes
Prepare a water bath and place the Sous Vide in it. Set to 138 F.   Combine all the ingredients and place them in a vacuum-sealable bag. Release air by the water displacement method, seal and submerge the bag in the water bath. Cook for 60 minutes. Once the timer has stopped, remove the bag and transfer to a serving bowl.

Mixed Beans In Tomato Sauce

INGREDIENTS for Servings: 4

1 pound trimmed green beans	1 (14-oz) can whole crushed tomatoes
1 pound trimmed snow beans	3 sliced garlic cloves
1 thinly sliced onion	3 tbsp olive oil

DIRECTIONS and Cooking Time: 3 Hours 10 Minutes
Prepare a water bath and place Sous Vide in it. Set to 183 F. Place the tomatoes, snow and green beans, garlic, and onion in a vacuum-sealable bag. Release air by water displacement method, seal and submerge in the water bath. Cook for 3 hours. Once done, transfer into a bowl. Sprinkle with olive oil.

White Cannellini Beans

INGREDIENTS for Servings: 5

1 cup cannellini beans (dried) soaked overnight in salty cold water	1 cup water
	1 quartered shallot
	4 crushed garlic cloves
½ cup extra-virgin olive oil	2 fresh rosemary sprigs
1 peeled carrot, cut up	2 bay leaves

into 1-inch dice 1 celery stalk, cut up into 1-inch dice	Kosher salt, and pepper to taste

DIRECTIONS and Cooking Time: 180 Minutes
Prepare the Sous Vide water bath using your Sous-vide immersion circulator and raise the temperature to 190-degrees Fahrenheit. Drain the soaked beans and rinse them. Transfer to a heavy duty resealable zip bag and add the olive oil, celery, water, carrot, shallot, garlic, rosemary, and bay leaves. Season with pepper and salt. Seal using the immersion method and cook for 3 hours. Once cooked, remove the beans and check for seasoning. Discard the rosemary and serve!

Nutrition Info: Per serving: Calories: 578 ; Carbohydrates: 77g ; Protein: 31g ; Fat: 18g ; Sugar: 5g ; Sodium: 519mg

Yogurt Caraway Soup
INGREDIENTS for Servings: 4

1 tbsp olive oil 1½ tsp caraway seeds 1 medium onion, diced 1 leek, halved and thinly sliced Salt to taste 2 pounds carrots, chopped	1 bay leaf 3 cups vegetable broth ½ cup whole milk yogurt Apple cider vinegar Fresh dill fronds

DIRECTIONS and Cooking Time: 2 Hours 20 Minutes
Prepare a water bath and place the Sous Vide in it. Set to 186 F. Heat olive oil in a large skillet over medium heat and add caraway seeds. Toast them for 1 minute. Add in onion, salt and leek, Sauté for 5-7 minutes or until tender. Combine the onion, bay leaf, carrots and 1/2 tbsp of salt into a large bowl. Distribute the mixture in a vacuum-sealable bag. Release air by the water displacement method, seal and submerge the bag in the water bath. Cook for 2 hours. Once the timer has stopped, remove the bag and pour into a bowl. Add in vegetable broth and blend. Stir in yogurt. Season the soup with some salt and vinegar and serve garnished dill fronds.

Pickled Fennel
INGREDIENTS for Servings: 5

1 cup white wine vinegar 2 tablespoons beet sugar Juice and zest from 1 lemon	1 teaspoon kosher salt 2 medium bulb fennels, trimmed up and cut into ¼ inch thick slices

DIRECTIONS and Cooking Time: 30 Minutes

Prepare the Sous Vide water bath using your immersion circulator and raise the temperature to 180-degrees Fahrenheit. Take a large bowl and add the vinegar, sugar, lemon juice, salt, lemon zest, and whisk them well. Transfer the mixture to your resealable zip bag. Add the fennel and seal using the immersion method. Submerge underwater and cook for 30 minutes. Transfer to an ice bath and allow the mixture to reach the room temperature. Serve!

Nutrition Info: Per serving: Calories: 156 ; Carbohydrates: 33g ; Protein: 5g ; Fat: 1g ; Sugar: 20g ; Sodium: 603mg

Long Green Beans In Tomato Sauce
INGREDIENTS for Servings: 4

1 pound, trimmed green beans 1 can, whole crushed tomatoes 1 thinly sliced onion	3 peeled and thinly sliced garlic clove Kosher salt as needed Extra virgin olive oil

DIRECTIONS and Cooking Time: 3 Hours
Prepare your Sous Vide water bath by dipping your immersion cooker and raising the temperature to 183ºF Take a heavy-duty zip bag and add tomatoes, green bean, garlic, and onion Submerge underwater and cook for 3 hours Remove the bag and transfer content to a large sized bowl Season with salt and drizzle a bit of olive oil Serve and enjoy!

Nutrition Info: Per serving: Calories 54, Carbohydrates 5 g, Fats 2 g, Protein 4 g

White Beans
INGREDIENTS for Servings: 8

1 cup dried and soaked navy beans 1 cup water ½ cup extra-virgin olive oil 1 peeled carrot, cut up into 1-inch dices 1 stalk celery, cut up into 1-inch dices	1 quartered shallot 4 cloves crushed garlic 2 sprigs fresh rosemary 2 pieces' bay leaves Kosher salt, to taste Freshly ground black pepper, to taste

DIRECTIONS and Cooking Time: 3-4 Hours
Prepare your Sous-vide water bath using your immersion circulator and raise the temperature to 190-degrees Fahrenheit. Carefully drain and rinse your beans and add them alongside the rest of the ingredients to a heavy-duty zip bag. Seal using the immersion method and submerge it underwater. Cook for about 3 hours. Once cooked, taste the beans. If they are firm, then cook for another 1 hour and pour them in a serving bowl. Serve!

Nutrition Info: Per serving: Calories: 210 ;Carbohydrates: 36g ;Protein: 14g ;Fat: 2g ;Sugar: 2g ;Sodium: 224mg

Hearty White Beans

INGREDIENTS for Servings: 8

1 cup, dried and soaked navy beans	1 quartered shallot
1 cup, water	4 cloves, crushed garlic
½ a cup, extra virgin olive oil	2 sprigs, fresh rosemary
1 peeled carrot cut up into 1-inch dices	2 pieces, bay leaves
1 stalk, celery cut up into 1-inch dices	Kosher salt
	Freshly ground black pepper

DIRECTIONS and Cooking Time: 3 Hours
Prepare your Sous Vide water bath by dipping your immersion cooker and raising the temperature to 190ºF Carefully drain and rinse your beans and add them to a heavy-duty zipper bag Seal it up using immersion method and submerge it underwater Let it cook for about 3 hours Once done, taste the beans If they are firm, then cook for another 1 hour, or cook for another hour and serve them on a bowl Serve!

Nutrition Info: Per serving: Calories 119, Carbohydrates 9 g, Fats 3 g, Protein 14 g

Buttered Asparagus With Thyme & Cheese

INGREDIENTS for Servings: 6

¼ cup shaved Pecorino Romano cheese	Salt to taste
16 oz fresh asparagus, trimmed	1 garlic clove, minced
4 tbsp butter, cubed	1 tbsp thyme

DIRECTIONS and Cooking Time: 21 Minutes
Prepare a water bath and place the Sous Vide in it. Set to 186 F. Place the asparagus in a vacuum-sealable bag. Add the butter cubes, garlic, salt, and thyme. Release air by the water displacement method, seal and submerge the bag in the water bath. Cook for 14 minutes. Once the timer has stopped, remove the bag and transfer the asparagus to a plate. Sprinkle with some cooking juices. Garnish with the Pecorino Romano cheese.

Fall Squash Cream Soup

INGREDIENTS for Servings: 6

¾ cup heavy cream	1 garlic clove, chopped
1 winter squash, chopped	1 tsp ground cumin
1 large pear	Salt and black pepper
½ yellow onion, diced	to taste
3 fresh thyme sprigs	4 tbsp crème fraîche

DIRECTIONS and Cooking Time: 2 Hours 20 Minutes
Prepare a water bath and place the Sous Vide in it. Set to 186 F. Combine the squash, pear, onion, thyme, garlic, cumin, and salt. Place in a vacuum-sealable bag. Release air by the water displacement method, seal and submerge in water bath. Cook for 2 hours. Once the timer has stopped, remove the bag and transfer all the contents into a blender. Puree until smooth. Add in cream and stir well. Season with salt and pepper. Transfer the mix into serving bowls and top with some créme fraiche. Garnish with pear chunks.

Garlic Tabasco Edamame Cheese

INGREDIENTS for Servings: 4

1 tbsp olive oil	1 tsp salt
4 cups fresh edamame in pods	1 tbsp red pepper flakes
1 garlic clove, minced	1 tbsp Tabasco sauce

DIRECTIONS and Cooking Time: 1 Hour 6 Minutes
Prepare a water bath and place the Sous Vide in it. Set to 186 F. Heat a pot with water over high heat and blanch the edamame pots for 60 seconds. Strain them and transfer into an ice water bath. Combine the garlic, red pepper flakes, Tabasco sauce, and olive oil. Place the edamame in a vacuum-sealable bag. Pour the Tabasco sauce. Release air by the water displacement method, seal and submerge the bag in the water bath. Cook for 1 hour. Once the timer has stopped, remove the bag and transfer into a bowl and serve.

Honey Apple & Arugula Salad

INGREDIENTS for Servings: 4

2 tbsp honey	Dressing
2 apples, cored, halved and sliced	¼ cup olive oil
½ cup walnuts, toasted and chopped	1 tbsp white wine vinegar
½ cup shaved Grana Padano cheese	1 tsp Dijon mustard
4 cups arugula	1 garlic clove, minced
Sea salt to taste	Salt to taste

DIRECTIONS and Cooking Time: 3 Hours 50 Minutes
Prepare a water bath and place the Sous Vide in it. Set to 158 F. Place the honey in a glass bowl and heat for 30 seconds, add the apples and mix well. Place it in a vacuum-sealable bag. Release air by the water displacement method, seal and submerge the bag in the water bath. Cook for 30 minutes. Once the timer has stopped, remove the bag and transfer into an ice-water bath for 5 minutes. Refrigerate for 3 hours. Combine all the dressing ingredients in a jar and shake

well. Allow cooling in the fridge for a moment. In a bowl, mix the arugula, walnuts, and Grana Padano cheese. Add the peach slices. Top with the dressing. Season with salt and pepper and serve.

Delicious Cardamom And Apricots

INGREDIENTS for Servings: 4

1 pint, mall and halved apricots	½ a teaspoon, ground ginger
1 tablespoon, unsalted butter	Just a pinch, smoked sea salt
1 teaspoon, cardamom seeds freshly ground	Chopped up fresh basil

DIRECTIONS and Cooking Time: 1 Hour
Prepare your Sous Vide water bath by increasing the temperature to a 180ºF using an immersion cooker Take a large sized heavy-duty plastic bag and add butter, apricots, ginger, cardamom, salt and mix the whole mixture well Seal up the bag using water displacement method and submerge it underwater Let it cook for 1 hour and remove the bag once done Take serving bowls and add the apricots to the bowl Garnish with a bit of basil and serve!

Nutrition Info:Per serving:Calories 28, Carbohydrates 6 g, Fats 0 g, Protein 1 g

Tangerine & Green Bean Platter With Hazelnuts

INGREDIENTS for Servings: 9

1 pound green beans, trimmed	2 tbsp butter
2 small tangerines	Salt to taste
	2 oz hazelnuts

DIRECTIONS and Cooking Time: 1 Hour 20 Minutes
Prepare a water bath and place the Sous Vide in it. Set to 186 F. Combine the green beans, butter and salt. Place in a vacuum-sealable bag. Zest one of the tangerines inside. Release air by the water displacement method, seal and submerge the bag in the water bath. Cook for 60 minutes. Once the timer has stopped, remove the bag. Preheat the oven yo 400 F. and toast the hazelnuts for 7 minutes. Peel and chop, and top the beans with hazelnuts and tangerine zest.

Radishes With "vegan" Butter

INGREDIENTS for Servings: 4

1 pound radishes, cut up in half lengthwise	3 tablespoons vegan butter
	½ teaspoon sea salt

DIRECTIONS and Cooking Time: 45 Minutes

Prepare your Sous Vide water bath using your immersion circulator and raise the temperature to 190-degrees Fahrenheit. Add your radish halves, butter, and salt in a resealable zipper bag and seal it up using the immersion method. Submerge underwater and cook for 45 minutes. Once cooked, strain the liquid and discard. Serve the radishes in a bowl!

Nutrition Info:Per serving:Calories: 134 ;Carbohydrates: 30g ;Protein: 1g ;Fat: 0g ;Sugar: 28g ;Sodium: 517mg

Lemon Collard Greens Salad With Cranberries

INGREDIENTS for Servings: 6

6 cups fresh collard greens, stemmed	4 tbsp lemon juice
6 tbsp olive oil	½ tsp salt
2 garlic cloves, crushed	¾ cup dried cranberries

DIRECTIONS and Cooking Time: 15 Minutes
Prepare a water bath and place the Sous Vide in it. Set to 196 F. Combine the collard greens with 2 tbsp of olive oil. Place it in a vacuum-sealable bag. Release air by the water displacement method, seal and submerge the bag in the water bath. Cook for 8 minutes. Stir the remaining olive oil, garlic, lemon juice and salt. Once the timer has stopped, remove the collard greens and transfer onto a serving plate. Sprinkle with the dressing. Garnish with cranberries.

Sweet Daikon Radishes With Rosemary

INGREDIENTS for Servings: 4

½ cup lemon juice	1 large size daikon radish, sliced
3 tbsp sugar	
1 tsp rosemary	

DIRECTIONS and Cooking Time: 40 Minutes
Prepare a water bath and place the Sous Vide in it. Set to 182 F. Combine the lemon juice, rosemary, salt, and sugar. Place the mixture and daikon radish in a vacuum-sealable bag. Release air by the water displacement method, seal and submerge the bag in the water bath. Cook for 30 minutes. Once the timer has stopped, remove the bag and transfer into an ice-water bath. Serve in a plate.

Coconut Potato Mash

INGREDIENTS for Servings: 4

1 ½ pounds Yukon gold potatoes, sliced	8 oz coconut milk
4 ounces butter	Salt and white pepper to taste

DIRECTIONS and Cooking Time: 45 Minutes
Prepare a water bath and place Sous Vide in it. Set to 193 F. Place the potatoes, coconut milk, butter, and salt in a vacuum-sealable bag. Release air by water displacement method, seal and submerge in the bath. Cook for 30 minutes. Once done, remove the bag and drain. Reserve butter juices. Mash the potatoes until soft and transfer to the butter bowl. Season with pepper and serve.

Radish & Basil Salad

INGREDIENTS for Servings: 2

20 small radishes, trimmed	½ cup feta cheese
1 tbsp white wine vinegar	1 tsp sugar
	1 tbsp water
¼ cup chopped basil	¼ tsp salt

DIRECTIONS and Cooking Time: 50 Minutes
Prepare a water bath and place the Sous Vide in it. Set to 200 F. Place the radishes in a large vacumm-sealable bag and add vinegar, sugar, salt and water. Shake to combine. Release air by the water displacement method, seal and submerge in water bath. Cook for 30 minutes. Once the timer has stopped, remove the bag and let cool in an ice bath. Serve warm. Serve tossed with the basil and feta.

Sous Vide Balsamic Onions

INGREDIENTS for Servings: 2

2 medium white onions, sliced julienne	1 tbsp, balsamic vinegar
2 tbsp, brown sugar	2 tbsp, olive oil
	Salt/Pepper to taste

DIRECTIONS and Cooking Time: 2 Hours
Prepare your Sous Vide water bath by attaching the immersion circulator and setting the temperature to 185ºF. Mix the onions with the rest of the ingredients in a sealable plastic bag and seal using a vacuum sealer or the water displacement method. Submerge into the bath water and allow cooking for 2 hours. Remove, transfer into a mason jar, cool and keep in the fridge for up to 12 hours before serving.

Nutrition Info: Per serving:Calories 186.7, Carbohydrates 15.5 g, Fats 13.5 g, Protein 0.8 g

Garlicky Snow Bean Sauce

INGREDIENTS for Servings: 4

4 cups halved snow beans	2 tsp rice wine vinegar
3 minced garlic cloves	1½ tbsp prepared black bean sauce
1 tbsp olive oil	

DIRECTIONS and Cooking Time: 1 Hour 50 Minutes
Prepare a water bath and place the Sous Vide in it. Set to 172 F. Combine well all the ingredients with the snow beans and place them in a vacuum-sealable bag. Release air by the water displacement method, seal and submerge the bag in the water bath. Cook for 1 hour and 30 minutes. Once the timer has stopped, remove the bag and serve warm.

Maple Beet Salad With Cashews & Queso Fresco

INGREDIENTS for Servings: 8

6 large beets, peeled and cut into chunks	1 tbsp olive oil
Salt and black pepper to taste	½ tsp cayenne pepper
	1½ cups cashews
3 tbsp maple syrup	6 cup arugula
2 tbsp butter	3 tangerines, peeled and segmented
Zest of 1 large orange	1 cup queso fresco, crumbled

DIRECTIONS and Cooking Time: 1 Hour 35 Minutes
Prepare a water bath and place the Sous Vide in it. Set to 186 F. Place the beet chunks in a vacuum-sealable bag. Season with salt and pepper. Add 2 tbsp of maple syrup, butter, and orange zest. Release air by the water displacement method, seal and submerge the bag in the water bath. Cook for 1 hour and 15 minutes. Preheat the oven to 350 F. Mix the remaining maple syrup, olive oil, salt, and cayenne. Add in cashews and stir well. Transfer the cashew mixture into a baking tray, previously lined with wax pepper and bake for 10 minutes. Set aside and allow to cool. Once the timer has stopped, remove the beets and discard the cooking juices. Put the arugula on a serving plate, beets and tangerine wedges all over. Scatter with queso fresco and cashew mix to serve.

Buttery Summer Squash

INGREDIENTS for Servings: 4

2 tbsp butter	¾ cup onion, chopped
1½ pounds summer squash, sliced	½ cup whole milk
	2 large whole eggs
Salt and black pepper to taste	½ cup crumbled plain potato chips

DIRECTIONS and Cooking Time: 1 Hour 35 Minutes
Prepare a water bath and place the Sous Vide in it. Set to 175 F   Meanwhile, grease a few jars. Heat a large skillet over medium heat and melt the butter. Add in onions and sauté for 7 minutes. Add the squash, season with salt and pepper and sauté for 10 minutes. Divide the mix in the jars. Allow it cool and set aside. Whisk the milk, salt and eggs in a bowl. Season with pepper. Pour the mixture over the jars, seal and submerge the jars in the water bath. Cook for 60 minutes. Once the timer has stopped, remove the jars and allow cooling for 5 minutes. Serve over potato chips.

Radish With Herb Cheese

INGREDIENTS for Servings: 3

10 oz goat cheese	3 tsp lemon juice
4 oz cream cheese	2 tbsp parsley
¼ cup red bell pepper, minced	2 clove garlic
3 tbsp pesto	9 large radishes, sliced.

DIRECTIONS and Cooking Time: 1 Hour 15 Minutes
Make a water bath, place Sous Vide in it, and set to 181 F. Place the radish slices in a vacuum-sealable bag, release air and seal it. Submerge the bag in the water bath and set the timer for 1 hour.   In a bowl, mix the remaining listed ingredients and pour the mixture into a piping bag. Set aside. Once the timer has stopped, remove the bag and unseal. Arrange the radish slices on a serving platter and pipe the cheese mixture on each slice. Serve as a snack.

Bell Pepper Rice Pilaf With Raisins

INGREDIENTS for Servings: 6

2 cups white rice	2 tbsp sour cream
2 cups veggie stock	1 bell pepper, chopped
⅔ cup water	
3 tbsp raisins, chopped	Salt and black pepper to taste
½ cup chopped red onion	1 tsp thyme

DIRECTIONS and Cooking Time: 3 Hours 10 Minutes
Prepare a water bath and place the Sous Vide in it. Set to 180 F.   Place all the ingredients in a vacumm-sealable bag. Stir to combine well. Release air by the water displacement method, seal and submerge the bag in water bath.Set the timer for 3 hours. Once the timer has stopped, remove the bag. Serve warm.

Balsamic Braised Cabbage Currants

INGREDIENTS for Servings: 4

1 and ½ pound, red cabbage	1 tablespoon, balsamic vinegar
¼ cup, currants	1 tablespoon, unsalted butter
1 thinly sliced shallot	
3 thinly sliced garlic clove	½ teaspoon, kosher salt

DIRECTIONS and Cooking Time: 2 Hours
Prepare your Sous Vide water bath by dipping your immersion cooker and raising the temperature to 185ºF   Slice up your cabbage into quarters and remove the core   Chop up the cabbage into 1 and ½ inch pieces   Take 2 large sized heavy-duty zip bag and divide the cabbages between the bags   Divide the dry ingredients between the bags as well   Seal up the bags using immersion method   Submerge the bag underwater and let them cook for 2 hours   Once the cooking is done, remove the bag from the water and transfer it to a serving bowl   Add the juices   Season with some salt and vinegar and serve!

Nutrition Info: Per serving:Calories 204, Carbohydrates 9 g, Fats 16 g, Protein 6 g

Garlicky Truffled Potatoes

INGREDIENTS for Servings: 4

8 oz red potato wedges	Salt and black pepper to taste
3 tbsp white truffle butter	1 garlic clove, minced
1 tbsp truffle oil	

DIRECTIONS and Cooking Time: 1 Hour 50 Minutes
Prepare a water bath and place the Sous Vide in it. Set to 182 F.   Place the truffle butter, red potatoes and truffle oil in a vacuum-sealable bag. Season with salt and pepper. Shake well. Release air by the water displacement method, seal and submerge the bag in the water bath. Cook for 90 minutes. Once the timer has stopped, remove the potatoes and transfer to a hot skillet. Cook for 5 minutes more until the liquid evaporated.

Beetroot & Goat Cheese Salad

INGREDIENTS for Servings: 3

1 lb beetroot, cut into wedges	1 tsp lemon zest
	Salt to taste
½ cup almonds, blanched	½ cup goat cheese, crumbled
2 tbsp hazelnuts, skinned	Fresh mint leaves to garnish

2 tsp olive oil	Dressing:
1 clove garlic, finely minced	2 tbsp olive oil
	1 tbsp apple cider
1 tsp cumin powder	vinegar

DIRECTIONS and Cooking Time: 2 Hours 20 Minutes
Make a water bath, place the Sous Vide in it, and set to
183 F.   Place the beetroots in a vacuum-sealable bag.
Release air by the water displacement method, seal
and submerge the bag in the water bath and set the
timer for 2 hours. Once the timer has stopped, remove
and unseal the bag. Place the beetroot aside.   Put a
pan over medium heat, add almonds and hazelnuts,
and toast for 3 minutes. Transfer to a cutting board
and chop. Add oil to the same pan, place garlic and
cumin. Cook for 30 seconds. Turn heat off. In a bowl,
add the goat cheese, almond mixture, lemon zest, and
garlic mixture. Mix. Whisk olive oil and vinegar and set
aside. Serve as a side dish.

VEGETABLES & SIDES

Chinese Black Bean Sauce

INGREDIENTS for Servings: 4

4 cups halved green beans	1½ tablespoons prepared black bean sauce
3 minced garlic cloves	
2 teaspoons rice wine vinegar	1 tablespoon olive oil

DIRECTIONS and Cooking Time: 90 Minutes
Prepare the Sous-vide water bath using your immersion circulator and raise the temperature to 170-degrees Fahrenheit. Add all the listed ingredients into a large mixing bowl alongside the green beans. Coat everything evenly. Take a heavy-duty zip bag and add the mixture. Zip the bag using the immersion method and submerge it underwater. Cook for about 1 hour and 30 minutes. Once cooked, take it out and serve immediately!

Nutrition Info: Calories: 375 Carbohydrates: 14g Protein: 12g Fat: 12g Sugar: 5g Sodium: 485mg

Southern Sweet Potatoes & Pecans

INGREDIENTS for Servings: 2

1 lb. sweet potatoes sliced up into ¼ inch thick rounds	½ teaspoon kosher salt
¼ cup pecans	1 tablespoon coconut oil

DIRECTIONS and Cooking Time: 180 Minutes
Prepare the Sous Vide water bath using your immersion circulator and raise the temperature to 145-degrees Fahrenheit. Add the potatoes and salt to your resealable bag and seal using the immersion method Transfer the bag to the water bath and let it cook for 3 hours. Toast the pecans in a dry skillet over medium heat. Once done, transfer the pecans to a cutting board and chop them up. Preheat your oven to 375-degrees Fahrenheit and line a rimmed baking sheet with parchment paper. Once the potatoes are cooked, move them to a bowl and toss with the coconut oil. Then, spread the potatoes on the baking sheet and bake for 20-30 minutes, making sure to flip them once. Transfer to serving platter and serve with a sprinkle of toasted pecans.

Nutrition Info: Calories: 195 Carbohydrates: 30g Protein: 6g Fat: 6g Sugar: 9g Sodium: 346mg

Caramelized Onions

INGREDIENTS

1 tablespoon cooking oil	2 tablespoons butter
2 pound yellow onions, thinly sliced	1 garlic clove, crushed
	¼ Teaspoon salt

DIRECTIONS and Cooking Time: 24 Hours Cooking Temperature: 186°f
Attach the sous vide immersion circulator to a Cambro container or pot with water using an adjustable clamp and preheat water to 186°F. In a skillet, heat oil and butter over medium heat and cook onions and salt until translucent. Add garlic and cook for about 1 minute. Remove from heat and set aside to cool completely. Place cooled onions in a cooking pouch. Seal pouch tightly after squeezing out the excess air. Place pouch in sous vide bath and set the cooking time for about 24 hours. Cover the sous vide bath with plastic wrap to minimize water evaporation. Add water intermittently to maintain the proper water level. Remove pouch from the sous vide bath and carefully open it. Transfer onions to a container. Onions can be stored in a refrigerator for up to 3 days.

Easy Garden Green Beans

INGREDIENTS for Servings: 4

1 ½ pounds fresh green beans, trimmed and snapped in half	Flaky salt and lemon pepper, to taste
2 tablespoons olive oil	3 cloves garlic, minced

DIRECTIONS and Cooking Time: 45 Minutes
Preheat a sous vide water bath to 183 degrees F. Place the green beans, 1 tablespoon of olive oil, salt, and lemon pepper in a large cooking pouch; seal tightly. Submerge the cooking pouch in the water bath; cook for 40 minutes. In the meantime, heat the remaining tablespoon of olive oil in a pan; sauté the garlic for 1 minute or until aromatic. Add the green beans to the pan with garlic, stir, and serve immediately. Enjoy!

Nutrition Info:100 Calories; 6g Fat; 1g Carbs; 1g Protein; 4g Sugars

Cardamom Apricots

INGREDIENTS for Servings: 4

1 pint small apricots, halved	½ teaspoon ground ginger
1 tablespoon unsalted butter	A pinch of smoked sea salt
1 teaspoon cardamom seeds, freshly ground	Fresh basil for garnishing, chopped

DIRECTIONS and Cooking Time: 1 Hour

Prepare your Sous Vide water bath by increasing the temperature to 180-degrees Fahrenheit using an immersion circulator   Put the butter, apricots, ginger, cardamom, and salt in a large, heavy-duty plastic bag, and mix them well   Carefully seal the bag using the immersion method and submerge it in the hot water   Let it cook for 60 minutes and remove the bag once done   Put the apricots in serving bowls   Garnish by topping it up with basil   Serve!

Nutrition Info: Per serving:Calories: 270 ;Carbohydrate: 60g ;Protein: 1g ;Fat: 0g ;Sugar: 49g ;Sodium: 33mg

Strawberry Jam

INGREDIENTS for Servings: 10

2 cups strawberries, coarsely chopped	1 cup white sugar 2 tbsp orange juice

DIRECTIONS and Cooking Time: 1 Hour 30 Minutes
Put the ingredients into the vacuum bag and seal it. Cook for 1 hour 30 minutes in the water bath, previously preheated to 180ºF.   Serve over ice cream or cheese cake, or store in the fridge in an airtight container.

Nutrition Info: Per serving:Calories 131, Carbohydrates 13 g, Fats 7 g, Protein 4 g

Beet Salad With Pecans

INGREDIENTS for Servings: 4

1 ½ pounds beets, peeled and sliced 1/4-inch thick 1 medium-sized leek 2 garlic cloves, minced 1 cup baby arugula 1/4 cup mayonnaise 1 teaspoon grainy mustard	Salt and ground black pepper, to taste 1/3 teaspoon cumin seeds 2 teaspoons balsamic vinegar 1 tablespoon honey 1/4 cup pecan halves, roasted

DIRECTIONS and Cooking Time: 1 Hour 5 Minutes
Preheat a sous vide water bath to 185 degrees F. Place the beets in a cooking pouch; seal tightly. Submerge the cooking pouch in the water bath; cook for 1 hour. Remove from the cooking pouch.   Add the leeks, garlic, and baby arugula; toss to combine. Then, toss your salad with the mayo, mustard, salt, pepper, cumin, vinegar, and honey; toss again to combine well.   Serve topped with roasted pecan halves and enjoy!

Nutrition Info:206 Calories; 7g Fat; 24g Carbs; 1g Protein; 12g Sugars

Tomato Confit

INGREDIENTS for Servings: 4

1.25lb. cherry tomatoes 1 pinch Fleur de sel 6 black peppercorns	1 teaspoon cane sugar 2 tablespoons Bianco Aceto Balsamico 2 sprigs rosemary

DIRECTIONS and Cooking Time: 20 Minutes
Preheat Sous Vide to 126°F.   Heat water in a pot and bring to simmer.   Make a small incision at the bottom of each tomato.   Place the tomatoes into simmering water and simmer 30 seconds.   Remove from the water and peel their skin.   Divide the tomatoes between two Souse Vide bags.   Sprinkle the tomatoes with salt, peppercorns, sugar, and Aceto Balsamico. Add 1 sprig rosemary per bag.   Vacuum-seal the bags, but just to 90%. Tomatoes are soft, and they can turn into mush.   Submerge tomatoes in water and cook 20 minutes.   Remove the tomatoes from Sous Vide cooker and submerge in ice-cold water for 5 minutes.   Transfer the tomatoes to a bowl, and serve with fresh mozzarella.

Nutrition Info: Per serving:Calories 34.3, Carbohydrates 6.6 g, Fats 0.3 g, Protein 1.3 g

Vanilla Poached Peaches

INGREDIENTS for Servings: 4

4 peaches, halved, stone removed ½ cup white rum ¾ cup brown sugar 2 tablespoons lemon juice	½ vanilla bean, seeds scraped ¼ cup Greek yogurt 2 tablespoons honey ¼ cup chopped pistachios

DIRECTIONS and Cooking Time: 1 Hour
Heat Sous Vide cooker to 165ºF.   In a Sous Vide bag, combine peaches, rum, ¼ cup brown sugar, lemon juice, and vanilla.   Vacuum seal the bag and cook the peaches in the cooker for 1 hour.   In a small bowl, combine Greek yogurt and honey.   Open the bag and pour the poaching liquid into a saucepan. Add brown sugar and simmer 6-7 minutes or until thickened. Serve peaches on a plate. Fill the cavities with Greek yogurt and drizzle all with the syrup.   Serve.

Nutrition Info: Per serving:Calories 240, Carbohydrates 51 g, Fats 2.5 g, Protein 3.5 g

Mashed Potatoes With Garlic

INGREDIENTS

2 pound russet potatoes, peeled and cut into 1/8-inch pieces 1 cup whole milk 1 cup unsalted butter	3 fresh rosemary sprigs 5 garlic cloves, smashed 2 teaspoons kosher salt

DIRECTIONS and Cooking Time: 1 Hour 30 Mins
Cooking Temperature: 194°f

Attach the sous vide immersion circulator to a Cambro container or pot with water using an adjustable clamp and preheat water to 194°F. Place all ingredients in a cooking pouch. Seal pouch tightly after squeezing out the excess air. Place pouch in sous vide bath and set the cooking time for about 1½ hours. Remove pouch from the sous vide bath and carefully open it. Remove potatoes from pouch, reserving cooking liquid in a bowl. Discard rosemary sprigs. Transfer potatoes into a large bowl and mash well. Gently beat reserved cooking liquid. Add reserved liquid into mashed potatoes and stir to combine. Serve immediately.

Blueberry Jam

INGREDIENTS for Servings: 10

2 cups blueberries	2 tbsp lemon juice
1 cup white sugar	

DIRECTIONS and Cooking Time: 1 Hour 30 Minutes
Preheat the water bath to 180ºF. Put the ingredients into the vacuum bag and seal it. Cook for 1 hour 30 minutes in the water bath. Serve over ice cream or cake, or store in the fridge in an airtight container.

Nutrition Info: Per serving:Calories 74, Carbohydrates 13 g, Fats 2 g, Protein 1 g

Corn On The Cob

INGREDIENTS

4 ears corn, in the husk, both ends trimmed	Kosher salt, to taste Fresh cilantro, chopped, as required
2 tablespoons butter, plus extra for serving	Garlic cloves, minced, as required

DIRECTIONS and Cooking Time: 30 Mins Cooking Temperature: 183°f
Attach the sous vide immersion circulator to a Cambro container or pot with water using an adjustable clamp and preheat water to 183°F. In 2 cooking pouches, divide all ingredients evenly. Seal pouch tightly after squeezing out the excess air. Place pouches in sous vide bath and set the cooking time for about 30 minutes. Remove pouches from the sous vide bath and carefully open them. Remove corn ears from pouches. Carefully, remove corn from husks. Discard husks. Serve corn with extra butter.

Currant & Braised Cabbage

INGREDIENTS for Servings: 4

1 ½ pounds red cabbage	1 tablespoon apple balsamic vinegar
¼ cup currants	1 tablespoon unsalted butter
1 thinly sliced shallot	

3 thinly sliced garlic clove	½ a teaspoon kosher salt

DIRECTIONS and Cooking Time: 120 Minutes
Prepare the Sous-vide water bath using your immersion circulator and raise the temperature to 185-degrees Fahrenheit. Take the cabbage and slice the cabbage into quarters, make sure to discard the core. Chop them up into 1 ½-inch pieces. Take 2 heavy-duty resealable zipper bags and divide the cabbages between the two bags. Divide as well the remaining ingredients equally between the bags Seal using the immersion method. Submerge underwater and cook for 2 hours. Once done, remove the bag and transfer to a bowl. Add the cooking juices and season with a bit of salt and vinegar. Serve!

Nutrition Info: Calories: 172 Carbohydrates: 6g Protein: 7g Fat: 14g Sugar: 3g Sodium: 342mg

Garlic & Paprika Sweet Potatoes

INGREDIENTS

7 tablespoons salted butter, softened	2 teaspoons fresh thyme, chopped
4½ tablespoons maple syrup	2 teaspoons smoked paprika
10 roasted, smoked garlic cloves	2 pounds /1 kg sweet potatoes, peeled and chopped
Sea salt, to taste	

DIRECTIONS and Cooking Time: 1 Hour Cooking Temperature: 185°f
Attach the sous vide immersion circulator to a Cambro container or pot with water using an adjustable clamp and preheat water to 185°F. In a bowl, add all ingredients except sweet potatoes and mix until well combined. Place sweet potatoes and butter mixture in a cooking pouch. Seal pouch tightly after squeezing out the excess air. Place pouch in sous vide bath and set the cooking time for about 45-60 minutes. Remove pouch from the sous vide bath and carefully open it. Remove sweet potatoes from pouch. Heat a sauté pan and cook sweet potatoes until golden brown.

Rosemary Potato Soup

INGREDIENTS for Servings: 4

1 pound potatoes, peeled and cubed	1/4 teaspoon ground allspice
2 sprigs fresh rosemary	Coarse salt and freshly ground black pepper, to your liking
2 garlic cloves, smashed	1 cup broth, preferably homemade
2 tablespoons butter	
1/2 small white onion, peeled and chopped	1/3 cup double cream

DIRECTIONS and Cooking Time: 1 Hour 10 Minutes

Preheat a sous vide water bath to 183 degrees F. Place the potatoes, fresh rosemary, and garlic in a cooking pouch; seal tightly. Submerge the cooking pouch in the water bath; cook for 1 hour. Remove the potatoes from the cooking pouch, reserving cooking liquid. In a pot, melt the butter over medium-high heat. Sauté the onions until translucent. Add ground allspice, salt, pepper, and reserved potatoes with cooking liquid. Add broth and bring it to a boil. Now, reduce the heat to medium-low; allow the soup to simmer until heated through. Remove from the heat. Fold in double cream and stir until well combined. Ladle into four soup bowls and serve immediately. Bon appétit!

Nutrition Info:178 Calories; 4g Fat; 39g Carbs; 3g Protein; 8g Sugars

Simple Apple And Pear Winter Compote

INGREDIENTS for Servings: 4

2 apples, cored and diced	1 teaspoon vanilla essence
2 pears, cored and diced	2 cinnamon sticks
1/2 cup stock syrup	5 green cardamom pods

DIRECTIONS and Cooking Time: 1 Hour
Preheat a sous vide water bath to 185 degrees F. Add all of the above ingredients to a large cooking pouch; seal tightly. Submerge the cooking pouch in the water bath; cook for 1 hour. Serve warm or cold. Bon appétit!

Nutrition Info:226 Calories; 5g Fat; 59g Carbs; 9g Protein; 58g Sugars

Whiskey Infused Apples

INGREDIENTS for Servings: 4

4 Gala apples	2 tablespoons maple whiskey
2 tablespoons brown sugar	

DIRECTIONS and Cooking Time: 1 Hour
Preheat your Sous Vide cooker to 175ºF Peel, core, and slice apples. Place the apple slices, sugar, and whiskey into Sous Vide bag. Vacuum seal and submerge in water. Cook 1 hour. Remove the bag from the water. Serve apples with ice cream while hot.

Nutrition Info: Per serving:Calories 86.9, Carbohydrates 20.4 g, Fats 0.5 g, Protein 0.2 g

Curried Apples

INGREDIENTS for Servings: 4

2 tart apples, cored, peeled and sliced	2 tablespoons coconut cream
1 tablespoon Madras curry powder	

DIRECTIONS and Cooking Time: 1 Hour
Prepare your Sous Vide water bath using your immersion circulator and raise the temperature to 185-degrees Fahrenheit Put all the ingredients into a heavy-duty resealable bag and seal it using the immersion method Submerge and cook for 60 minutes Remove the apples and transfer to a large bowl Divide them among the serving plates and serve!

Nutrition Info: Per serving:Calories: 368 ;Carbohydrate: 70g ;Protein: 6g ;Fat: 8g ;Sugar: 17g ;Sodium: 450mg

Szechuan Style Green Beans

INGREDIENTS

12 ounces /3/4 pound fresh, long green beans	1 teaspoon sesame oil, toasted
1 tablespoon dried onions, minced	½ Teaspoon garlic salt
1 tablespoon red chili flakes	1 tablespoon sesame seeds, toasted
1 tablespoon Sriracha chili sauce	Chopped scallions, for garnishing

DIRECTIONS and Cooking Time: 1 Hour Cooking Temperature: 186°f
Attach the sous vide immersion circulator to a Cambro container or pot with water using an adjustable clamp and preheat water to 186°F. Place beans, onions, chili flakes, Sriracha, sesame oil, and garlic salt in a cooking pouch. Seal pouch tightly after squeezing out the excess air. Place pouch in sous vide bath and set the cooking time for about 45-60 minutes. Remove pouch from the sous vide bath and carefully open it. Transfer beans onto a serving platter. Garnish with sesame seeds and scallions and serve.

Whiskey & Poached Peaches

INGREDIENTS for Servings: 4

2 peaches, pitted and quartered	1 teaspoon vanilla extract
½ cup rye whiskey	A pinch of salt
½ cup ultrafine sugar	

DIRECTIONS and Cooking Time: 30 Minutes
Prepare your Sous Vide water bath using your immersion circulator and raise the temperature to 180-degrees Fahrenheit Place all the ingredients in a heavy-duty zip bag Seal it using immersion method and submerge it in the hot water Let it cook

for about 30 minutes   Once the timer runs out, take the bag out and transfer it to an ice bath   Serve!

Nutrition Info:Per serving:Calories: 656 ;Carbohydrate: 162g ;Protein: 13g ;Fat: 3g ;Sugar: 147g ;Sodium: 8mg

Wine Maple Poached Fruits

INGREDIENTS for Servings: 4

1 pound ripe peaches, peeled, pitted and halved	1 cup maple syrup
1 cup white wine	1 teaspoon whole cloves
2 cups water	1 vanilla pod
1 /1-inch piece fresh ginger, peeled	2 sticks cinnamon
	1/3 cup almonds, blanched

DIRECTIONS and Cooking Time: 1 Hour
Preheat a sous vide water bath to 170 degrees F. Place all ingredient, except for almonds, in a large-sized cooking pouch; seal tightly.   Submerge the cooking pouch in the water bath; cook for 50 minutes. Pour the cooking liquid into a pan that is preheated over a moderate flame. Bring to a rolling boil. Immediately turn the heat to medium.   Continue to cook an additional 6 minutes, or until the sauce is slightly thickened and syrupy.   To serve, arrange peach on a serving plate; spoon the wine/maple syrup over them; garnish with blanched almonds. Bon appétit!

Nutrition Info:294 Calories; 3g Fat; 71g Carbs; 9g Protein; 64g Sugars

Pickled Carrots

INGREDIENTS for Servings: 1

1 cup white wine vinegar	½ cup beet sugar
3 tablespoons kosher salt	10-12 pieces' petite carrots, peeled with the stems trimmed
1 teaspoon black peppercorns	4 sprigs fresh thyme
1/3 cup ice cold water	2 peeled garlic cloves

DIRECTIONS and Cooking Time: 90 Minutes
Prepare the Sous-vide water bath using your immersion circulator and raise the temperature to 190-degrees Fahrenheit.   Take a medium-sized saucepan and add the vinegar, salt, sugar, and peppercorns and place it over medium heat.   Then, let the mixture reach the boiling point and keep stirring until the sugar has dissolved alongside the salt Remove the heat and add the cold water.   Allow the mixture to cool down to room temperature.   Take a resealable bag and add the thyme, carrots, and garlic alongside the brine solution and seal it up using the immersion method.   Submerge underwater and cook for 90 minutes.   Once cooked, remove the bag from the water bath and place into an ice bath.   Carefully take the carrots out from the bag and serve !

Nutrition Info:Calories: 127 Carbohydrates: 24g Protein: 2g Fat: 1g Sugar: 16g Sodium: 54mg

Brown Rice Pilaf

INGREDIENTS

1 tablespoon extra-virgin olive oil	Kosher salt, to taste
1 medium leek /white and light green portion, halved and thinly sliced	¼ Cup currants
	1 cup brown rice, rinsed
	2 cups vegetable broth
1 garlic clove, minced	¼ Cup walnuts, toasted and chopped

DIRECTIONS and Cooking Time: 3 Hours Cooking Temperature: 180°f
Attach the sous vide immersion circulator to a Cambro container or pot with water using an adjustable clamp and preheat water to 180°F.   In a small pan, heat the olive oil over medium heat and cook leek, garlic, and ½ teaspoon of salt until fragrant, stirring occasionally. Remove from heat and stir in currants and rice. Place rice mixture and broth in a cooking pouch. Seal pouch tightly after squeezing out the excess air. Place pouch in sous vide bath and set the cooking time for about 3 hours.   Remove pouch from the sous vide bath and carefully open it. Transfer rice mixture into a serving bowl and season with salt.   Sprinkle with walnuts and serve.

Okra With Chili Yogurt

INGREDIENTS for Servings: 6

4 tablespoons olive oil	2.5lb. fresh okra
1 ½ tablespoon lime zest	Yogurt:
	1 cup Greek yogurt
2 cloves garlic, crushed	2 teaspoons chili powder
Salt and white pepper, to taste	¼ cup chopped cilantro

DIRECTIONS and Cooking Time: 1 Hour
Preheat your Sous Vide to 178ºF.   Divide the fresh okra among two cooking bags.   Drizzle the okra with 2 ½ tablespoons olive oil (divided per bag), lime zest, and season to taste. Add one clove garlic per pouch.   Vacuum seal the bags and submerge in water.   Cook the okra 1 hour. Remove from a water bath and drain the accumulated liquid in a bowl. Place the okra in a separate bowl.   In a medium bowl, combine Greek yogurt, chili powder, cilantro, and accumulated okra water. Stir to combine.   Heat remaining olive oil in a skillet over medium-high heat. Fry okra in the heated oil for 2 minutes.   Serve warm, with chili yogurt.

Nutrition Info:Per serving:Calories 189.3, Carbohydrates 16.5 g, Fats 10.5 g, Protein 7.2 g

Pear & Walnut Salad

INGREDIENTS for Servings: 4

2 tablespoons honey	4 cups arugula
2 pears, cored, halved and thinly sliced	Garlic Dijon Dressing
½ cup walnuts, lightly toasted and roughly chopped	¼ cup olive oil
	1 tablespoon white wine vinegar
½ cup shaved parmesan	1 teaspoon Dijon mustard
Sea salt and pepper as needed	1 garlic clove, minced
	Salt as needed

DIRECTIONS and Cooking Time: 30 Minutes
Prepare your Sous Vide water bath using your immersion circulator and raise the temperature to 159-degrees Fahrenheit   Put the honey in a heat-proof bowl   Heat for 20 seconds   Put the pears in the honey and mix well   Put them in a heavy-duty resealable bag and seal using the immersion method   Cook for 30 minutes and plunge the bag into an ice water bath for 5 minutes   Chill in your fridge for 3 hours   Add all of the dressing ingredients and give the jar a nice shake   Leave it in your fridge for a while   Serve by placing the walnuts, arugula, and parmesan in a large bowl   Add your drained pear slices and the dressing   Toss everything well and season with pepper and salt

Nutrition Info:Calories: 377 Carbohydrate: 56g Protein: 5g Fat: 14g Sugar: 35g Sodium: 165mg

Garlic & Herb Potatoes

INGREDIENTS

1 stick butter, melted	½ Teaspoon oregano
2 garlic cloves, chopped	½ Teaspoon paprika
½ Teaspoon basil	½ Teaspoon salt
Pinch of dried rosemary	5 pounds russet potatoes, peeled and cubed

DIRECTIONS and Cooking Time: 1 Hour Cooking Temperature: 183°f
Attach the sous vide immersion circulator to a Cambro container or pot with water using an adjustable clamp and preheat water to 183°F.   In a bowl, add all ingredients except potatoes and mix until well combined.   In 2 cooking pouch, divide potatoes and butter mixture. Seal pouch tightly after squeezing out the excess air. Place pouch in sous vide bath and set the cooking time for about 1 hour.   Preheat the broiler of oven to high.   Remove pouch from the sous vide bath and carefully open them. Transfer carrot mixture onto a broiler pan.   Broil for about 2-3 minutes.

Garlic & Rosemary Mashed Potatoes

INGREDIENTS for Servings: 4

2 lbs. Russet potatoes	8 oz. unsalted butter, melted
5 pieces' garlic cloves, peeled and mashed	3 sprigs rosemary
1 cup whole milk	Kosher salt as needed
	White pepper as needed

DIRECTIONS and Cooking Time: 90 Minutes
Prepare your water bath using your Sous Vide immersion circulator and raise the temperature to 194-degrees Fahrenheit   Rinse the potatoes well under cold water   Peel the potatoes and slice them into ⅛ inch thick rounds   Put the potatoes, garlic, butter, 2 teaspoons of salt, and rosemary into a heavy-duty, resealable bag and seal using the immersion method   Cook for 1½ hours   Strain the mixture and pour into a medium-sized bowl   Transfer the potatoes to a large-sized bowl and mash them using a potato masher   Stir the melted butter and milk into your mashed potatoes   Season with salt and pepper   Garnish with rosemary and serve!

Nutrition Info:Per serving:Calories: 184 ;Carbohydrate: 6g ;Protein: 6g ;Fat: 6g ;Sugar: 3g ;Sodium: 449mg

Pickled Mixed Veggies

INGREDIENTS for Servings: 4

12 oz. beets, cut up into ½-inch slices	2/3 cup white vinegar
½ Serrano pepper, seeds removed	2/3 cup filtered water
	2 tablespoons pickling spice
1 garlic clove, diced	

DIRECTIONS and Cooking Time: 40 Minutes
Prepare the Sous-vide water bath using your immersion circulator and raise the temperature to 190-degrees Fahrenheit.   Take 4-6 ounces' mason jar and add the Serrano pepper, beets, and garlic cloves   Take a medium stock pot and add the pickling spice, filtered water, white vinegar, and bring the mixture to a boil   Remove the stock and strain the mix over the beets in the jar.   Fill them up.   Seal it loosely and submerge it underwater. Cook for 40 minutes.   Allow the jars to cool and serve!

Nutrition Info:Calories: 174 Carbohydrates: 34g Protein: 4g Fat: 2g Sugar: 19g Sodium: 610mg

Spring Vegetables & Risotto

INGREDIENTS

For Risotto:	½ Teaspoon butter
1 cup Arborio rice	Salt and freshly
2 4-ounce cans	ground black pepper,

mushroom stems and pieces, chopped Leaves from 1 fresh rosemary sprig, minced 3 cups vegetable broth 1 pound spring vegetables /asparagus, broccoli, peppers, summer squash, cut into bite sized pieces	to taste For Vegetables: Salt and freshly ground black pepper, to taste 1-2 tablespoons butter Fresh herbs of choice For Garnishing: Freshly grated Parmesan cheese, for serving

DIRECTIONS and Cooking Time: 40 Mins Cooking Temperature: 183°f

Attach the sous vide immersion circulator to a Cambro container or pot with water using an adjustable clamp and preheat water to 183°F. Place all risotto ingredients in a cooking pouch and all vegetable ingredients in a second pouch. Seal pouches tightly after squeezing out the excess air. Place pouches in sous vide bath and set the cooking time for about 40 minutes. Remove pouches from the sous vide bath and carefully open them. Transfer rice mixture into a serving bowl. With a fork, fluff the rice. Transfer vegetable mixture into another bowl. Divide rice into serving plate and top with vegetables evenly. Sprinkle with cheese and serve.

Spinach Cheese Dip

INGREDIENTS

1 pound cream cheese, cubed ½ Cup beer 2 ounces smoked Gouda cheese, grated ½ Medium red bell pepper, seeded and chopped ½ Cup fresh baby spinach leaves, chopped	1 garlic clove, peeled and pressed 1 tablespoon Dijon mustard 1 teaspoon Herbs de Provence 1 teaspoon salt ½ Teaspoon ground white pepper 1 sourdough round loaf, for serving

DIRECTIONS and Cooking Time: 1 Hour Cooking Temperature: 180°f

Attach the sous vide immersion circulator to a Cambro container or pot with water using an adjustable clamp and preheat water to 180°F. Place all ingredients except bread in a cooking pouch. Seal pouch tightly after squeezing out the excess air. Place pouch in sous vide bath and set the cooking time for about ½-1 hour. Remove the pouch from the sous vide bath and carefully massage it to mix the dip mixture. Return pouch to sous vide bath until cheese melts completely. Meanwhile, with a bread knife, remove the top from the loaf of bread. Carefully hollow out the middle of loaf to make a bread bowl. Cut the interior bread into bite-sized pieces. Remove the pouch from the sous

vide bath and carefully open it. Immediately, transfer dip into the bread bowl. Serve with bread pieces.

Greek-style Eggplant With Sour Cream

INGREDIENTS for Servings: 4

2 pounds eggplant 1/4 cup tomato puree 1 teaspoon red chili paste 1 tablespoon garlic paste	1 cup sour cream 1/2 cup fresh cilantro, chopped 1/2 cup Kalamata olives, pitted and sliced

DIRECTIONS and Cooking Time: 1 Hour 35 Minutes

Heat a nonstick skillet over a high heat; blister the skin of your eggplants until they are charred. In a small mixing bowl, whisk tomato puree, red chili paste, and garlic paste. Slice your eggplants lengthwise into halves. Now, divide the paste among eggplant halves. Preheat a sous vide water bath to 185 degrees F. Place the eggplant in cooking pouches; seal tightly. Submerge the cooking pouches in the water bath; cook for 1 hour 30 minutes. Serve with sour cream topped with fresh cilantro and Kalamata olives. Bon appétit!

Nutrition Info: 162 Calories; 3g Fat; 23g Carbs; 7g Protein; 9g Sugars

Biscuits

INGREDIENTS

1 cup all-purpose flour ½ Teaspoon granulated sugar 1 teaspoon baking powder ¼ Teaspoon salt	¼ Teaspoon baking soda ½ Cup chilled buttermilk 4 tablespoons unsalted butter, melted

DIRECTIONS and Cooking Time: 2 Hours Cooking Temperature: 195°f

Attach the sous vide immersion circulator to a Cambro container or pot with water using an adjustable clamp and preheat water to 195°F. Grease 5 half-pint canning jars generously. In a medium bowl, mix together flour, sugar, baking powder, baking soda, and salt. In another bowl, add buttermilk and butter and stir until butter forms distinct clumps in the buttermilk. Add buttermilk mixture into flour mixture and stir until just combined. Divide dough between prepared jars evenly. With a damp towel, wipe off sides and tops of jars. Cover each jar with the lid just tight. /Do not over-tighten jars; air will need to escape. Place jars in sous vide bath and set the cooking time for about 2 hours. Remove the jars from the sous vide bath and carefully remove the lids. Place jars onto a wire rack to cool for about 5 minutes. Carefully remove biscuits from jars and serve warm.

Herby Braised Leeks

INGREDIENTS for Servings: 4

1 pound leeks, discard outer leaves and halved lengthwise 1 cup vegetable stock 2 tablespoons sesame oil	2 garlic cloves, sliced 2 thyme sprigs Sea salt and ground black pepper, to taste

DIRECTIONS and Cooking Time: 40 Minutes
Preheat a sous vide water bath to 185 degrees F. Place all of the above ingredients in a cooking pouch; seal tightly. Submerge the cooking pouch in the water bath; cook for 35 minutes. Taste, adjust the seasonings and serve with mashed potatoes. Bon appétit!

Nutrition Info: 139 Calories; 2g Fat; 13g Carbs; 9g Protein; 8g Sugars

Brussels Sprouts With Garlic

INGREDIENTS

1 tablespoon olive oil 2 garlic cloves, smashed and minced Pinch of salt	Freshly ground black pepper, to taste 1 pound Brussels sprouts, trimmed

DIRECTIONS and Cooking Time: 1 Hour Cooking Temperature: 180°f
Attach the sous vide immersion circulator to a Cambro container or pot with water using an adjustable clamp and preheat water to 180°F. In a bowl, add all ingredients except Brussels sprouts and mix until well combined. Place Brussels sprouts and oil mixture in a cooking pouch. Seal pouch tightly after squeezing out the excess air. Place pouch in sous vide bath and set the cooking time for about 1 hour. Preheat a grill to medium heat. Remove pouch from the sous vide bath and carefully open it. Remove Brussels sprouts from pouch. Thread Brussels sprouts onto pre-soaked bamboo skewers. Grill for about 2-3 minutes per side.

Marinated Eggplant

INGREDIENTS

2 pound eggplant, cut into ½-inch slices Sea salt, to taste 1 tablespoon garlic, chopped 2 teaspoons fresh lemon zest, grated	Handful of fresh oregano, chopped Dash of olive oil 1 tablespoon smoked paprika Freshly cracked black pepper, to taste

DIRECTIONS and Cooking Time: 1 Hour 40 Mins Cooking Temperature: 185°f
Season eggplant slices with salt generously. Arrange eggplant slices onto a large flat tray, smaller round down. Sprinkle with more salt and set aside for about 2 hours. Attach the sous vide immersion circulator to a Cambro container or pot with water using an adjustable clamp and preheat water to 185°F. Rinse the eggplant slices completely and pat dry with paper towels. In a large bowl, add remaining ingredients and mix until well combined. Add eggplant slices and coat generously with mixture. In 2-3 cooking pouches, place eggplant slices in a single layer. Seal pouches tightly after squeezing out the excess air. Place the pouches in the sous vide bath and set the cooking time for about 1½ hours. Remove pouches from the sous vide bath and immediately immerse in a bowl of ice water. After cooling, remove eggplant slices from pouch. With paper towels, pat dry eggplant slices completely. Coat the eggplant slices with a coating of your choice, such as breadcrumbs, sesame seeds, or Parmesan cheese. Fry the coated slices in some butter and olive oil over low heat until golden brown. Serve alongside tomato salsa, goat cheese, and basil.

Green Beans & Mandarin Hazelnuts

INGREDIENTS for Servings: 9

1 lb. green beans, trimmed 2 small mandarin oranges	2 tablespoons butter ½ teaspoon salt 2 oz. toasted hazelnuts

DIRECTIONS and Cooking Time: 60 Minutes
Prepare the Sous Vide water bath using your immersion circulator and increase the temperature to 185-degrees Fahrenheit Put the green beans, butter, and salt in a zip bag Zest one of the mandarins into the bag and keep the other for later use Cut the zested mandarin in half and squeeze the juice into the bag Use the immersion method to seal the bag Submerge and cook for 60 minutes Pre-heat your oven to 400-degrees Fahrenheit and toast the hazelnuts for 7 minutes Remove the skin and chop roughly Serve by putting the beans on a platter and topping them up with a garnish of toasted hazelnut and the remaining mandarin zest

Nutrition Info: Calories: 520 Carbohydrate: 48g Protein: 40g Fat: 18g Sugar: 8g Sodium: 131mg

Sesame Broccoli And Cauliflower

INGREDIENTS for Servings: 4

1 pound cauliflower, cut into florets 1 pound broccoli, cut	1/4 teaspoon ground black pepper 2 teaspoons extra-

into florets 1 teaspoon dried parsley flakes Sea salt, to taste	virgin olive oil 1 tablespoon black sesame seeds

DIRECTIONS and Cooking Time: 45 Minutes
Preheat a sous vide water bath to 185 degrees F. Place the cauliflower, broccoli, parsley flakes, black pepper, sea salt, and 1 teaspoon of olive oil in cooking poaches; seal tightly. Submerge the cooking pouches in the water bath; cook for 40 minutes. Remove your veggies form the cooking pouches. Drizzle the remaining teaspoon of olive oil over your veggies. Sprinkle with black sesame seeds just before serving. Enjoy!

Nutrition Info:86 Calories; 3g Fat; 2g Carbs; 2g Protein; 6g Sugars

Sweet Potato Casserole

INGREDIENTS for Servings: 6

2 pounds sweet potatoes, peeled and cut into 1-inch cubes 1/4 teaspoon ground allspice Salt and white pepper, to taste 4 tablespoons sour cream	1 teaspoon vanilla 1/4 cup butter, softened 1/2 cup finely chopped pecans, divided 2 cups miniature marshmallows

DIRECTIONS and Cooking Time: 2 Hours
Preheat a sous vide water bath to 180 degrees F. Add sweet potatoes, allspice, vanilla, salt, and white pepper to a large cooking pouch; seal tightly. Submerge the cooking pouch in the water bath; cook for 1 hour 45 minutes. Then, mix sweet potatoes with sour cream. Spoon the mixture into a casserole dish. Combine the butter with pecans; top the casserole with this butter mixture. Spread miniature marshmallows over the top. Preheat the oven to 380 degrees F. Bake for 15 minutes or until the top is golden brown. Bon appétit!

Nutrition Info:307 Calories; 16g Fat; 48g Carbs; 5g Protein; 12g Sugars

Apple & Cauliflower Soup

INGREDIENTS for Servings: 8

2 tablespoons extra-virgin olive oil 1 large onion, diced 2 garlic cloves, thinly sliced 1/8 teaspoon crushed red chili flakes	Kosher salt as needed 1 large cauliflower head, chopped into medium florets 1 apple, peeled and diced 4-6 cups vegetable broth

DIRECTIONS and Cooking Time: 1 Hour

Prepare the Sous Vide water bath using your immersion circulator and increase the temperature to 183-degrees Fahrenheit Place a medium-sized skillet over a medium heat, add the oil and allow the oil to shimmer Add the onion, ¼ teaspoon of salt, and garlic and sauté for 7 minutes until they are tender Add the chili flakes and stir well Once done, turn-off the heat and allow the mixture to cool Divide the apple, the onion mix, cauliflower, and ¼ teaspoon of salt between two individual resealable bags Seal the bags using the immersion method, submerge and cook for 1 hour Once done, remove the bag and place the contents in a large pot Add the vegetable broth and blend well using an immersion blender Add a bit more broth for a thicker consistency Season with salt and serve

Nutrition Info: Calories: 192 Carbohydrate: 19g Protein: 8g Fat: 11g Sugar: 11g Sodium: 11mg

Momofuku Styled Brussels

INGREDIENTS for Servings: 8

2 lbs. Brussels sprouts, stems trimmed and slice in half 2 tablespoons extra-virgin olive oil ¼ teaspoon kosher salt ¼ cup fish sauce 1½ tablespoons granulated sugar	2 tablespoons water 1 tablespoon rice vinegar 1½ teaspoons lime juice 12 pieces thinly sliced Thai chilis 1 small minced garlic clove Chopped fresh mint Chopped fresh cilantro

DIRECTIONS and Cooking Time: 50 Minutes
Prepare the Sous Vide water bath using your immersion circulator and raise the temperature to 183-degrees Fahrenheit Put the Brussel sprouts, olive oil and salt in a heavy-duty, resealable bag Seal using the immersion method Cook for 50 minutes Put the fish sauce, sugar, water, rice vinegar, lime juice, garlic, and chilis in a small bowl and mix them to prepare the vinaigrette Once done, put the Brussels on an aluminum foil, lined baking sheet and heat up your broiler Broil the Brussels for 5 minutes until they are charred Transfer to a medium-sized bowl and add the vinaigrette Toss well and sprinkle with mint and cilantro

Nutrition Info: Calories: 610 Carbohydrate: 38g Protein: 10g Fat: 5g Sugar: 20g Sodium: 684mg

Mashed Potato

INGREDIENTS for Servings: 4

1 lb. russet potatoes, peeled and sliced 8 tablespoons butter	½ cup heavy cream 1 teaspoon kosher salt

DIRECTIONS and Cooking Time: 1 Hour

Prepare your water bath using your Sous Vide immersion circulator and raise the temperature to 190-degrees Fahrenheit   Add the heavy cream, russet potatoes, kosher salt, and butter into a heavy-duty zip bag and seal using the immersion method   Submerge and cook for 60 minutes   Pass the contents through a food processor into a large bowl   Mix them well and serve!

Nutrition Info: Per serving:Calories: 226 ;Carbohydrate: 34g ;Protein: 5g ;Fat: 7g ;Sugar: 3g ;Sodium: 93mg

Whiskey Sugared Sweet Potatoes

INGREDIENTS

½ Cup brown sugar	1 teaspoon salt
½ Teaspoon cinnamon	¼ cup American whiskey
½ Teaspoon ground allspice	4 sweet potatoes, peeled, and cut into
¼ Teaspoon cayenne pepper	½-inch cubes
Pinch of granulated onions	4 tablespoons butter
Pinch of granulated garlic	1 tablespoon cider vinegar

DIRECTIONS and Cooking Time: 1 Hour 25 Mins

Cooking Temperature: 150°f

Attach the sous vide immersion circulator to a Cambro container or pot with water using an adjustable clamp and preheat water to 150°F.   In a bowl, mix together sugar, spices, and salt. Set aside.   In a small pan, bring whiskey to a boil. Cook until it reduces by half. Add sugar mixture and cook until a paste is formed. Transfer sugar paste into a large bowl. Add sweet potato cubes and butter to the bowl and mix until well combined.   Place sweet potato mixture in a cooking pouch. Seal pouch tightly after squeezing out the excess air. Place pouch in sous vide bath and set the cooking time for about 1 hour.   Preheat oven to 400°F. Line a baking sheet with parchment paper. Remove pouch from the sous vide bath and carefully open it. Remove sweet potato cubes from pouch, reserving cooking liquid in a pan.   Place sweet potato cubes onto prepared baking sheet. Roast for about 25 minutes, stirring once after 15 minutes.   Meanwhile, cook reserved cooking liquid until desired thickness. Remove sweet potatoes from oven and transfer into a bowl. Add thickened sauce and vinegar and toss to coat well.   Serve immediately.

Persimmon Chutney

INGREDIENTS for Servings: 4

2 lbs. fuyu persimmons, peeled and diced into small	1½ teaspoons yellow mustard seeds
	1½ teaspoons
pieces	coriander seeds
1 small onion, diced	½ teaspoon kosher salt
½ cup light brown sugar	¼ teaspoon curry powder
¼ cup raisins	¼ teaspoon dried ginger
2 tablespoons apple cider vinegar	⅛ teaspoon cayenne
2 tablespoons freshly squeezed lemon juice	

DIRECTIONS and Cooking Time: 90 Minutes

Prepare your Sous Vide water bath using your immersion circulator and raise the temperature to 183-degrees Fahrenheit   Put all the ingredients into a large, heavy-duty resealable bag   Seal it using the immersion method and submerge   Cook for 90 minutes   Once done, remove the bag and transfer it to a storage container   Serve cool

Nutrition Info: Calories: 313 Carbohydrate: 79g Protein: 2g Fat: 1g Sugar: 28g Sodium: 509mg

Colorful Veggies With Tomato Sorbet

INGREDIENTS for Servings: 4

8 carrots, halved	2 tablespoons sugar
12 spears green asparagus	4 ripe tomatoes, peeled
1 cup fresh peas	2 tablespoons fresh lemon juice
3 tablespoons olive oil	1 tablespoon tomato paste
Salt and pepper, to taste	
Sorbet:	Salt and black pepper, to taste
¼ cup water	

DIRECTIONS and Cooking Time: 12 Minutes

Make the sorbet; in a food blender, blend the tomatoes until pureed.   Bring water, sugar, and basil to a boil in a saucepan. Remove from heat and allow to cool. Pour in the tomatoes and add tomato paste. Stir to combine.   Season to taste with salt and pepper.   Place the sorbet into a freezer. Freeze 2-4 hours or until firm.   Make the vegetables; peel and trim asparagus.   Place the asparagus in one Souse vide bag and add 1 tablespoon olive oil.   In a separate bag, place carrots and peas. Drizzle with olive oil. Vacuum seal both bags.   Set the Sous Vide to 190ºF. Cook the carrots and peas 12 minutes in heated water. After the carrots have been cooked 8 minutes, add asparagus.   Remove the bags from Sous Vide. Unpack the bags and arrange veggies onto a serving plate. Season to taste.   Serve veggies with a scoop of tomato sorbet.

Nutrition Info: Per serving:Calories 243.4, Carbohydrates 30.8 g, Fats 11 g, Protein 5.3 g

Orange Compote

INGREDIENTS for Servings: 4

4 blood oranges, quartered and thinly sliced 2 cups granulated sugar ½ vanilla seed pod	1 lemon, juice and zest 1 teaspoon beef gelatin powder or agar agar

DIRECTIONS and Cooking Time: 3 Hours
Set the Sous Vide cooker to 190ºF. Combine all ingredients in a Sous Vide bag. Seal using water immersion technique. Cook the oranges 3 hours. Remove the bag from the cooker and place into an ice-cold water bath. Once cooled transfer into a food processor. Add the gelatin and process until smooth. Allow cooling completely before serving.

Nutrition Info: Per serving:Calories 502.7, Carbohydrates 123.1 g, Fats 0.3 g, Protein 1.9 g

Pickled Jalapeño Peppers

INGREDIENTS

1 cup white wine vinegar 3 tablespoons ultrafine sugar 2 teaspoons kosher salt	6 jalapeño peppers, sliced crosswise ¼-inch thick ½ White onion, thinly sliced

DIRECTIONS and Cooking Time: 30 Mins Cooking Temperature: 180°f
Attach the sous vide immersion circulator to a Cambro container or pot with water using an adjustable clamp and preheat water to 180°F. In a large bowl, add vinegar, sugar, and salt and beat until sugar is dissolved. Place jalapeño peppers, onion, and vinegar mixture in a cooking pouch. Seal pouch tightly after squeezing out the excess air. Place pouch in sous vide bath and set the cooking time for about 30 minutes. Remove pouch from the sous vide bath and immediately immerse in a large bowl of ice water to cool. Remove peppers from pouch and serve immediately.

Peach And Orange Jam

INGREDIENTS for Servings: 10

2 cups peaches, coarsely chopped 1 ½ cup white sugar	1 cup water Zest and juice of 1 orange

DIRECTIONS and Cooking Time: 2 Hours
Put the ingredients into the vacuum bag and seal it. Cook for 2 hours in the water bath, previously preheated to 190ºF. Serve over ice cream or cake, or store in the fridge in an airtight container.

Nutrition Info: Per serving:Calories 135, Carbohydrates 14 g, Fats 7 g, Protein 4 g

Queso Blanco Dip

INGREDIENTS

1½ cups Asadero or Chihuahua cheese, shredded finely ¼ Cup half-and-half cream 4 ounces /1/4 pound green chilies, chopped	1 Serrano pepper, stemmed and chopped finely 2 tablespoons onion, grated 2 teaspoons ground cumin ½ Teaspoon salt

DIRECTIONS and Cooking Time: 30 Mins Cooking Temperature: 175°f
Attach the sous vide immersion circulator to a Cambro container or pot with water using an adjustable clamp and preheat water to 175°F. Place all ingredients except bread in a cooking pouch. Seal pouch tightly after squeezing out the excess air. Place pouch in sous vide bath and set the cooking time for about 30 minutes. Remove pouch from bath occasionally and massage mixture to mix. Remove the pouch from the sous vide bath and carefully open it. Immediately, transfer dip into a bowl and serve.

Root Vegetables With Brown Butter

INGREDIENTS

8 baby carrots, cut into 1-inch pieces 1 medium rutabaga, peeled and cut into 1-inch pieces 1 medium turnip, peeled and cut into 1-inch pieces 1 medium parsnip, peeled and cut into 1-inch pieces 4 garlic cloves, crushed	½ Medium red onion, cut into 1-inch pieces 4 fresh rosemary sprigs 2 tablespoons extra-virgin olive oil Kosher salt and freshly ground black pepper, to taste 2 tablespoons butter

DIRECTIONS and Cooking Time: 3 Hours 10 Minutes Cooking Temperature: 185°f
Attach the sous vide immersion circulator to a Cambro container or pot with water using an adjustable clamp and preheat water to 185°F. In a large bowl, add vegetables and mix. In 2 cooking pouches, divide vegetable mixture, rosemary sprigs, olive oil, salt, and black pepper. Seal pouch tightly after squeezing out the excess air. Place pouch in sous vide bath and set the cooking time for about 3 hours. Remove pouches from the sous vide bath and carefully open them. Remove vegetables from pouches, reserving cooking liquid. Heat a large sauté pan over high heat and

cook vegetables with reserved cooking liquid for about 5 minutes. Stir in butter and cook for an additional 5 minutes, stirring occasionally. Serve warm.

Cinnamon Poached Pears

INGREDIENTS for Servings: 8

4 Bosc pears /firm yet ripe	1 cup tawny port
½ cup granulated sugar	2 wide strips lemon zest, 2 inches long and ½ inch wide
2 wide strips orange zest, 2 inches long and ½ inch wide	½ teaspoon ground cinnamon
	Ice cream for flavor

DIRECTIONS and Cooking Time: 30 Minutes
Set your Sous Vide immersion circulator to a temperature of 180-degrees Fahrenheit, and prepare your water bath Peel the pears and add them in a heavy-duty zip bag, together with the remaining ingredients Seal using the immersion method and cook for 30 minutes Cool for 30 minutes and pour the liquid into a pan. Place it over medium heat and reduce the liquid by 2/3 Remove the heat and wait until the liquid is cooled Core the pears diagonally and create fan shapes Carefully transfer the pears to your serving plate and pour the previously prepared sauce on top Serve with a topping of your favorite ice cream

Nutrition Info: Calories: 383 Carbohydrate: 97g Protein: 1g Fat: 0g Sugar: 85g Sodium: 12mg

Pomme Purée

INGREDIENTS for Servings: 4

1½ lb. potatoes, peeled	A pinch of salt
15-ounce vegan butter	White pepper as needed
8-ounce coconut milk	

DIRECTIONS and Cooking Time: 30 Minutes
Prepare your Sous-vide water bath using your immersion circulator and raise the temperature to 194-degrees Fahrenheit. Slice the potatoes to 1 cm thick slices Take your heavy-duty resealable zipper bag and add the potatoes, coconut milk, vegan butter and salt Submerge underwater and let it cook for 30 minutes Strain the mixture through a metal mesh/sieve and allow the butter mixture to pour into a bowl Puree the potatoes by blending them or mashing them using a spoon Pour the puree into the butter bowl Season with pepper and serve!

Nutrition Info: Calories: 56 Carbohydrates: 2g Protein: 1g Fat: 5g Sugar: 0g Sodium: 56mg

Stuffed Apples

INGREDIENTS for Servings: 4

4 golden apples	1/3 cup organic apple juice
¼ cup palm sugar + 1 ½ tablespoons	1 ½ tablespoons whipping cream
1 tablespoon chopped dates	To garnish:
3 tablespoons raisins	A handful of chopped walnuts
2 tablespoons butter	
¼ teaspoon cinnamon	

DIRECTIONS and Cooking Time: 90 Minutes
Preheat your Sous Vide cooker to 185ºF. Core the apples, leaving the bottom intact. In a bowl, combine sugar, raisins, dates, butter, and cinnamon. Fill the apples with prepared mixture. Place each apple in Sous Vide bag and vacuum seal. Cook the apples 90 minutes. Combine the remaining sugar with apple juice in a saucepan. Simmer until sauce is thick, for 10 minutes. Stir in the whipping cream. Remove the apples from bags and serve on a plate. Drizzle with sauce and sprinkle with walnuts.

Nutrition Info: Per serving:Calories 153.2, Carbohydrates 20.7 g, Fats 7.6 g, Protein 0.5 g

Ma Po Tofu

INGREDIENTS for Servings: 6

2 tablespoons tomato paste	1 cup vegetable broth
1 tablespoon grated ginger	2 teaspoons sriracha sauce
1 tablespoon rice wine vinegar	3 cloves minced garlic
1 tablespoon agave nectar	1 teaspoon soy sauce
	2 boxes cubed silken tofu

DIRECTIONS and Cooking Time: 90 Minutes
Prepare the Sous Vide water bath using your immersion circulator and increase the temperature to 185-degrees Fahrenheit Whisk all of the listed ingredients in a bowl, except the tofu Put the tofu in a zip bag and add the mixture Seal the bag using the immersion method and cook for 1½ hours Serve!

Nutrition Info: Calories: 560 Carbohydrate: 83g Protein: 33g Fat: 14g Sugar: 1g Sodium: 402mg

Sweet Curried Winter Squash

INGREDIENTS for Servings: 6

1 medium winter squash	½ teaspoon kosher salt
2 tablespoons unsalted vegan butter	Fresh cilantro for serving
1 to 2 tablespoons Thai curry paste	Lime wedges for serving

DIRECTIONS and Cooking Time: 90 Minutes

Prepare the Sous-vide water bath using your immersion circulator and raise the temperature to 185-degrees Fahrenheit. Slice up the squash into half lengthwise and scoop out the seeds alongside the inner membrane. Keep the seeds for later use. Slice the squash into wedges of about 1 ½-inch thickness. Take a large heavy-duty bag resealable zip bags and add the squash wedges, curry paste, butter and salt and seal it using the immersion method. Submerge it underwater and let it cook for 1 ½ hour. Once cooked, remove the bag from water and give it a slight squeeze until it is soft. If it is not soft, then add to the water once again and cook for 40 minutes more. Transfer the cooked dish to a serving plate and drizzle with a bit of curry butter sauce from the bag. Top your squash with a bit of cilantro, lime wedges and serve!

Nutrition Info: Calories: 185 Carbohydrates: 27g Protein: 2g Fat: 9g Sugar: 5g Sodium: 422mg

Green Beans In Tomato Sauce

INGREDIENTS for Servings: 4

1 lb. trimmed green beans	1 can whole crushed tomatoes
1 thinly sliced onion	Kosher salt, to taste
3 garlic clove, peeled and thinly sliced	Extra-virgin olive oil

DIRECTIONS and Cooking Time: 180 Minutes
Prepare the Sous-vide water bath using your immersion circulator and raise the temperature to 183-degrees Fahrenheit Take a large heavy-duty resealable zip bag and add the tomatoes, green beans, garlic, and onion Seal using the immersion method. Submerge underwater and let it cook for 3 hours. Once cooked, transfer the contents of the bag to a large bowl. Serve with a seasoning of salt and a drizzle of olive oil.

Nutrition Info: Calories: 277 Carbohydrates: 6g Protein: 20g Fat: 19g Sugar: 2g Sodium: 470mg

Daikon Radishes

INGREDIENTS for Servings: 4

½ cup white winger vinegar	3 tablespoons beet sugar
1 large size Daikon radish, trimmed and sliced up	2 teaspoons kosher salt

DIRECTIONS and Cooking Time: 30 Minutes
Prepare the Sous-vide water bath using your immersion circulator and raise the temperature to 180-degrees Fahrenheit. Take a large bowl and mix in vinegar, salt, and beet sugar. Transfer to a Sous-vide zip bag and seal using the immersion method. Submerge underwater and cook for 30 minutes

Once cooked, remove the bag and transfer to an ice bath. Serve!

Nutrition Info: Calories: 141 Carbohydrates: 19g Protein: 5g Fat: 6g Sugar: 6g Sodium: 87mg

Pickle In A Jar

INGREDIENTS for Servings: 6

1 cup white wine vinegar	½ cup beet sugar
2 teaspoons kosher salt	2 English cucumbers sliced up into ¼ inch thick slices
1 tablespoon pickling spice	½ white onion, thinly sliced

DIRECTIONS and Cooking Time: 15 Minutes
Prepare the Sous-vide water bath using your immersion circulator and raise the temperature to 180-degrees Fahrenheit. Take a large bowl and add the vinegar, sugar, salt, pickling spice and whisk them well. Transfer to a heavy-duty resealable zipper bag alongside the cucumber and sliced onions and seal using the immersion method. Submerge underwater and let it cook for 15 minutes. Transfer the bag to an ice bath Pour the mixture into a 4-6 ounce mason jar Serve or store!

Nutrition Info: Calories: 117 Carbohydrates: 27g Protein: 1g Fat: 1g Sugar: 19g Sodium: 304mg

Gnocchi Pillows With Parmesan

INGREDIENTS for Servings: 2

1 pack store-bought gnocchi	Salt and black pepper as needed
1 tablespoon unsalted butter	¼ cup heavy cream
½ thinly sliced sweet onion	½ cup grated parmesan
½ cup frozen peas	Salt and pepper as needed

DIRECTIONS and Cooking Time: 1 Hour 30 Min
Prepare your water bath using your Sous Vide immersion circulator and raise the temperature to 183-degrees Fahrenheit Put the gnocchi in a heavy-duty resealable bag Seal using the immersion method and cook for 1½ hours Once done, place a cast iron skillet over a medium heat Add the butter and allow to melt Add the onion and season with salt. Sauté for 3 minutes Add the frozen peas and cream, and bring to a simmer Stir in the gnocchi and grated parmesan, to coat with the cream sauce Season with pepper and salt Transfer to a plate and serve!

Nutrition Info: Calories: 189 Carbohydrate: 16g Protein: 9g Fat: 12g Sugar: 5g Sodium: 517mg

Buttered Beets & Orange

INGREDIENTS for Servings: 4

1 lb. medium red beets, peeled and quartered 2 tablespoons unsalted butter 2 peeled oranges, cut into Supreme 3 tablespoons balsamic vinegar 4 tablespoons extra virgin olive oil	1 tablespoon honey Kosher salt and black pepper as needed 6 oz. baby romaine leaves ½ cup pistachios, chopped and roasted ½ cup Parmigiano Reggiano/Parmesan Cheese

DIRECTIONS and Cooking Time: 90 Minutes

Prepare the Sous Vide water bath using your immersion circulator and increase the temperature to 180-degrees Fahrenheit   Put the beets in a plastic zip bag and add the butter   Seal using the immersion method, and cook for 90 minutes   Once cooked, take the beets out from the bag and discard the cooking liquid   Whisk the honey, oil and vinegar, with a seasoning of salt and pepper, in a bowl   Toss the romaine leaves, orange, beets and vinaigrette, and divide the whole mixture amongst four platters   Top the servings with pistachio and Parmigiano Reggiano cheese and serve!

Nutrition Info: Calories: 130 Carbohydrate: 17g Protein: 3g Fat: 6g Sugar: 12g Sodium: 591mg

Italian-style Fruit Toast

INGREDIENTS for Servings: 6

1 ½ cups granulated sugar 1 ½ cups water 2 tablespoons fresh cilantro, chiffonade 2 tablespoons freshly squeezed orange juice 1 cup banana, sliced 1 cup cherries 1 cup pears, cored and sliced	2 tablespoons coconut oil, melted 1/2 teaspoon pure vanilla extract 1/4 cup honey 8 slices ciabatta, cut on the bias 1 cup ricotta, at room temperature 1/4 teaspoon ground cinnamon

DIRECTIONS and Cooking Time: 1 Hour 20 Minutes

In a saucepan, cook the sugar, water, cilantro, and orange juice over medium-low heat; allow it to simmer about 8 minutes.   Preheat a sous vide water bath to 183 degrees F.   Separate fruits in individual cooking pouches by type; divide the prepared syrup among cooking pouches, seal tightly, and let it sit for 30 minutes.   Submerge the cooking pouches in the water bath; cook for 15 minutes.   Remove the pouches with banana and cherries from the water bath and reserve the liquid. Cook the pears an additional 25 minutes.   Toss the sous vide fruit with coconut oil, vanilla extract, and honey. Serve on ciabatta slices topped with the reserved syrup, ricotta and ground cinnamon. Bon appétit!

Nutrition Info:282 Calories; 2g Fat; 49g Carbs; 8g Protein; 37g Sugars

Creamy And Cheesy Kale

INGREDIENTS for Servings: 4

2 pounds Tuscan kale, stems discarded, torn into pieces 2 tablespoons butter 2 shallots, chopped 2 cloves garlic, minced	1 cup half-and-half 4 ounces cheddar cheese, shredded Salt and black pepper, to taste 1/2 teaspoon cayenne pepper

DIRECTIONS and Cooking Time: 15 Minutes

Preheat a sous vide water bath to 190 degrees F. Place the kale in a cooking pouch; seal tightly. Submerge the cooking pouch in the water bath; cook for 9 minutes. Remove from the cooking pouch.   Melt the butter in a saucepan over a moderate flame. Now, sauté the shallots and garlic until tender.   Add half-and-half and bring to a simmer. Remove from heat; stir in cheddar cheese, salt, black pepper, and cayenne pepper.   Fold in sous vide kale, stir and serve warm. Bon appétit!

Nutrition Info:252 Calories; 12g Fat; 24g Carbs; 13g Protein; 14g Sugars

Cauliflower Mash

INGREDIENTS for Servings: 4

1 lb. trimmed cauliflower ½ teaspoon garlic powder 1 tablespoon butter	1 teaspoon kosher salt 1 tablespoon heavy whipping cream

DIRECTIONS and Cooking Time: 2 Hours

Prepare the Sous Vide water bath using your immersion circulator and increase the temperature to 183-degrees Fahrenheit   Add the cauliflower, salt, garlic powder, and heavy whipping cream in a large resealable bag and seal using the immersion method   Cook for about 2 hours   Pour the contents into a blender and purée   Season and serve!

Nutrition Info: Per serving:Calories: 307 ;Carbohydrate: 14g ;Protein: 7g ;Fat: 28g ;Sugar: 3g ;Sodium: 206mg

Buttered Brussels Sprouts

INGREDIENTS for Servings: 4

1 ½ pounds Brussels sprouts, halved 1 leek, sliced 2 garlic cloves, smashed	Celery salt and freshly cracked black pepper, to taste 1 stick butter

DIRECTIONS and Cooking Time: 50 Minutes

Preheat a sous vide water bath to 183 degrees F. Place Brussels sprouts, leek, garlic, celery salt, and black pepper in cooking pouches; seal tightly. Submerge the cooking pouches in the water bath; cook for 40 minutes.   Melt the butter in a large-sized pan. Stir in the vegetables and sauté for 5 minutes, coating them well with melted butter. Taste, adjust the seasonings and serve.

Nutrition Info:296 Calories; 25g Fat; 19g Carbs; 6g Protein; 3g Sugars

Vanilla Apricots In Syrup

INGREDIENTS for Servings: 4

1 cup water	4 cloves
1 cup sugar syrup	1 star anise
1 vanilla pod, seeds scraped	1/2 pound apricots, pitted and halved

DIRECTIONS and Cooking Time: 30 Minutes
Preheat a sous vide water bath to 183 degrees F. Place the water, sugar syrup, and vanilla, cloves, and anise in a saucepan over a moderate heat. Bring to a rapid boil and immediately remove from the heat. Add the syrup and the apricot halves to a cooking pouch; seal tightly.   Submerge the cooking pouch in the water bath; cook for 25 minutes.   Serve with whipped cream and enjoy!

Nutrition Info:234 Calories; 3g Fat; 64g Carbs; 9g Protein; 57g Sugars

Marinated Mushrooms

INGREDIENTS

10 ounces white mushrooms, quartered	½ Teaspoon dried thyme, crushed
3 tablespoons olive oil	1 bay leaf
2 tablespoons dry sherry	Pinch of garlic powder
1 teaspoon Worcestershire sauce	Salt and freshly ground black pepper, to taste
1 lemon peel strip	

DIRECTIONS and Cooking Time: 1 Hour Cooking Temperature: 185°f
Attach the sous vide immersion circulator to a Cambro container or pot with water using an adjustable clamp and preheat water to 185°F.   Place all ingredients in a cooking pouch. Seal pouch tightly after squeezing out the excess air. Place pouch in sous vide bath and set the cooking time for about 1 hour.   Remove pouch from the sous vide bath and let mushrooms cool in pouch. Drain and serve.

Basic Risotto

INGREDIENTS

1 cup Arborio rice	1 teaspoon extra-virgin olive oil
1/3 cup Romano cheese, grated	3 cups vegetable broth
Leaves from 1 fresh rosemary sprig, minced	Salt and freshly ground black pepper, to taste
2 tablespoons jarred roasted minced garlic	

DIRECTIONS and Cooking Time: 45 Mins Cooking Temperature: 183°f
Attach the sous vide immersion circulator to a Cambro container or pot with water using an adjustable clamp and preheat water to 183°F.   Place all ingredients in a cooking pouch. Seal pouch tightly after squeezing out the excess air. Place pouch in sous vide bath and set the cooking time for about 45 minutes.   Remove pouch from the sous vide bath and carefully open it. Transfer rice mixture into a serving bowl. With a fork, fluff the rice and serve.

Apricot Dates Compote

INGREDIENTS for Servings: 4

10oz. fresh apricots	1 tablespoon Pernod
6oz. pitted dates	1 tablespoon unsalted butter
1-star anise	
4 tablespoons brown sugar	2 tablespoons maple syrup

DIRECTIONS and Cooking Time: 30 Minutes
Set the Sous Vide cooker to 180ºF.   In a large Sous Vide bag, combine all ingredients.   Shake gently. Vacuum seal the bag and submerge in water.   Cook the figs and dates 30 minutes.   Remove the bag from the Sous Vide cooker.   Open the bag and transfer the content to the bowl.   Allow cooling before serving.

Nutrition Info: Per serving:Calories 260.3, Carbohydrates 55.2 g, Fats 3.5 g, Protein 2 g

Cheesy Grits

INGREDIENTS

1 cup old fashioned grits	4 ounces /1/4 pound cheddar cheese, grated, plus extra for garnish
3 cups vegetable broth	
1 cup cream	
2 tablespoons cold butter, cut into small pieces	Salt and freshly ground black pepper, to taste
	Paprika for garnish

DIRECTIONS and Cooking Time: 3 Hours Cooking Temperature: 180°f
Attach the sous vide immersion circulator to a Cambro container or pot with water using an adjustable clamp and preheat water to 180°F.   In a large bowl, add grits, broth, and cream and beat until well combined. Add butter and gently stir.   Place grits mixture in a

cooking pouch. Seal pouch tightly after squeezing out the excess air. Place pouch in sous vide bath and set the cooking time for about 2-3 hours. Remove pouch from the sous vide bath and carefully open it. Transfer grits into a bowl. Immediately, add cheese and beat until well combined. Stir in salt and black pepper. Serve immediately with a sprinkling of extra cheese and paprika.

Honey Poached Pears

INGREDIENTS for Servings: 2

1 pear, thinly sliced	2 cups rocket leaves
1 lb. honey	2 tablespoons lemon
½ cup of walnuts	juice
4 tablespoons shaved	2 tablespoons extra-
Parmesan	virgin olive oil
Salt and pepper as	
needed	

DIRECTIONS and Cooking Time: 45 Minutes
Prepare your water bath using your Sous Vide immersion circulator and raise the temperature to 158-degrees Fahrenheit Put the honey, smeared pears in a heavy-duty resealable bag Seal using the immersion method and submerge Cook for 45 minutes Put the contents of the bag in a bowl Add the remaining dressing ingredients and toss well Serve!

Nutrition Info: Calories: 189 Carbohydrate: 16g Protein: 9g Fat: 12g Sugar: 5g Sodium: 437mg

Root Vegetables Mix

INGREDIENTS for Servings: 4

1 peeled rutabaga, cut up into 1-inch pieces	1 peeled turnip, cut up into 1-inch pieces
8 pieces petite carrots peeled up and cut into 1-inch pieces	4 pieces' garlic, crushed
1 peeled parsnip, cut up into 1-inch pieces	4 sprigs fresh rosemary
½ red onion, cut up into 1-inch pieces and peeled	2 tablespoons extra-virgin olive oil
	Kosher salt, and black pepper to taste
	2 tablespoons unsalted vegan butter

DIRECTIONS and Cooking Time: 180 Minutes
Prepare the Sous-vide water bath using your immersion circulator and raise the temperature to 185-degrees Fahrenheit. Take two large heavy-duty resealable zipper bags and divide the vegetables and the rosemary between the bags. Add 1 tablespoon of oil to the bag and season with some salt and pepper. Seal the bags using the immersion method. Submerge underwater and cook for 3 hours Take a skillet and place it over high heat and add in the oil. Once done, add the contents of your bag to the skillet. Cook the

mixture for about 5-6 minutes until the liquid comes to a syrupy consistency. Add the butter to your veggies and toss them well. Keep cooking for another 5 minutes until they are nicely browned. Serve!

Nutrition Info: Calories: 268 Carbohydrates: 43g Protein: 6g Fat: 10g Sugar: 16g Sodium: 612mg

Sous-vide Pennies

INGREDIENTS for Servings: 4

1 pound carrots, peeled up and sliced into ¼ inch thick rounds	1/4 cup dried apricots, thinly sliced up
¼ cup freshly squeezed orange juice	½ a teaspoon kosher salt
2 tablespoons freshly squeezed lemon juice	¼ teaspoon orange zest
1 tablespoon unsalted vegan butter	¼ teaspoon freshly ground black pepper
2 teaspoons beet sugar	1/8 teaspoon ground cinnamon

DIRECTIONS and Cooking Time: 180 Minutes
Prepare the Sous-vide water bath using your immersion circulator and raise the temperature to 183-degrees Fahrenheit. Add the listed ingredients to your resealable zip bag and seal using the immersion method. Submerge underwater and cook for 3 hours. Transfer the carrots to a serving platter with cooking liquid and season with salt and pepper. Garnish with the additional lemon juice and serve!

Nutrition Info: Calories: 256 Carbohydrates: 35g Protein: 2g Fat: 12g Sugar: 23g Sodium: 117mg

Cauliflower Puree

INGREDIENTS for Servings: 4

1 head cauliflower	1 cup chicken stock
3 tablespoons unsalted butter	¾ teaspoon salt

DIRECTIONS and Cooking Time: 45 Minutes
Prepare the Sous Vide water bath using your immersion circulator and increase the temperature to 185-degrees Fahrenheit Remove a few leaves from the bottom part of the cauliflower core and cut into ¼ inch small slices Put the cauliflower, butter and chicken stock in a heavy-duty, resealable bag Seal using the immersion method Submerge underwater and cook for 45 minutes Once cooked, remove the bag and strain the contents through a metal mesh Save the cooking liquid Put the cauliflower to a blender and puree until smooth Add some of the cooking liquid, season with salt and serve!

Nutrition Info: Calories: 171 Carbohydrate: 29g Protein: 7g Fat: 5g Sugar: 4g Sodium: 6mg

Broccoli With Roasted Red Peppers

INGREDIENTS

2 canned roasted red peppers, rinse, seeded and cut into strips lengthwise	½ Teaspoon salt
	¼ Teaspoon freshly ground black pepper
	1 tablespoon butter
2 cups broccoli florets	¼ cup Parmesan
1 garlic clove, minced	cheese, grated freshly

DIRECTIONS and Cooking Time: 50 Minutes Cooking Temperature: 183°f

Attach the sous vide immersion circulator to a Cambro container or pot with water using an adjustable clamp and preheat water to 183°F.   Place red pepper strips in a cooking pouch.   In a bowl, mix together broccoli, garlic, salt, and black pepper. In another cooking pouch, place broccoli mixture and butter.   Seal pouches tightly after squeezing out the excess air. Place the pouch of broccoli in sous vide bath and set the cooking time for about 30 minutes. After 10-15 minutes, add pouch of red peppers to the sous vide bath.   Remove pouches from the sous vide bath and carefully open them. Remove vegetables from pouch and discard cooking liquid.   Transfer vegetables into warm serving bowls evenly. Garnish with Parmesan cheese and serve immediately.

Pickled Radishes

INGREDIENTS

2/3 cup water	½ Teaspoon yellow mustard seeds
2/3 cup white wine vinegar	¼ Teaspoon coriander seeds
2 garlic cloves, sliced in half lengthwise	½ Teaspoon whole peppercorns
3 tablespoons sugar	12 ounces /3/4 pound of radishes, trimmed and quartered
1 bay leaf	
1 tablespoon salt	

DIRECTIONS and Cooking Time: 45 Mins Cooking Temperature: 190°f

Attach the sous vide immersion circulator to a Cambro container or pot with water using an adjustable clamp and preheat water to 190°F.   In a pot, add all ingredients except radishes and bring to a boil, stirring continuously until sugar melts.   Place radishes in a single layer in a cooking pouch. Pour sugar mixture over radishes. Seal pouch tightly after squeezing out the excess air. Place pouch in sous vide bath and set the cooking time for about 45 minutes. Remove pouch from the sous vide bath and immediately immerse in a bowl of ice water. After cooling, remove radishes from pouch and serve immediately.   Radishes can be stored in the refrigerator in an airtight container.

Root Vegetable Soup With Pita Chips

INGREDIENTS for Servings: 4

2 shallots, peeled and chopped	1 cup turnip, chopped
2 parsnips, chopped	2 tablespoons olive oil
2 celery stalks, chopped	2 cups baby spinach
	2 heaping tablespoons fresh parsley, chopped
2 carrots, chopped	1 sprig fresh rosemary, chopped
2 cloves garlic, minced	1 cup pita chips
4 cups vegetable broth, preferably homemade	

DIRECTIONS and Cooking Time: 55 Minutes

Preheat a sous vide water bath to 185 degrees F. Place the shallots, parsnips, celery, carrots, turnip, garlic, vegetable broth, and olive oil in cooking pouches; seal tightly.   Submerge the cooking pouches in the water bath; cook for 50 minutes. Now, empty the contents into a serving bowl; add baby spinach, parsley, and rosemary. Serve with pita chips and enjoy!

Nutrition Info:178 Calories; 9g Fat; 23g Carbs; 3g Protein; 6g Sugars

Poached Mixed Berries With Mascarpone Cream

INGREDIENTS for Servings: 4

1 pound mixed berries, halved	3/4 cup double cream
1/2 cup water	1/4 cup mascarpone cheese
1/2 cup Semillon wine	2 tablespoons agave syrup
1/2 cup apple juice	
Mascarpone Cream:	

DIRECTIONS and Cooking Time: 50 Minutes

Preheat a sous vide water bath to 183 degrees F. Place mixed berries, water, Semillon wine, and apple juice in a cooking pouch; seal tightly.   Submerge the cooking pouch in the water bath; cook for 40 minutes. Meanwhile, beat the double cream using an electric mixer until fairly thick. Now, add cheese and continue beating until soft peaks form.   Add agave syrup and mix well.   Arrange berries and syrup in serving bowls; top with a dollop of mascarpone cream. Bon appétit!

Nutrition Info:202 Calories; 16g Fat; 27g Carbs; 2g Protein; 19g Sugars

Carrots With Butter

INGREDIENTS

Baby carrots	Pinch of salt
Olive oil, as required	Butter, as required

DIRECTIONS and Cooking Time: 25 Mins Cooking Temperature: 185°f
Attach the sous vide immersion circulator to a Cambro container or pot with water using an adjustable clamp and preheat water to 185°F. Place carrots in a single layer in a cooking pouch. Add a little olive oil and salt. Seal pouch tightly after squeezing out the excess air. Place pouch in sous vide bath and set the cooking time for about 25 minutes. Remove pouch from the sous vide bath and carefully open it. Remove carrots from pouch. With paper towels, pat dry carrots completely Serve immediately with a topping of butter.

Tangerine Ice Cream
INGREDIENTS for Servings: 6

1 cup mandarin (only juice and pulp) 2 cups heavy cream 6 fresh egg yolks ½ cup milk	½ cup white sugar ¼ cup sweet condensed milk A pinch of salt

DIRECTIONS and Cooking Time: 24 Hours And 30 Minutes
In a big bowl, combine all ingredients and whisk well until even. Carefully pour the mixture into the vacuum bag and seal it. Cook for 30 minutes in the water bath, previously preheated to 185ºF. When the time is up, quick chill the vacuum bag without opening it. To do this, put it into big bowl or container, filled with ice and water. Refrigerate the vacuum bag with ice-cream for 24 hours. Carefully transfer the mixture to an ice-cream machine and cook according to the instructions.

Nutrition Info: Per serving:Calories 152, Carbohydrates 17 g, Fats 8 g, Protein 3 g

Steak Fries
INGREDIENTS

¼ Cup butter, melted ½ Teaspoon paprika ¼ Teaspoon cayenne pepper ¼ Teaspoon onion powder	¼ Teaspoon garlic powder ¼ Teaspoon salt 5 russet potatoes, cut in half lengthwise

DIRECTIONS and Cooking Time: 1 Hour 30 Mins Cooking Temperature: 190°f
Attach the sous vide immersion circulator to a Cambro container or pot with water using an adjustable clamp and preheat water to 190°F. In a bowl, add all ingredients except potatoes and mix well. Place potatoes in a single layer in a cooking pouch. Pour butter mixture over potatoes evenly. Seal pouch tightly after squeezing out the excess air. Place pouch in sous vide bath and set the cooking time for about 1½ hours. Preheat the broiler of oven to high.

Remove pouch from the sous vide bath carefully open it. Remove potatoes from pouch. With paper towels, pat potatoes completely dry. Arrange potatoes in a single layer on a baking sheet and broil for about 2-3 minutes per side. Serve immediately.

Mexican Street Corn
INGREDIENTS for Servings: 2

2 ears of corn, shucked 2 tablespoons cold butter Kosher salt as needed Fresh ground pepper ½ tablespoon Mexican style chili powder	¼ cup mayonnaise ½ teaspoon grated lime zest ¼ cup crumbled Queso Fresco ¼ cup chopped, fresh cilantro

DIRECTIONS and Cooking Time: 30 Minutes
Prepare the Sous Vide water bath using your immersion circulator and increase the temperature to 183-degrees Fahrenheit Put the corn ears and butter in a zip bag Season with salt and pepper and seal using the immersion method Cook for 30 minutes Once done, remove the corn Add the mayo, lime zest, and chili powder into a small bag and mix Place the Queso Fresco on a small plate Spread 1 tablespoon of mayonnaise mixture on top of the corn ears, and roll them on the cheese Sprinkle with salt and fresh cilantro and serve!

Nutrition Info: Calories: 373 Carbohydrate: 30g Protein: 15g Fat: 24g Sugar: 9g Sodium: 587mg

Squash Casserole
INGREDIENTS

2 tablespoons unsalted butter ¾ Cup onion, chopped 1½ pound summer squash, quartered lengthwise and cut into ¼-inch-thick pieces	Kosher salt, to taste 2 large eggs ½ Cup whole milk Freshly ground black pepper, to taste ½ Cup plain potato chips, crumbled

DIRECTIONS and Cooking Time: 1 Hour 17 Mins Cooking Temperature: 176°f
Attach the sous vide immersion circulator to a Cambro container or pot with water using an adjustable clamp and preheat water to 176°F. Grease 4 half-pint canning jars generously. In a large skillet, melt butter over medium-high heat and sauté onion for about 5-7 minutes. Add squash and a generous pinch of salt and sauté for an additional 10 minutes. Season with salt and black pepper and remove from heat. Divide squash mixture into prepared jars evenly and set aside at room temperature to cool. In a bowl, add eggs, milk, a pinch of salt, and a few grinds of black pepper and beat until well combined. Place milk

mixture over squash mixture in each jar evenly. With a damp towel, wipe off sides and tops of jars. Tap the jars on a counter firmly to remove air bubbles. Cover each jar with the lid. /Do not over-tighten jars because air will need to escape. Place jars in sous vide bath and set the cooking time for about 1 hour. Remove the jars from the sous vide bath and carefully remove the lids. Place jars onto a wire rack to cool for about 5 minutes. Top with potato chips and serve immediately.

Miso Roasted Celeriac

INGREDIENTS for Servings: 6

1 tablespoon miso paste	1 tablespoon mustard seeds
1 whole celeriac, carefully peeled and cut into small bite-sized pieces	Juice of ¼ a large lemon
6 cloves garlic	5 cherry tomatoes roughly cut
5 sprigs thyme	Chopped up parsley
1 teaspoon onion powder	8-ounce vegan butter
3 tablespoon feta cheese	1 tablespoon olive oil
	8 ounce cooked quinoa

DIRECTIONS and Cooking Time: 2 Hours
Prepare the Sous Vide water bath using your immersion circulator and raise the temperature to 185-degrees Fahrenheit   Take a large-sized pan and place it over medium heat, add the garlic, thyme, feta cheese, and dry fry them for 1 and a ½ minute   Add the butter and keep stirring until slightly browned   Add the onion powder and keep the mixture on the side and allow it to cool at room temperature   Add the celeriac to a zip bag alongside the cooled butter mixture   Submerge and cook for 1½ to 2 hours   Transfer the mixture to a hot pan (place over medium heat) and stirring it until golden brown   Season with miso paste   Add the oil to another pan and place it over medium heat, add the tomatoes, mustard seeds and re-heat the quinoa   Carefully add the lemon and parsley to the previously made tomato mixture   Assemble your platter by transferring the celeriac and tomato mix   Serve!

Nutrition Info: Per serving:Calories: 200 ;Carbohydrate: 5g ;Protein: 12g ;Fat: 15gt ;Sugar: 1g ;Sodium: 36mg

Sous Vide Ratatouille

INGREDIENTS for Servings: 4

2 red bell peppers, seeded, sliced	6 small tomatoes, sliced
2 yellow bell peppers, seeded, sliced	2 tablespoons soy sauce
2 green bell peppers, seeded, sliced	4 tablespoons chopped mixed herbs,

4 small green zucchinis, sliced	parsley, coriander, mint
4 yellow zucchinis, sliced	2 pinches sugar
4 shallots, sliced	2 pinches black pepper
4 cloves garlic	½ cup olive oil
10 brown mushrooms	Salt, to taste

DIRECTIONS and Cooking Time: 30 Minutes
Before you start, cut the vegetables into equal-size pieces. This way you will ensure all ingredients are cooked at the same time.   Preheat your Sous Vide to 150ºF.   Combine all ingredients in a large bowl. Toss gently to coat with oil.   Divide the veggies between four cooking bags.   Vacuum seal the bags and submerge underheated water.   Cook the vegetables 30 minutes.   Heat some oil in a wok pan.   Add in the veggies and stir-fry 30 seconds.   Serve warm.

Nutrition Info: Per serving:Calories 366.7, Carbohydrates 25.5 g, Fats 26.3 g, Protein 7 g

Crunchy Apple Salad With Almonds

INGREDIENTS for Servings: 4

3 crisp eating apples, cored, and sliced	1/4 cup mayonnaise
2 tablespoons honey	1 teaspoon yellow mustard
1/2 cup dried cranberries	1/2 tablespoon lime juice
1 cup almonds	1 tablespoon sugar
6 ounces package mixed spring greens	Salt and white pepper, to your liking
1/4 cup sour cream	

DIRECTIONS and Cooking Time: 40 Minutes + Chilling Time
Preheat a sous vide water bath to 160 degrees F. Add the apples and honey to a cooking pouch; seal tightly.   Submerge the cooking pouches in the water bath; cook for 35 minutes. Remove the apples from the cooking pouch and let them cool completely. Transfer the apples to a nice salad bowl. Add the cranberries, almonds, and greens.   In a mixing bowl, whisk the sour cream, mayonnaise, mustard, lime juice, sugar, salt, and pepper. Whisk until sugar is dissolved.   Dress the salad and serve well-chilled. Bon appétit!

Nutrition Info:193 Calories; 9g Fat; 39g Carbs; 3g Protein; 28g Sugars

Yogurt & Caraway Soup

INGREDIENTS for Servings: 4

1 tablespoon extra-virgin olive oil	2 pounds red beets, peeled and chopped
1½ teaspoons caraway seeds	1 bay leaf
	3 cups chicken broth

1 medium onion, diced	½ cup whole milk yogurt
1 leek, halved and thinly sliced	Apple cider vinegar
Kosher salt as needed	Fresh dill fronds

DIRECTIONS and Cooking Time: 2 Hours 8 Minutes
Prepare your Sous Vide water bath using your immersion circulator and raise the temperature to 185-degrees Fahrenheit   Add the oil in a large skillet and heat it over medium heat   When the oil is shimmering, add your caraway seeds   Toast them for about 1 minute   Put the onion, pinch of salt and leek, and sauté them for 5-7 minutes until the leek and onion are tender   Put the bay leaf, beets, and ½ teaspoon of salt into a large bowl and mix them well   Divide the mixture between two heavy-duty, resealable zipper bags and seal them using the displacement/water immersion method   Submerge the bag under water for about 2 hours   Once done, take the bags out and pour the contents to a large-sized bowl or pot.   Add the chicken broth and blend the whole mixture using an immersion blender   Stir in the yogurt, with some extra water or broth if you want a different consistency   Season the soup with some salt and vinegar   Serve with a garnish of dill fronds!

Nutrition Info: Per serving:Calories: 189 ;Carbohydrate: 16g ;Protein: 9g ;Fat: 12g ;Sugar: 5g ;Sodium: 325mg

Asian-style Noodle With Fennel

INGREDIENTS for Servings: 4

1 ½ pounds fennel bulb, cut into wedges	1 teaspoon grated ginger
2 bay leaves	1/2 teaspoon Japanese curry powder
1 tablespoon sesame oil	
1 teaspoon garlic, minced	16 ounces soba noodles
Salt and freshly ground black pepper, to taste	1 teaspoon Harissa paste
	4 tablespoons Ponzu sauce

DIRECTIONS and Cooking Time: 1 Hour 10 Minutes

Preheat a sous vide water bath to 185 degrees F. Place the fennel and bay leaves in a cooking pouch; seal tightly.   Submerge the cooking pouch in the water bath; cook for 25 minutes. Remove the fennel wedges from the cooking pouch and pat it dry with kitchen towels; discard bay leaves.   Heat the oil in a wok over a moderately high heat. Then, cook the garlic and ginger for 40 seconds or until aromatic.   Stir in the reserved fennel. Cook the fennel until nice and browned on all sides. Season with salt, black pepper, and curry powder.   Next, cook the noodles according to package instructions. Drain and rinse noodles; add the prepared fennel.   Stir in Harissa paste and Ponzu sauce; toss to combine well. Serve right away.

Nutrition Info:471 Calories; 6g Fat; 97g Carbs; 18g Protein; 4g Sugars

Steamed Asparagus With Hollandaise Sauce

INGREDIENTS for Servings: 3

20 spears white asparagus, trimmed	2 eggs
2 tablespoons butter	¼ cup butter
¼ cup orange juice	½ tablespoon lemon juice
2 orange slices	Salt and pepper, to taste
1 teaspoon salt	
Hollandaise sauce:	

DIRECTIONS and Cooking Time: 25 Minutes
Set the cooker to 185ºF.   Place the asparagus, butter, orange juice, orange slices, and salt in a vacuum seal bag.   Seal the bag and submerge in a water bath. Cook 25 minutes.   Heat large skillet over medium-high heat.   Remove the asparagus from the bag and transfer to the skillet. Cook 30 seconds and remove. Make the sauce; place the egg yolks in a heat-proof bowl. Set the bowl over simmering water.   Melt butter over medium heat. Gradually add butter to egg yolks, whisking rapidly. Continue until all butter is incorporated.   Stir in the lemon juice. Season to taste.   Serve asparagus and drizzle with sauce.

Nutrition Info: Per serving:Calories 132.5, Carbohydrates 5.6 g, Fats 10.1 g, Protein 4.8 g

POULTRY RECIPES

Yummy Chicken Legs With Lime-sweet Sauce

INGREDIENTS for Servings: 8

¼ cup olive oil	12 chicken legs
4 red bell peppers, chopped	¼ cup lime juice
6 spring onions, chopped	2 tbsp lime zest
4 garlic cloves, minced	2 tbsp sugar
1 oz fresh ginger, chopped	2 tbsp fresh thyme leaves
½ cup Worcestershire sauce	1 tbsp allspice
	Salt and black pepper to taste
	1 tsp ground nutmeg

DIRECTIONS and Cooking Time: 14 Hours 30 Minutes

Put in a food processor the peppers, onions, garlic, ginger, Worcestershire sauce, olive oil, lime juice and zest, sugar, thyme, allspice, salt, black pepper, and nutmeg. and blend. Reserve 1/4 cup of sauce. Place the chicken and lime sauce in a vacuum-sealable bag. Release air by the water displacement method. Transfer into the fridge and allow to marinade for 12 hours. Prepare a water bath and place the Sous Vide in it. Set to 152 F. Seal and submerge the bag in the water bath. Cook for 2 hours. Once the timer has stopped, remove the chicken and pat dry with kitchen towel. Discard the cooking juices. Brush the chicken with the reserved lime sauce. Heat a skillet over high heat and sear the chicken for 30 seconds per side.

Oregano Chicken Meatballs

INGREDIENTS for Servings: 4

1 pound ground chicken	1 tbsp cumin
1 tbsp olive oil	½ tsp grated lemon zest
2 garlic cloves, minced	½ tsp black pepper
1 tsp fresh oregano, minced	¼ cup panko breadcrumbs
Salt to taste	Lemon wedges

DIRECTIONS and Cooking Time: 2 Hours 20 Minutes

Prepare a water bath and place Sous Vide in it. Set to 146 F. Combine in a bowl ground chicken, garlic, olive oil, oregano, lemon zest, cumin, salt, and pepper. Using your hands make at least 14 meatballs. Place the meatballs in a vacuum-sealable bag. Release air by the water displacement method, seal and submerge the bag in the water bath. Cook for 2 hours. Once the timer has stopped, remove the bag and transfer the meatballs to a baking sheet, lined with foil. Heat a skillet over medium heat and sear the meatballs for 7 minutes. Top with lemon wedges.

Cheesy Turkey Burgers

INGREDIENTS for Servings: 6

1½ pounds ground turkey	6 tsp olive oil
16 cream crackers, crushed	½ tbsp soy sauce
2½ tbsp chopped fresh parsley	½ tsp garlic powder
2 tbsp chopped fresh basil	1 egg
½ tbsp Worcestershire sauce	6 buns, toasted
	6 tomato slices
	6 Romaine lettuce leaves
	6 slices Monterey Jack cheese

DIRECTIONS and Cooking Time: 1 Hour 45 Minutes

Prepare a water bath and place the Sous Vide in it. Set to 148 F. Combine the turkey, crackers, parsley, basil, soy sauce and garlic powder. Add the egg and mix using your hands. In a baking sheet with wax pepper, with the mixture create 6 patties and place them. Cover and transfer to the fridge Remove the patties from the fridge and place in three vacuum-sealable bag. Release air by the water displacement method, seal and submerge the bags in the water bath. Cook for 1 hour and 15 minutes. Once the timer has stopped, remove the patties. Discard cooking juices. Heat olive oil in a skillet over high heat and place the patties. Sear for 45 seconds per side. Place the patties over the toasted buns. Top with tomato, lettuce and cheese. Serve.

Teriyaki Chicken

INGREDIENTS

For Chicken Bowl:	Salt, to taste
1 teaspoon garlic, minced	1 tablespoon corn flour
1 teaspoon fresh ginger, minced	1 tablespoon water
4 tablespoons sake	4 eggs
4 tablespoons soy sauce	2 cups white rice
2 tablespoons rice wine vinegar	For Pickled Veggies:
1 tablespoon brown sugar	3 cups veggies (2-parts carrot and cucumber, 1-part red onion and daikon), sliced finely
¼ teaspoon chili powder	1 cup water
Freshly ground black pepper, to taste	1 cup vinegar
4 medium chicken thighs	2 tablespoons brown sugar
	1 tablespoon salt

DIRECTIONS and Cooking Time: 56 Minutes Cooking Temperature: 145°f

Attach the sous vide immersion circulator to a Cambro container or pot with water using an adjustable clamp and preheat water to 145°F. In a bowl, add garlic, ginger, sake, soy sauce, vinegar, brown sugar, chili powder, and black pepper and mix until well combined. Place chicken thighs in a cooking pouch with the ginger mixture. Seal pouch tightly after removing the excess air. Place pouch in sous vide bath and set the cooking time for 50 minutes. Gently place the eggs in the same sous vide bath for 50 minutes. Prepare white rice according to the package's directions For pickled veggies: add all ingredients in a pan over high heat and bring to a boil. Remove from heat and set aside until chicken cooks, keeping the pan covered. Remove pouch and eggs from the sous vide bath. Carefully open pouch and remove chicken thighs, reserving the cooking liquid in a bowl. Pat dry chicken thighs with paper towels. Lightly season chicken thighs with salt. In a small bowl, dissolve corn flour into water. Add the flour mixture to the bowl of reserved cooking liquid and stir to combine. Heat a non-stick skillet over medium heat and sear chicken thighs for 2 minutes on each side. Add reserved liquid mixture to the skillet for the last minute of cooking and toss chicken thighs to coat. With a slotted spoon, transfer chicken thighs to a platter. Continue cooking sauce in the skillet, stirring continuously, until it reaches desired thickness. Remove sauce from heat. Drain pickled veggies and cut chicken thighs into desired slices. Divide cooked rice into serving bowls and top with chicken slices. Pour sauce over chicken slices and place pickled veggies on the side. Crack the egg over rice and chicken. Season with salt and pepper and serve.

Chicken Thighs With Carrot Puree

INGREDIENTS for Servings: 5

2 pounds chicken thighs 1 cup carrots, thinly sliced ¼ cup finely chopped onion 2 cups of chicken broth	2 tbsp olive oil 2 tbsp fresh parsley, finely chopped 2 crushed garlic cloves Salt and black pepper to taste

DIRECTIONS and Cooking Time: 60 Minutes
Make a water bath, place Sous Vide in it, and set to 167 F. Wash the chicken thighs under cold running water and pat dry with a kitchen paper. Set aside. In a bowl, combine 1 tablespoon of olive oil, parsley, salt, and pepper. Stir well and generously brush the thighs with the mixture. Place in a large vacuum-sealable bag and add chicken broth. Press the bag to remove the air. Seal the bag and put in the water bath and set the timer for 45 minutes. Once the timer has stopped, remove the thighs from the bag and pat them dry. Reserve the cooking liquid. Meanwhile, prepare the

carrots. Transfer to a blender and process until pureed. Set aside. Heat up the remaining olive oil in a large skillet over a medium heat. Add garlic and onion and stir-fry for about 1-2 minutes, or until soft. Add chicken thighs and cook for 2-3 minutes, turning occasionally. Taste for doneness, adjust the seasonings and then add broth. Bring it to a boil and remove from the heat. Transfer the thighs to a serving plate and top with carrot puree, and sprinkle with parsley.

Sweet Chili Chicken

INGREDIENTS for Servings: 2

4 chicken thighs 2 tablespoons olive oil Salt and pepper as needed 1 garlic clove, crushed 3 tablespoons fish sauce ¼ cup lime juice	1 tablespoon palm sugar 3 tablespoons Thai basil, chopped 3 tablespoons cilantro, chopped 2 red chilies /deseeded, chopped 1 tablespoon sweet chili sauce

DIRECTIONS and Cooking Time: 120 Minutes
Prepare your water bath using your Sous Vide immersion circulator, and increase the temperature to 150-degrees Fahrenheit Cover the chicken thighs with cling film and chill them for a while Place them in a zip bag along with the olive oil, salt and pepper, and seal using the immersion method Cook for 2 hours Once done, heat the olive oil in a pan and chop the chicken into 4-5 pieces Dip them in the veggie oil and cook until crispy Combine all the above dressing ingredients in a bowl and place to one side Sprinkle with salt on top and serve with the sauce

Nutrition Info:Calories: 721 Carbohydrate: 9g Protein: 46g Fat: 54g Sugar: 4g Sodium: 572mg

Layered Cheese Chicken

INGREDIENTS for Servings: 2

2 chicken breasts, boneless, skinless Salt and black pepper to taste 2 tsp butter 4 cups lettuce 1 large tomato, sliced	1 oz cheddar cheese cheese, sliced 2 tbsp red onion, diced Fresh basil leaves 1 tbsp olive oil 2 lemon wedges for serving

DIRECTIONS and Cooking Time: 60 Minutes
Prepare a water bath and place the Sous Vide in it. Set to 146 F. Place the chicken in a vacuum-sealable bag. Season with salt and pepper. Release air by the water displacement method, seal and submerge the bag in the water bath. Cook for 45 minutes. Once the timer has stopped, remove the chicken and discard cooking

juices. Heat a skillet over high heat with butter. Sear the chicken until browned. Transfer to a serving plate. Put the lettuce among the chicken and top with tomato, red onion, cheddar cheese, and basil. Sprinkle with olive oil, salt and pepper. Serve with lemon wedges.

Mirin Teriyaki Wings

INGREDIENTS for Servings: 4

5lb. chicken wings, sliced into flats and drumettes	1 tablespoon hoisin sauce
Salt and freshly ground black pepper	¼ teaspoon minced fresh ginger
1 teaspoon teriyaki sauce	Vegetable oil, for frying
½ teaspoon mirin	Wasabi for garnish

DIRECTIONS and Cooking Time: 45 Minutes
Set the Sous Vide cooker to 140F. Season chicken wings, lightly with salt and pepper. Place wings in a zip-lock bag and seal using immersion water technique. Place the bag in a water bath and set the timer to 45 minutes. Meanwhile, prepare the sauce; combine teriyaki sauce, hoisin sauce, mirin and ginger in a bowl. Finishing steps: When the timer goes off, remove the bag and take the chicken out. Pour around 2-inches of oil in large pan and heat over medium-high heat. Fry wings for 1-2 minutes and transfer to bowl with prepared sauce; toss to combine. Serve wings on a platter, with wasabi paste.

Nutrition Info: Calories 335 Total Fat 18g Total Carb 4g Dietary Fiber 1g Protein 44g

Caesar Salad Tortilla Rolls With Turkey

INGREDIENTS for Servings: 4

2 garlic cloves, minced	1 cup mayonnaise
2 skinless, boneless turkey breasts	1 tsp anchovy paste
Salt and black pepper to taste	1 tsp Dijon mustard
	1 tsp soy sauce
2 tbsp freshly squeezed lemon juice	4 cups iceberg lettuce
	4 tortillas

DIRECTIONS and Cooking Time: 1 Hour 40 Minutes
Prepare a water bath and place the Sous Vide in it. Set to 152 F. Season the turkey breast with salt and pepper and put in a vacuum-sealable bag. Release air by the water displacement method, seal and submerge the bag in the water bath. Cook for 1 hour and 30 minutes. Combine the mayonnaise, garlic, lemon juice, anchovy paste, mustard, soy sauce, and remaining salt and pepper. Allow to rest in the fridge. Once the timer has stopped, remove the turkey and pat dry. Slice the turkey. Mix the lettuce with the cold

dressing. Pour one-quarter of the turkey mixture into each tortilla and fold. Cut by the half and serve with the dressing.

Cheesy Chicken Salad With Chickpeas

INGREDIENTS for Servings: 2

6 chicken breast tenderloins, boneless, skinless	½ cup crumbled feta cheese
4 tbsp olive oil	½ cup crumbled queso fresco cheese
2 tbsp hot sauce	½ cup torn basil
1 tsp ground cumin	½ cup freshly torn mint
1 tsp light brown sugar	4 tsp pine nuts, toasted
1 tsp ground cinnamon	2 tsp honey
Salt and black pepper to taste	2 tsp freshly squeezed lemon juice
1 can drained chickpeas	

DIRECTIONS and Cooking Time: 1 Hour 30 Minutes
Prepare a water bath and place the Sous Vide in it. Set to 138 F. Place the chicken breasts, 2 tbsp of olive oil, hot sauce, brown sugar, cumin, and cinnamon in a vacuum-sealable bag. Season with salt and pepper. Release air by the water displacement method, seal and submerge the bag in the water bath. Cook for 75 minutes. Meanwhile, combine in a bowl the chickpeas, basil, queso fresco, mint, and pine nuts. Pour in honey, lemon juice and 2 tbsp of olive oil. Season with salt and pepper. Once the timer has stopped, remove the chicken and chop in bites. Discard cooking juices. Stir the salad and chicken, mix well and serve.

Cilantro Chicken With Peanut Butter Sauce

INGREDIENTS for Servings: 2

4 chicken breasts	2 tbsp chopped cilantro
1 bag mixed salad	3 cloves garlic
1 bunch cilantro	2 tbsp fresh ginger
2 cucumbers	½ cup water
2 carrots	2 tbsp white vinegar
1 pack wonton wrappers	1 tbsp soy sauce
Oil for frying	1 tsp fish sauce
¼ cup peanut butter	1 tsp sesame oil
Juice of 1 lime	3 tbsp canola oil

DIRECTIONS and Cooking Time: 1 Hour 40 Minutes
Prepare a water bath and place the Sous Vide in it. Set to 149 F. Season the chicken with salt and pepper and place in a vacuum-sealable bag. Release air by the

water displacement method, seal and submerge the bag in the water bath. Cook for 60 minutes. Chop the cucumber, cilantro and carrots and combine with the salad- Heat a pot to 350 F. and fill with oil. Slice the wonton wrappers in pieces and fry until crispy. In a food processor, put peanut butter, lime juice, fresh ginger, cilantro, water, white vinegar, fish sauce, soy sauce, sesame, and canola oil. Blend until smooth. Once the timer ends, remove the chicken and transfer to a hot skillet. Sear for 30 seconds per side. Mix the wonton strips with the salad. Slice the chicken. Serve on top of the salad. Drizzle with the dressing.

Pesto Chicken Mini Bites With Avocado

INGREDIENTS for Servings: 2

1 chicken breast, boneless, skinless, butterflied	3 tbsp olive oil
	1 tbsp pesto
	1 zucchini, sliced
Salt and black pepper to taste	1 avocado
1 tbsp sage	1 cup fresh basil leaves

DIRECTIONS and Cooking Time: 1 Hour 40 Minutes
Prepare a water bath and place the Sous Vide in it. Set to 138 F. Pound the chicken breast until thin. Season with sage, pepper and salt. Place in a vacuum-sealable bag. Add 1 tbsp of oil and pesto. Release air by the water displacement method, seal and submerge the bag in the water bath. Cook for 75 minutes. After 60 minutes, heat 1 tbsp of olive oil in a skillet over high heat, add the zucchini and ¼ cup water. Cook until the water has evaporated. Once the timer has stopped, remove the chicken. Heat the remaining olive oil in a skillet over medium heat and sear the chicken for 2 minutes per side. Set aside and allow cooling. Cut the chicken in tiny slices just like the zucchini. Slice the avocado as well. Serve the chicken with slices of avocado on the top. Garnish with zucchini slices and basil.

Bacon & Nut Stuffed Turkey Wrapped In Ham

INGREDIENTS for Servings: 6

1 white onion, chopped	4 tbsp chopped parsley
3 tbsp butter	¾ cup bread crumbs
1 cup bacon cubes	1 egg, beaten
4 tbsp pine nuts	4 lb boneless turkey breast, butterflied
2 tbsp chopped thyme	
4 garlic cloves, minced	Salt and black pepper to taste
Zest of 2 lemons	16 slices ham

DIRECTIONS and Cooking Time: 3 Hours 45 Minutes

Prepare a water bath and place the Sous Vide in it. Set to 146 F. Heat 2 tbsp of butter in a skillet over medium heat and sauté the onion for 10 minutes until softened. Set aside. In the same skillet, add the bacon and cook for 5 minutes until brown. Stir in pine nuts, thyme, garlic, and lemon zest and cook for 2 minutes more. Add in parsley and mix. Return the onion to the skillet, stir in bread crumbs and egg. Take out the turkey and cover it with plastic wrap. With a meat hammer pound it to the thickness. Place ham in an aluminium foil. Put the turkey on the ham and smash the center to create a strip. Roll the turkey tightly from one side to other until is completely wrapped. Cover with plastic wrap and place in a vacuum-sealable bag. Release air by the water displacement method, seal and submerge the bag in the water bath. Cook for 3 hours. Once the timer has stopped, remove the turkey and discard the plastic. Heat the remaining butter in a skillet over medium heat and put the breast. Sear the ham for 45 seconds per side. Roll the turkey and sear for 2-3 minutes more. Cut the breast into medallions and serve.

Panko Crusted Chicken

INGREDIENTS for Servings: 4

4 boneless chicken breasts	Small bunch of thyme
	2 eggs
1 cup panko bread crumbs	Salt and pepper as needed
1 lb. sliced mushrooms	Canola oil as needed

DIRECTIONS and Cooking Time: 60 Minutes
Prepare your water bath using your Sous Vide immersion circulator, and increase the temperature to 150-degrees Fahrenheit Season the chicken with salt, and thyme Place the breast in a resealable bag and seal using the immersion method and cook for 60 minutes Then, place a pan over medium heat, add the mushrooms and cook them until the water has evaporated Add 3-4 sprigs of thyme and stir Once cooked, remove the chicken from the bag and pat dry Add the oil and heat it up over medium-high heat. Add the eggs into a container and dip the chicken in egg wash until well coated. Add the panko bread crumbs in a shallow container and add some salt and pepper. Put the chicken to bread crumbs and coat until well covered. Fry the chicken for 1-2 minutes per side and serve with the mushrooms

Nutrition Info: Per serving:Calories: 394 ;Carbohydrate: 71g ;Protein: 19g ;Fat: 5g ;Sugar: 5g ;Sodium: 59mg

Spice Turkey Dish

INGREDIENTS for Servings: 4

1 turkey leg	1 tsp black pepper
1 tbsp olive oil	3 sprigs of thyme
1 tbsp garlic salt	1 tbsp rosemary

DIRECTIONS and Cooking Time: 14 Hours 15 Minutes

Prepare a water bath and place the Sous Vide in it. Set to 146 F. Season the turkey with garlic, salt and pepper. Place it in a vacuum-sealable bag. Release air by the water displacement method, seal and submerge the bag in the bath. Cook for 14 hours. Once done, remove the legs and pat dry.

Mediterranean Chicken

INGREDIENTS for Servings: 2

2 chicken breast fillets	2 tablespoons oil,
½ cup sun-dried	from the sun-dried
tomatoes, packed in	tomatoes
oil	1 sprig basil
Salt and black pepper,	1 tablespoon olive oil
to taste	

DIRECTIONS and Cooking Time: 90 Minutes

Preheat the Sous Vide Cooker to 140ºF. Season the chicken with salt and pepper. Heat the olive oil in a skillet. Add chicken breasts and cook for 1 minute per side. Transfer immediately into Sous Vide bag, and add remaining ingredients. Vacuum seal the bag and submerge in water. Cook the chicken 90 minutes. Remove the bag with chicken from the Cooker. Open the bag and transfer the chicken to a warmed plate. Serve.

Nutrition Info: Per serving: Calories 400, Carbohydrates 17.8 g, Fats 21.7 g, Protein 33.4 g

Cherry Tomatoes, Avocado & Chicken Salad

INGREDIENTS for Servings: 2

1 chicken breast	1 tbsp lime juice
1 avocado, sliced	1 garlic clove, crushed
10 pieces of halved	Salt and black pepper
cherry tomatoes	to taste
2 cups chopped	2 tsp maple syrup
lettuce	
2 tbsp olive oil	

DIRECTIONS and Cooking Time: 1 Hour 30 Minutes

Prepare a water bath and place the Sous Vide in it. Set to 138 F. Place the chicken in a vacuum-sealable bag. Season with salt and pepper. Release air by the water displacement method, seal and submerge the bag in the water bath. Cook for 75 minutes. Once the timer has stopped, remove the chicken. Heat oil in a pan over medium heat. Sear the breasts for 30 seconds and slice. In a bowl, combine the garlic, lime juice, maple syrup, and olive oil. Add in lettuce, cherry tomatoes and avocado. Mix well. Plate the salad and top with chicken.

Duck Breast A La Orange

INGREDIENTS

2 (6-ounce) duck	4 fresh thyme sprigs
breasts	Salt and freshly
1 shallot, quartered	ground black pepper,
4 garlic cloves,	to taste
crushed	1 tablespoon sherry
Juice and zest of 1	vinegar
orange	1 cup chicken broth
1 tablespoon black	2 tablespoons cold,
peppercorns	unsalted butter

DIRECTIONS and Cooking Time: 3 Hours 40 Minutes Cooking Temperature: 135°f

Attach the sous vide immersion circulator to a Cambro container or pot with water using an adjustable clamp and preheat water to 135°F. Place duck breasts, shallot, garlic, thyme, orange zest, juice from orange, and the peppercorns in a cooking pouch. Seal pouch tightly after removing the excess air. Place pouch in sous vide bath and set the cooking time for 3½ hours. Remove pouch from the sous vide bath and open carefully. Remove the duck breasts from pouch, reserving the remaining pouch ingredients and liquid. Pat dry the duck breasts with paper towels. Using a sharp knife, score a wide crisscross pattern on the top skin of both breasts. Season breasts evenly with salt and pepper. Heat a non-stick sauté pan over medium heat and sear breasts for 5 minutes. Transfer the duck breasts to a plate, discarding the duck fat left in the pan. For sauce: in the same pan, add vinegar over medium-high heat and scrape browned bits from bottom of pan. Add the broth and the reserved orange mixture from pouch and simmer until sauce reduces to ¼ cup. Add cold butter and beat until well combined. Stir in desired amount of salt and black pepper and remove from heat. Cut duck breasts into desired slices and serve alongside orange sauce.

Orange Chicken Thighs

INGREDIENTS for Servings: 4

2 pounds chicken	1 onions, chopped
thighs	1 tsp orange extract,
2 small chili peppers,	liquid
finely chopped	2 tbsp vegetable oil
1 cup chicken broths	1 tsp barbecue
½ cup freshly	seasoning mix
squeezed orange juice	Fresh parsley to
	garnish

DIRECTIONS and Cooking Time: 2 Hours

Make a water bath, place Sous Vide in it, and set to 167 F. Heat olive oil in a large saucepan. Add in chopped onions and stir-fry for 3 minutes, over a medium temperature, until translucent. In a food processor, combine the orange juice with chili pepper, and orange extract. Pulse until well combined. Pour the mixture into a saucepan and reduce the heat. Simmer for 10 minutes. Coat chicken with barbecue seasoning mix and place in a saucepan. Add in chicken broth and cook until half of the liquid evaporates. Remove to a large vacuum-sealable bag and seal. Submerge the bag in the water bath and cook for 45 minutes. Once the timer has stopped, remove the bag from the water bath and open it. Garnish with fresh parsley and serve.

Chicken Salad

INGREDIENTS

2 pounds chicken breast	1 tablespoon honey
2 tarragon sprigs	1 celery stalk, minced
2 garlic cloves, smashed	1 garlic clove, minced
Zest and juice of 1 lemon	½ Serrano Chile, stemmed, seeded, and minced
Kosher salt and freshly ground black pepper, to taste	2 tablespoons fresh tarragon leaves, minced
½ cup mayonnaise	

DIRECTIONS and Cooking Time: 2 Hours Cooking Temperature: 150°f
Attach the sous vide immersion circulator to a Cambro container or pot with water using an adjustable clamp and preheat water to 150°F. Place chicken breasts, tarragon sprigs, smashed garlic cloves, lemon zest, salt, and pepper in a cooking pouch. Seal pouch tightly after removing the excess air. Place pouch in sous vide bath and set the cooking time for 2 hours. Remove pouch from the sous vide bath and immediately plunge into a large bowl of ice water. Once cooled completely, remove chicken breasts from pouch and transfer to a cutting board, discarding the tarragon sprigs, garlic, and lemon zest. Roughly chop chicken and transfer place in a bowl. Add remaining ingredients and a little salt and black pepper and stir to combine. Serve immediately.

Chicken Roulade

INGREDIENTS for Servings: 2

1 x 8 oz chicken breast	Salt and pepper as needed
¼ cup goat cheese	1 tablespoon oil for searing
¼ cup julienned roasted red pepper	
½ cup loosely packed arugula	Tools Required:
6 slices prosciutto	Plastic wrap, wine/vinegar bottle

DIRECTIONS and Cooking Time: 90 Minutes

Prepare your water bath, using your Sous Vide immersion circulator, and raise the temperature to 155-degrees Fahrenheit Drain the chicken breast if needed, and place it between plastic wrap. Pound it using a mallet or the side of wine bottle, until it gets ¼ inch thick Cut in half and season both sides with pepper and salt Spread 2 tablespoons of goat cheese on top and top each half with roasted red peppers Top with half the arugula Roll both breasts like sushi Place 3 layers of prosciutto on your work surface /overlapping each other Put the rolled chicken at the base of the prosciutto and roll it all up to enclose the roulade Place in a zip bag and seal using the immersion method and cook for 90 minutes Take out of the bag and sear Slice and then serve

Nutrition Info:Calories: 513 Carbohydrate: 6g Protein: 47g Fat: 32g Sugar: 2g Sodium: 527mg

Pheasant With Mushrooms

INGREDIENTS

For Pheasant:	For Mushrooms:
2 pheasant breasts, trimmed	4 ounces of Beech mushrooms, trimmed
Kosher salt and freshly ground black pepper, to taste	½ cup red onion, finely chopped
2 tablespoons unsalted sweet butter	2 tablespoons fresh sage leaves, chopped
1 tablespoon extra-virgin olive oil	2 tablespoons unsalted butter
2 tablespoons extra-virgin olive oil	Kosher salt and freshly ground black pepper, to taste
	White truffle oil, to taste

DIRECTIONS and Cooking Time: 1 Hour Cooking Temperature: 145°f
Attach the sous vide immersion circulator to a Cambro container or pot with water using an adjustable clamp and preheat water to 145°F. Season pheasant breasts evenly with salt and black pepper. Place pheasant breasts and butter in a cooking pouch. Seal pouch tightly after removing the excess air. Place pouch in sous vide bath and set the cooking time for 45-60 minutes. Remove pouch from the sous vide bath and open carefully. Remove pheasant breasts from pouch, reserving cooking liquid, and pat dry pheasant breasts with paper towels. In a large, non-stick skillet, heat oil over medium heat. Place pheasant breasts skin side down and sear for 1 minute per side. Transfer pheasant breasts to a plate and set aside. For mushrooms: in the same skillet, heat oil over medium-high heat and sauté mushrooms and onion for 3-5 minutes. Stir in sage, butter, and reserved cooking liquid and bring to a boil. Season with salt and pepper then remove from heat. Place pheasant breasts onto a serving platter and top with the

mushroom sauce. Drizzle with truffle oil and serve immediately.

Rosemary Chicken Stew

INGREDIENTS for Servings: 2

2 chicken thighs	2 bay leaves
6 garlic cloves, crushed	¼ cup dark soy sauce
	¼ cup white vinegar
¼ tsp whole black pepper	1 tbsp rosemary

DIRECTIONS and Cooking Time: 4 Hours 15 Minutes
Prepare a water bath and place the Sous Vide in it. Set to 165 F. Combine the chicken thighs with all the ingredients. Place in a vacuum-sealable bag. Release air by the water displacement method, seal and submerge in water bath. Cook for 4 hours. Once the timer has stopped, remove the chicken, discard bay leaves and reserve the cooking juices. Heat canola oil in a skillet over medium heat and sear the chicken. Add in cooking juices and cook until you have reached the desired consistency. Filter the sauce and top the chicken.

Turkey Breast With Orange Rosemary Butter

INGREDIENTS

For Butter Mixture:	⅛ teaspoon red pepper flakes, crushed
¼ cup unsalted butter, softened	For Turkey Breast:
1 tablespoon honey	2 (1½-2-pound) skin-on, boneless turkey breast halves
Zest of navel orange	
1 teaspoon fresh rosemary, chopped	1½ teaspoons kosher salt
½ teaspoon salt	
⅛ teaspoon ground black pepper	2 fresh rosemary sprigs

DIRECTIONS and Cooking Time: 2 Hours 35 Minutes
Cooking Temperature: 145°f
Attach the sous vide immersion circulator to a Cambro container or pot with water using an adjustable clamp and preheat water to 145. For butter mixture: add all butter mixture ingredients to a small bowl and mix until well combined. Gently separate skin from each turkey breast half, leaving one side of skin attached to the breast. Sprinkle each exposed breast half with kosher salt. Evenly rub butter mixture under and on top of the skin . Place turkey breast halves and rosemary sprigs in a large cooking pouch. Seal pouch tightly after removing the excess air. Place pouch in sous vide bath and set the cooking time for 2½ hours. Preheat the oven broiler to high. Remove pouch from the sous vide bath and open carefully. Remove turkey breast halves from pouch and pat dry with paper towels. Place on a roasting tray. Broil for 5

minutes. Remove turkey breast halves from the oven. Cut into desired slices and serve.

Extra Spicy Habanero Chicken Wings

INGREDIENTS

For Sauce:	For Wings:
6 habanero peppers	40 split chicken wings
3 tablespoons white vinegar	Salt and freshly ground black pepper, to taste
1 teaspoon butter or oil	

DIRECTIONS and Cooking Time: 4 Hours 15 Minutes
Cooking Temperature: 160°f
Attach the sous vide immersion circulator to a Cambro container or pot with water using an adjustable clamp and preheat water to 160°F. For sauce: add all sauce ingredients in a blender and pulse until smooth. Reserve 1 tablespoon of sauce in a bowl. Season chicken wings lightly with salt and black pepper. In a cooking pouch, place chicken wings and all but the 1 tablespoon of reserved sauce. Seal pouch tightly after removing the excess air. Place pouch in sous vide bath and set the cooking time for 4 hours. Preheat the oven broiler to high. Line a baking sheet with parchment paper. Remove pouch from the sous vide bath and open carefully, removing chicken wings from pouch. Arrange chicken wings onto the prepared baking sheet in a single layer. Broil for 10-15 minutes, flipping once halfway through the cooking time. Remove from oven and transfer into bowl of reserved sauce. Toss to coat well and serve immediately.

Chicken & Walnut Salad

INGREDIENTS for Servings: 4

2 skinless chicken breasts, boneless	1 stick rib celery, diced
Salt and black pepper to taste	1/3 cup mayonnaise
1 tbsp corn oil	2 tsp Chardonnay wine
1 apple, cored and diced	1 tsp Dijon mustard
1 tsp lime juice	1 head Romaine lettuce
½ cup white grapes, cut in half	½ cup walnuts, toasted and chopped

DIRECTIONS and Cooking Time: 2 Hours 20 Minutes
Prepare a water bath and place the Sous Vide in it. Set to 146 F. Place the chicken in a vacuum-sealable bag and season with salt and pepper. Release air by the water displacement method, seal and submerge the bag in the water bath. Cook for 2 hours. Once the timer has stopped, remove the bag and discard cooking juices. In a large bowl, toss apple slices with lime juice. Add in celery and white grapes. Mix well.

In another bowl, stir the mayonnaise, Dijon mustard and Chardonnay wine. Pour the mixture over the fruit and mix well. Chop the chicken and put in a medium bowl, season with salt and combine well. Put the chicken in the salad bowl. Colocate the romaine lettuce in salad bowls and place salad on top. Garnish with walnuts.

Sage Turkey Roulade

INGREDIENTS for Servings: 6

3 tbsp olive oil	3 tbsp ground sage
2 small yellow onions, diced	3 cups turkey stuffing mix
2 stalks celery, diced	2 cups turkey or chicken stock
2 lemons' zest and juice	5 pounds halved turkey breast

DIRECTIONS and Cooking Time: 5 Hours 15 Minutes
Place a pan over medium heat, add olive oil, onion, and celery. Sauté for 2 minutes. Add the lemon juice, zest, and sage until the lemon juice reduce. In a bowl, pour the stuffing mixture and add the cooked sage mixture. Mix with your hands. Add in stock, while mixing with your hand until ingredients hold together well and are not runny. Gently remove the turkey skin and lay it on a plastic wrap. Remove bones and discard. Place the turkey breast on the skin and lay a second layer of plastic wrap on the turkey breast. Flatten it to 1 - inch of thickness using a rolling pin. Remove the plastic wrap on top and spread the stuffing on the flattened turkey, leaving ½ inch space around the edges. Starting at the narrow side, roll the turkey like a pastry roll and drape the extra skin on the turkey. Secure the roll with butcher's twine. Wrap the turkey roll in the broader plastic wrap and twist the ends to secure the roll, which should form a tight cylinder. Place the roll in a vacuum-sealable bag, release air and seal the bag. Refrigerate for 40 minutes. Make a water bath, place Sous Vide in it, and set to 155 F. Place the turkey roll in the water bath and set the timer for 4 hours. Once the timer has stopped, remove the bag and unseal it. Preheat an oven to 400 F, remove the plastic wrap from the turkey and place on a baking dish with skin side up. Roast for 15 minutes. Slice in rounds. Serve with a creamy sauce and steamed low carb vegetables.

Thai Green Curry Noodle Soup

INGREDIENTS for Servings: 2

1 chicken breast, boneless and skinless	1½ tablespoons palm sugar
Salt and pepper as needed	½ cup Thai basil leaves, roughly chopped
1 can /15 oz. coconut milk	2 oz cooked egg noodle nests
2 tablespoons Thai	

Green Curry Paste	1 cup cilantro, roughly chopped
1¾ cups chicken stock	
1 cup enoki mushrooms	1 cup bean sprouts
5 kaffir lime leaves, torn in half	2 tablespoons fried noodles
2 tablespoons fish sauce	2 red Thai chilis, roughly chopped

DIRECTIONS and Cooking Time: 90 Minutes
Prepare your water bath using your Sous Vide immersion circulator, and raise the temperature to 140-degrees Fahrenheit   Take the chicken and season it generously with salt and pepper and place it in a medium-sized, resealable bag with 1 tablespoon of coconut milk   Seal it using the immersion method and submerge. Cook for 90 minutes   After 35 minutes, place a medium-sized saucepan over a medium heat   Add the green curry paste and half the coconut milk   Bring the mix to a simmer and cook for 5-10 minutes until the coconut milk starts to show a beady texture   Add the chicken stock and the rest of the coconut milk and bring the mixture to a simmer once again, keep cooking for about 15 minutes   Add the kaffir lime leaves, enoki mushrooms, palm sugar and fish sauce   Lower the heat to medium-low and simmer for about 10 minutes   Remove from the heat and season with palm sugar and fish sauce, stir in the basil   Once the chicken is cooked fully, transfer it to a cooking board. Let it cool for few minutes and then cut into slices   Serve the chicken with the curry sauce and a topping of cooked egg noodles   Garnish the chicken with some bean sprouts, cilantro, Thai chilies and fried noodles. Serve!

Nutrition Info: Calories: 237 Carbohydrate: 21g Protein: 15g Fat: 11g Sugar: 5g Sodium: 567mg

Minted Chicken & Pea Salad

INGREDIENTS for Servings: 2

6 chicken breast tenderloins, boneless	4 tbsp olive oil
Salt and black pepper to taste	½ cup crumbled queso fresco cheese
2 cups snow peas, blanched	1 tbsp freshly squeezed lemon juice
1 cup mint, freshly torn	2 tsp honey
	2 tsp red wine vinegar

DIRECTIONS and Cooking Time: 1 Hour 30 Minutes
Prepare a water bath and place the Sous Vide in it. Set to 138 F. Place the chicken with olive oil in a vacuum-sealable bag. Season with salt and pepper. Release air by the water displacement method, seal and submerge the bag in the water bath. Cook for 75 minutes. In a bowl, combine the peas, queso fresco and mint. Mix the lemon juices, red wine vinegar, honey and 2 tbsp of olive oil. Season with salt and

pepper.   Once ready, remove the chicken and slice in bites. Discard the cooking liquids. Serve.

Chicken Caprese

INGREDIENTS for Servings: 2

2 chicken breasts, boneless, skinless Salt and pepper as needed 2 teaspoons unsalted butter 1 large tomato, sliced 1 oz fresh mozzarella, sliced	4 cups lettuce 2 tablespoons red onion, diced Fresh basil leaves 1 tablespoon extra-virgin olive oil 2 lemon wedges for serving

DIRECTIONS and Cooking Time: 45 Minutes
Prepare your Sous Vide water bath, using your immersion circulator, and raise the temperature to 145-degrees Fahrenheit   Season the chicken with pepper and salt   Add them in a large zip bag and seal using the immersion method and cook for 45 minutes   Once cooked, remove the chicken from the bag and discard the cooking liquid   Place a large skillet over a medium/high heat   Add the butter and allow to heat   Add the chicken breasts and sear until they turn golden brown   Transfer to a serving platter   Divide the lettuce among the breasts and top up with tomato, red onion, mozzarella, and basil   Season with pepper and salt and then drizzle the olive oil over the top   Serve with lemon wedges

Nutrition Info: Calories: 440 Carbohydrate: 5g Protein: 30g Fat: 33g Sugar: 3g Sodium: 524mg

Sous Vide Poached Chicken

INGREDIENTS for Servings: 4

1 whole bone-in chicken, trussed 1-quart low sodium chicken stock 2 tablespoons soy sauce 5 sprigs fresh thyme 2 dried bay leaves 2 cups thickly sliced carrots	Salt and pepper as needed ½ tablespoon olive oil 2 cups thickly sliced celery ½ oz. dried mushrooms 3 tablespoons unsalted butter

DIRECTIONS and Cooking Time: 6 Hours
Prepare your Sous Vide water bath using your immersion circulator and raise the temperature to 150-degrees Fahrenheit   Add the soy sauce, chicken, stock, herbs and veggies in a heavy-duty zip bag and seal using the immersion method and cook for 6 hours   Remove the chicken and strain the veggies   Pat dry and season with the olive oil, pepper and salt   Roast in your oven for 10 minutes at 450-degrees Fahrenheit   Simmer the cooking liquid in a large saucepan   Once done, turn off the heat and whisk in

the butter   Carve the chicken, making sure to discard the skin   Divide the veggies and chicken between the platters and serve with the sauce on top

Nutrition Info: Per serving:Calories: 435 ;Carbohydrate: 17g ;Protein: 34g ;Fat: 26g ;Sugar: 5g ;Sodium: 342mg

Korean Chicken Wings

INGREDIENTS for Servings: 3

12 chicken wings Salt and pepper as needed 1 cup Korean fried chicken batter ½ cup water ½ cup soy sauce ½ minced onion 4-5 garlic cloves, minced 2 teaspoons ginger powder	2 tablespoons brown sugar ¼ cup mirin Sesame seeds for garnishing Cornstarch slurry (make mixing 1 tablespoon of cornstarch, and 2 tablespoons of water) Olive oil as needed for frying

DIRECTIONS and Cooking Time: 2 Hours
Prepare your Sous Vide water bath, using your immersion circulator and raise the temperature to 147-degrees Fahrenheit   Season the wings with pepper and salt   Put the wings in the Sous Vide zip bag and seal using the immersion method and cook for 2 hours   Once the cooking is done, take the bag out of the water and remove the wings, transfer the wings to a kitchen towel and dry them   Pre-heat the oil to 475-degrees Fahrenheit   Mix ½ cup of Korean fried chicken batter mix, and ½ cup of water in a bowl   Put the other ½ cup of batter mix onto another plate   Drench the wings in the wet batter, then dredge them through the dry batter   Flash fry for 1-2 minutes until golden brown and crispy   Mix all the ingredients for the sauce and heat over a saucepan until boiling   Add the wings to the sauce and coat well   Garnish with sesame seeds and serve!

Nutrition Info: Per serving:Calories: 915 ;Carbohydrate: 15g ;Protein: 41g ;Fat: 279g ;Sugar: 1g ;Sodium: 813mg

Fried Chicken

INGREDIENTS for Servings: 4

8 pieces chicken, legs or thighs Salt and pepper as needed Lemon wedges for serving For Wet Mix 2 cups soy milk 1 tablespoon lemon juice	For Dry Mix 1 cup plain, high protein flour 1 cup rice flour ½ cup cornstarch 2 tablespoons paprika 2 tablespoons salt 2 tablespoons ground black pepper

DIRECTIONS and Cooking Time: 1 Hour

Prepare your sous vide water bath to a temperature of 154-degrees Fahrenheit, using your immersion circulator Season your chicken pieces well with pepper and salt and seal them in a resealable bag using the water immersion method Cook them in the water bath for 1 hour Remove the chicken and place it to one side. Allow it to sit for 15-20 minutes Take a pan and place it on the stove, pour in some oil and pre-heat to a temperature of 400-425-degrees Fahrenheit Take a large-sized bowl and add the soy milk and lemon juice, whisk them well Use another bowl to mix the protein flour, rice flour, cornstarch, paprika, salt and ground black pepper Gently dip the cooked chicken in the dry mix, then dip into the wet mixture Repeat 2-3 times then place the prepared chickens on a wire rack Keep repeating until all the chicken has been used Fry the chicken in small batches for about 3-4 minutes for each batch Once done, allow the chicken to cool on the wire rack for 10-15 minutes Serve with some lemon wedges and sauce!

Nutrition Info: Calories: 251 Carbohydrate: 10g Protein: 28g Fat: 11g Sugar: 4g Sodium: 458mg Special Tips It is wise to rub the turkey legs with olive oil before searing them. This will allow them to take on a much crispier texture and help avoid burning.

Coq Au Vin

INGREDIENTS

1 bottle red wine, reserving 1 glass	4 bay leaves
1/2 cup bacon, crumbled	10 shallots or small onions
3 large carrots, peeled and chopped	Sea salt and freshly ground black pepper, to taste
3 celery stalks, finely chopped	A few thyme sprigs
4 garlic cloves, pressed	2 tablespoons all-purpose flour
7 tbsp unsalted butter, divided	Vegetable oil*
1 chicken, jointed into 2 breasts on the bone with wings and 2 legs attached	7 ounces button mushrooms
	Finely chopped fresh parsley, for garnishing

DIRECTIONS and Cooking Time: 12 Hours 30 Minutes Cooking Temperature: 151°f

Add wine, bacon, carrots, celery, garlic, and bay leaves to a pan and bring to a gentle boil. Cook for 25 minutes, stirring occasionally. Remove from heat and allow to cool completely. Meanwhile in another pan, melt 1 tbsp butter and sauté onions for 4-5 minutes. Remove from heat and set aside. Attach the sous vide immersion circulator to a Cambro container or pot with water using an adjustable clamp and preheat

water to 151°F. Season the jointed chickens evenly with salt and black pepper. Divide chicken pieces, sautéed onions, and thyme sprigs between two cooking pouches. Seal pouches tightly after removing excess air. Place pouches in sous vide bath and set the cooking time for 12 hours. Preheat the oven to 355°F. Remove pouches from the sous vide bath and open carefully. Remove chicken pieces from pouches, reserving cooking liquid in a pan. Pat dry chicken pieces with paper towels. Season chicken lightly with salt and pepper. In a large frying pan, heat oil and 2 tablespoons butter. Add chicken, skin side down, and fry for 6-8 minutes on each side. Move chicken pieces to a baking sheet, skin side up, and bake for 10 minutes. While the chicken is baking, remove thyme sprigs from cooking liquid and bring liquid to a gentle boil, adding reserved wine. In a bowl, combine flour and 2 tablespoons unsalted butter and mix well. Add flour mixture to pan with cooking liquid, stirring continuously. Stir in salt and black pepper and simmer until desired consistency is reached. Move baked chicken pieces to a different pan on the stove. Add 2 tablespoons of butter and stir fry with mushrooms for 6-7 minutes or until browned on both sides. Place chicken on a serving platter and top with sauce, followed by mushrooms. Garnish with parsley and serve.

Crispy Chicken With Mushrooms

INGREDIENTS for Servings: 4

4 boneless chicken breasts	Small bunch of thyme
1 cup panko bread crumbs	2 eggs
1 pound sliced Portobello mushrooms	Salt and black pepper to taste
	Canola oil to taste

DIRECTIONS and Cooking Time: 1 Hour 15 Minutes

Prepare a water bath and place the Sous Vide in it. Set to 149 F. Place the chicken in a vacuum-sealable bag. Season with salt and thyme. Release air by the water displacement method, seal and submerge in water bath. Cook for 60 minutes. Meanwhile, heat a skillet over medium heat. Cook the mushrooms until the water has evaporated. Add in 3-4 sprigs of thyme. Season with salt and pepper. Once the timer has stopped, remove the bag. Heat a frying pan with oil over medium heat. Mix the panko with salt and pepper. Layer the chicken in panko mix. Fry for 1-2 minutes per side. Serve with mushrooms.

Chicken Mint Pea Feta

INGREDIENTS for Servings: 8

6 chicken breast tenderloins, boneless	1 cup mint, freshly torn
4 tablespoons extra	½ cup crumbled feta

virgin-olive oil Salt and pepper as needed 2 cups green peas, blanched 2 teaspoons honey	cheese 1 tablespoon freshly squeezed lemon juice 2 teaspoons red wine vinegar

DIRECTIONS and Cooking Time: 75 Minutes

Prepare your water bath, using your Sous Vide immersion circulator, and increase the temperature to 140-degrees Fahrenheit Put the chicken and 2 tablespoons of olive oil in a zip bag Season with pepper and salt Seal using the immersion method, and cook for 75 minutes Add the peas, feta cheese and mint in a large bowl Whisk the lemon juice, red wine vinegar, honey and 2 tablespoons of olive oil in a small bowl Season with salt and pepper Once cooked, take the chicken out from the bag and chop it into bite sized pieces Discard the cooking liquid and toss the salad with the chicken and the dressing Serve!

Nutrition Info: Calories: 252 Carbohydrate: 29g Protein: 16g Fat: 8g Sugar: 10g Sodium: 534mg

Duck A La Orange

INGREDIENTS for Servings: 2

2 5oz. duck breast fillets, skin on 1 orange, sliced 4 cloves garlic 1 shallot, chopped 1 teaspoon black peppercorns	4 sprigs thyme 1 tablespoon sherry vinegar ¼ cup red wine 2 tablespoons butter Salt, to taste

DIRECTIONS and Cooking Time: 2 Hours 30 Minutes

Preheat Sous Vide cooker to 135F. Place the duck breast fillets into a Sous Vide bag. Top the breasts with orange slices, garlic, shallot, thyme, and peppercorns. Vacuum seal the bag and submerge in water. Cook the breasts 2 ½ hours. Finishing steps: Remove the bag from a water bath. Open the bag and remove the breasts. Heat a large skillet over medium-high heat. Sear the duck, skin side down, for 30 seconds. Place the breasts aside and keep warm. In the same skillet, add sherry vinegar and wine. Add the bag content and bring to simmer. Simmer 5 minutes. Stir in the butter and simmer 1 minute. Serve the duck with prepared sauce.

Nutrition Info: Calories 466 Total Fat 24g Total Carb 11g Dietary Fiber 6g Protein 35g

Orange Balsamic Chicken

INGREDIENTS

1 large, whole, boneless chicken breast Salt and freshly	1 orange 1 small sprig fresh oregano or rosemary

ground black pepper, to taste	3 tablespoons balsamic vinegar

DIRECTIONS and Cooking Time: 1 Hour 35 Minutes
Cooking Temperature: 146°f

Attach the sous vide immersion circulator to a Cambro container or pot with water using an adjustable clamp and preheat water to 146°F. Season chicken breasts lightly with salt and black pepper. Cut 2 (¼-inch) slices from orange. Extract juice from remaining orange into a small bowl. Add vinegar and mix together with the juice of the orange. Place chicken breast in a cooking pouch and top breast with orange slices and herb sprig. Carefully pour vinegar mixture into pouch. Seal pouch tightly after removing the excess air. Place pouch in sous vide bath and set the cooking time for 1½ hours. Remove pouch from the sous vide bath and open carefully. Remove chicken breast from the pouch, reserving the cooking liquid. Add the cooking liquid to a small pan and cook until slightly thickened. Serve chicken with sauce.

Turkey Breast With Pecans

INGREDIENTS for Servings: 6

2 pounds turkey breast, thinly sliced 1 tbsp lemon zest 1 cup pecans, finely chopped 1 tbsp thyme, finely chopped	2 garlic cloves, crushed 2 tbsp fresh parsley, finely chopped 3 cups chicken broth 3 tbsp olive oil

DIRECTIONS and Cooking Time: 2 Hours 15 Minutes

Rinse the meat under cold running water and drain in a colander. Rub with lemon zest and transfer to a large vacuum-sealable bag along with chicken broth. Cook en Sous Vide for 2 hours at 149 F. Remove from the water bath and set aside. Heat olive oil in a medium-sized skillet and add garlic, pecan nuts, and thyme. Give it a good stir and cook for 4-5 minutes. Finally, add chicken breast to the frying pan and briefly brown on both sides. Serve immediately.

Turkey Breast With Spiced Sage Rub

INGREDIENTS

For Brine: 8 cups water 2 tablespoons light brown sugar ¼ cup kosher salt 1 teaspoon black peppercorns ½ teaspoon allspice berries 1 whole skin-on,	For Turkey: For Rub: 2 tablespoons fresh sage leaves, minced 2 garlic cloves, minced 1½ teaspoon fennel seeds, crushed ¼ teaspoon red pepper flakes, crushed

boneless turkey breast, about 4 pounds	For Searing: Olive oil, as required

DIRECTIONS and Cooking Time: 4 Hours 5 Minutes
Cooking Temperature: 133°f
For brine: add all brine ingredients to a large bowl and mix until brown sugar and salt dissolve. Place turkey breast in the bowl and refrigerate, covered, for 6-8 hours.   For rub: add all rub ingredients in a bowl and mix until well combined.   Attach the sous vide immersion circulator to a Cambro container or pot with water using an adjustable clamp and preheat water to 133°F.   Remove turkey breast from brine and pat dry with paper towels.   Arrange turkey breast on a smooth surface so that it is flat. Spread rub mixture evenly over breast. Roll up breast into a cylinder and tie with kitchen twine at 1-inch intervals. Place turkey roll in a cooking pouch. Seal pouch tightly after removing the excess air. Place pouch in sous vide bath and set the cooking time for 4 hours.   Remove pouch from the sous vide bath and open carefully. Remove turkey roll from pouch and pat dry with paper towels.   Heat oil in a skillet. Place turkey roll skin side down in skillet and sear until browned completely.   Remove from heat and carefully remove kitchen twine. Cut into slices of the desired size and serve immediately.

Singaporean Chicken Wings
INGREDIENTS for Servings: 2

¾ teaspoon soy sauce	½ inch fresh ginger
¾ teaspoon Chinese rice wine	1 clove garlic, smashed
¾ teaspoon honey	Sliced scallions for serving
¼ teaspoon five-spice	
2 whole chicken wings	

DIRECTIONS and Cooking Time: 120 Minutes
Prepare your Sous Vide water bath using your immersion circulator, and raise the temperature to 160-degrees Fahrenheit   Add the soy sauce, rice wine, honey and five spice in a bowl and mix well Place the chicken wings, garlic, ginger in a zip bag Seal using the immersion method and cook for 120 minutes   Heat your broiler to high heat and line a broil-safe baking sheet with aluminum foil   Remove the wings and transfer to your broiling pan   Broil for 3-5 minutes   Then, arrange on a serving platter and sprinkle some sliced scallions over it   Serve!

Nutrition Info: Calories: 402 Carbohydrate: 11g
Protein: 21g Fat: 18g Sugar: 6g Sodium: 340mg

Sweet Spicy Chicken Drumsticks
INGREDIENTS for Servings: 3

½ tbsp sugar	½ cup soy sauce
2 ½ tsp ginger,	2 tbsp olive oil

chopped	2 tbsp sesame seeds to garnish
2 ½ tsp garlic, chopped	1 scallion, chopped to garnish
2 ½ tsp red chili puree	Salt and black pepper to taste
¼ lb small chicken drumsticks, skinless	

DIRECTIONS and Cooking Time: 2 Hours 20 Minutes
Make a water bath, place Sous Vide in it, and set to 165 F. Rub chicken with salt and pepper. Put chicken in a vacuum-sealable bag, release air by water displacement method and seal it.   Put the bag in the water bath and set the timer for 2 hours. Once the timer has stopped, remove and unseal the bag. In a bowl, mix the remaining listed ingredients except for olive oil. Set aside. Heat oil in a skillet over medium heat, add chicken.   Once they brown slightly on both sides, add the sauce and coat the chicken. Cook for 10 minutes. Garnish with sesame and scallions. Serve with a side of cauliflower rice.

Whole Chicken
INGREDIENTS

4-pound whole chicken, trussed	2 cups leeks, chopped
4 cups chicken broth	1 dried bay leaf
2 cups celery stalk, chopped	1 teaspoon kosher salt
2 cups carrots, peeled and chopped	1 teaspoon whole black peppercorns

DIRECTIONS and Cooking Time: 6 Hours Cooking Temperature: 150°f
Attach the sous vide immersion circulator to a Cambro container or pot with water using an adjustable clamp and preheat water to 150°F.   In a large cooking pouch, mix together all ingredients. Seal the pouch tightly after removing the excess air. Place pouch in sous vide bath and set the cooking time to 6 hours. Cover the sous vide bath with plastic wrap to minimize water evaporation.   Add water intermittently to properly maintain the water level. Preheat the oven broiler to high and line a baking sheet with a piece of foil.   After 6 hours, remove pouch from the sous vide bath and open carefully. Remove the chicken from pouch and pat dry chicken completely with paper towels.   Arrange chicken on the prepared baking sheet. Broil for 5-7 minutes. Remove from oven and allow to sit for 10 minutes. Cut into desired pieces and serve.

Coconut Chicken
INGREDIENTS for Servings: 2

2 chicken breasts	4 tablespoons satay sauce
4 tablespoons coconut milk	2 tablespoons coconut
Salt and pepper as	

| needed | milk |
| For Sauce | Dash of fish sauce |

DIRECTIONS and Cooking Time: 60 Minutes
Prepare your Sous Vide water bath using your immersion circulator, and raise the temperature to 140-degrees Fahrenheit   Add the chicken in a zip bag and add the salt, pepper and 4 tablespoons of milk   Seal using the immersion method and cook for 60 minutes   Once done, mix the sauce ingredients in a bowl and microwave for 30 seconds   Slice the chicken and arrange on serving platter   Pour the sauce on top!   Serve

Nutrition Info: Calories: 923 Carbohydrate: 51g Protein: 71g Fat: 50g Sugar: 3g Sodium: 216mg

Thyme Duck Breast

INGREDIENTS for Servings: 3

| 3 (6 oz) duck breast, skin on | 2 tsp olive oil |
| 3 tsp thyme leaves | Salt and black pepper to taste |

DIRECTIONS and Cooking Time: 2 Hours 10 Minutes
Make crosswise strips on the breasts and without cutting into the meat. Season the skin with salt and the meat side with thyme, pepper, and salt. Place the duck breasts in 3 separate vacuum-sealable bags. Release air and seal the bags. Refrigerate for 1 hour.   Make a water bath, place Sous Vide in it, and set to 135 F. Remove the bags from the refrigerator and submerge in the water bath. Set the timer for 1 hour.   Once the timer has stopped, remove and unseal the bags. Set a skillet over medium heat, add olive oil. Once it has heated, add duck and sear until skin renders and meat is golden brown. Remove and let sit for 3 minutes and then slice. Serve.

Herby Chicken With Butternut Squash Dish

INGREDIENTS for Servings: 2

6 chicken tenderloin	2 tbsp olive oil
4 cups butternut squash, cubed and roasted	4 tbsp red onion, chopped
4 cups rocket lettuce	1 tbsp paprika
4 tbsp sliced almonds	1 tbsp turmeric
Juice of 1 lemon	1 tbsp cumin
	Salt to taste

DIRECTIONS and Cooking Time: 1 Hour 15 Minutes
Prepare a water bath and place the Sous Vide in it. Set to 138 F.   Place the chicken and all seasonings in a vacuum-sealable bag. Release air by the water displacement method, seal and submerge in water bath. Cook for 60 minutes.   Once the timer has stopped, remove the bag and transfer the chicken to a hot skillet. Sear for 1 minute per side. In a bowl,

combine the remaining ingredients. Serve the chicken with the salad.

Chicken & Avocado Salad

INGREDIENTS for Servings: 2

1 chicken breast	1 tablespoon lemon juice
1 avocado, sliced	
10 pieces of halved cherry tomatoes	1 garlic clove, crushed
2 cups chopped lettuce	Salt and pepper as needed
2 tablespoons olive oil	2 teaspoons honey

DIRECTIONS and Cooking Time: 75 Minutes
Prepare your Sous Vide water bath, using your immersion circulator, and raise the temperature to 140-degrees Fahrenheit   Add the breast to a Sous Vide zip bag and seal using the immersion method, submerge and cook for 75 minutes   Season the breast with salt and pepper   Pan fry 1 tablespoon of olive oil for 30 seconds   Slice the breasts   Add the garlic, lemon juice, honey and olive oil in a small bowl   Add the lettuce, cherry tomatoes and avocado and toss   Top the salad with chicken and season with pepper and salt   Serve!

Nutrition Info: Calories: 520 Carbohydrate: 13g Protein: 68g Fat: 22g Sugar: 5g Sodium: 214mg

Citrus Chicken Breasts

INGREDIENTS for Servings: 2

1½ tbsp freshly squeezed orange juice	Salt to taste
	¾ tsp black pepper
1½ tbsp freshly squeezed lemon juice	2 chicken breasts, bone-in, skin on
1½ tbsp brown sugar	1 fennel, trimmed, sliced
1 tbsp Pernod	
1 tbsp olive oil	2 clementines, unpeeled and sliced
1 tbsp whole grain	
1 tsp celery seeds	Chopped dill

DIRECTIONS and Cooking Time: 3 Hours
Prepare a water bath and place the Sous Vide in it. Set to 146 F.   Combine in a bowl the lemon juice, orange juice, Pernod, olive oil, celery seeds, brown sugar, mustard, salt, and pepper. Mix well. Place the chicken breast, sliced clementine and sliced fennel in a vacuum-sealable bag. Add the orange mixture. Release air by the water displacement method, seal and submerge the bag in the water bath. Cook for 2 hours and 30 minutes. Once the timer has stopped, remove the bag and transfer the contents to a bowl. Drain the chicken and put the cooking juices in a heated saucepan.   Cook for about 5 minutes, until bubbly. Remove and place in the chicken. Cook for 6 minutes until brown. Serve the chicken on a platter and glaze with the sauce. Garnish with dill and fennel fronds.

Whole Turkey

INGREDIENTS

8-10 pound whole turkey, rinsed	64 ounces chicken broth
Olive oil, as required	2 fresh thyme sprigs
4 chicken breasts	Salt and freshly ground black pepper, to taste
4 fresh rosemary sprigs, divided	

DIRECTIONS and Cooking Time: 7 Hours 30 Minutes Cooking Temperature: 185°f & 168°f

Before use, remove neck and giblets from turkey, reserving the turkey neck. Cover turkey & refrigerate until use. Cut turkey neck and chicken breasts into pieces. In a large pan, heat a little oil over medium heat and sear turkey neck and chicken breasts until browned. Add 2 rosemary sprigs and the chicken broth and bring to a boil. Skim the foam from the surface of the mixture. Reduce heat to low and simmer for 1 hour. Using a strainer, strain the liquid from the pan into a bowl, discarding the turkey neck and chicken pieces. Refrigerate the broth to chill it completely. Attach the sous vide immersion circulator to a Cambro container or pot with water using an adjustable clamp and preheat water to 185°F. Season turkey evenly with salt and pepper then cover both legs and neck bones with aluminum foil pieces. Place turkey neck side down in a large cooking pouch. Place chilled broth and 2 thyme sprigs into the turkey cavity. Arrange 2 rosemary sprigs on the top side of the turkey. Seal pouch tightly after removing the excess air. Place pouch in sous vide bath and set the cooking time for 1 hour. After 1 hour, set sous vide bath temperature to 168°F and set the cooking time for 5 hours. Remove pouch from the sous vide bath and immediately plunge the pouch into a large bowl of ice water. Set aside for 30 minutes to cool. Preheat conventional oven to 350°F. Remove turkey from pouch, reserving cooking liquid in a pan. Transfer turkey to a roasting pan with a raised grill. Roast for 1½ hours. For gravy: place the pan of reserved cooking liquid over medium heat and simmer until desired thickness. Remove turkey from oven and allow to cool on cutting board for 15-20 minutes before carving. Cut turkey into pieces of the desired size and serve alongside gravy.

Chicken Cacciatore

INGREDIENTS for Servings: 4

4 boneless, skinless chicken breasts	2 sprigs fresh thyme
	1 bay leaf
½ can /14 ounces whole tomatoes, crushed	3 cloves garlic, minced
	1 teaspoon salt
	1 teaspoon pepper to
1 small onion, sliced	Cooked pasta for serving

1 red bell pepper, cut into strips	

DIRECTIONS and Cooking Time: 3 Hours

Preheat the water bath to 145°F. Combine chicken, tomatoes, onion, bell pepper, thyme, bay leaf, garlic, and salt and pepper in a bag. Seal using water method. Place in water bath and cook 3 hours.

Nutrition Info: Calories – 336 Total Fat –87 g Total Carb – 128 g Dietary fiber – 3 g Protein –542 g

Chicken Breast With Mushroom Sauce

INGREDIENTS

For Chicken:	1 teaspoon olive oil
2 boneless, skinless chicken breasts	2 tablespoons butter
	1 cup button mushrooms, sliced
⅛ teaspoon salt	
1 teaspoon vegetable oil	2 tablespoons port wine
For Mushroom Sauce:	½ cup chicken broth
3 French shallots, finely chopped	1 cup cream
	Salt, to taste
2 large garlic cloves, finely chopped	¼ teaspoon cracked black pepper

DIRECTIONS and Cooking Time: 4 Hours Cooking Temperature: 140°f

Attach the sous vide immersion circulator to a Cambro container or pot with water using an adjustable clamp and preheat water to 140°F. Season chicken breasts lightly with salt. Place chicken breasts in a large cooking pouch. Seal pouch tightly after removing the excess air. Place pouch in sous vide bath and set the cooking time for 1½-4 hours. For the mushroom sauce: heat olive oil in a skillet over medium heat and sauté shallots for 2-3 minutes. Stir in butter and garlic and sauté for 1 minute. Increase the heat to medium-high. Stir in mushrooms and cook until all liquid is absorbed. Add wine. Cook until all liquid is absorbed then add broth and cook for 2 minutes. Stir in cream and reduce heat back to medium. Once the sauce becomes thick, stir in the black pepper and desired amount of salt and remove from heat. Remove pouch from the sous vide bath and open carefully. Remove chicken breasts from pouch and pat dry chicken breasts completely with paper towels. Coat chicken breasts evenly with vegetable oil. Heat a grill pan over high heat and cook chicken breasts for 1 minute per side. Divide onto serving plates once cooked, top with mushroom sauce, and serve.

Chicken Saltimbocca

INGREDIENTS for Servings: 4

4 small chicken breasts, boneless,	8 sage leaves
	1 tablespoon extra-

skinless 4 pieces of thinly sliced prosciutto Freshly ground black pepper	virgin olive oil 2 oz. grated provolone

DIRECTIONS and Cooking Time: 90 Minutes
Prepare your Sous Vide water bath using your immersion circulator, and increase the temperature to 145-degrees Fahrenheit   Transfer the chicken breast to a very clean flat surface and season with pepper and salt   Top each of the chicken breast with sage leaves and 1 slice of prosciutto   Place them in a zip bag and seal using the immersion method and cook for 90 minutes   Once cooked, remove the chicken from the bag and pat dry   Add some oil in a large skillet over a medium-high heat   Put the chicken and prosciutto and sear for 1 minute   Give the chicken pieces a flip and top each of the pieces with 1 tablespoon of provolone   Cover the skillet with lid and cook for 30 seconds to allow the cheese to melt   Add the chicken on a serving platter and garnish with sage leaves   Serve!

Nutrition Info: Calories: 299 Carbohydrate: 5g Protein: 24g Fat: 20g Sugar: 0g Sodium: 403mg

Chicken Breast Meal

INGREDIENTS for Servings: 2

1-piece boneless chicken breast Salt and pepper as needed	Garlic powder as needed

DIRECTIONS and Cooking Time: 60 Minutes
Prepare your water bath using your Sous Vide immersion circulator, and increase the temperature to 150-degrees Fahrenheit   Carefully drain the chicken breast and pat dry using a kitchen towel   Season the breast with garlic powder, pepper and salt   Place in a resealable bag and seal using the immersion method   Submerge and cook for 1 hour   Serve!

Nutrition Info: Per serving:Calories: 150 ;Carbohydrate: 0g ;Protein: 18g ;Fat: 8g ;Sugar: 0g ;Sodium: 257mg

Easy Spicy-honey Chicken

INGREDIENTS for Servings: 4

8 tbsp butter 8 garlic cloves, chopped 6 tbsp chili sauce 1 tsp cumin 4 tbsp honey	Juice of 1 lime Salt and black pepper to taste 4 boneless, skinless chicken breasts

DIRECTIONS and Cooking Time: 1 Hour 45 Minutes
Prepare a water bath and place the Sous Vide in it. Set to 141 F.   Heat a saucepan over medium heat and put the butter, garlic, cumin, chili sauce, sugar, lime juice, and a pinch of salt and pepper. Cook for 5 minutes. Set aside and allow to cool.   Combine the chicken with salt and pepper and place it in 4 vacuum-sealable bag with the marinate. Release air by the water displacement method, seal and submerge the bags in the water bath. Cook for 1 hour and 30 minutes. Once the timer has stopped, remove the chicken and pat dry with kitchen towel. Reserve the half of cooking juices from each bag and transfer into a pot over medium heat. Cook until the sauce simmer, then put chicken inside and cook for 4 minutes. Remove the chicken and cut into slices. Serve with rice.

Chicken Tikka Masala

INGREDIENTS for Servings: 4

2 boneless skinless chicken breasts 1 tablespoon ground cumin 1 tablespoon paprika ½ tablespoon ground coriander 1 teaspoon ground turmeric ¼ teaspoon cayenne 4 cloves garlic, minced 2 tablespoons ginger, minced	½ small onion, minced 1 cup plain Greek yogurt Juice of 2 limes 2 tablespoons butter ½ can /14 ounces whole peeled tomatoes, crushed ½ cup heavy cream ½ cup cilantro leaves, chopped Cooked white rice and/or naan for serving

DIRECTIONS and Cooking Time: 4 Hours 30 Minutes
Preheat the water bath to 140°F.   Combine the cumin, paprika, coriander, turmeric, cayenne, garlic, ginger, onion, yogurt, and lime juice in a bag. Add chicken and seal using the water method. Place bag in the water bath and cook 4 hours.   Remove chicken from bag. Heat butter in a pan. Brown chicken on both sides. Add tomatoes and bring to a simmer, then stir in cream. Transfer to a bowl.   Garnish with cilantro and serve with rice and naan.

Nutrition Info: Calories – 393 Total Fat –287 g Total Carb – 128 g Dietary fiber – 6 g Protein –32 g

Crunchy Homemade Fried Chicken

INGREDIENTS for Servings: 8

½ tbsp dried basil 2¼ cups sour cream 8 chicken drumsticks Salt and white pepper to taste ½ cup vegetable oil	3 cups flour 2 tbsp garlic powder 1 ½ tbsp Cayenne red pepper powder 1 tbsp dried mustard

DIRECTIONS and Cooking Time: 3 Hours 20 Minutes
Prepare a water bath and place the Sous Vide in it. Set to 156 F. Season the chicken salt and place in a vacuum-sealable bag. Release air by the water

displacement method, seal and submerge in the water bath. Cook for 3 hours. Once the timer has stopped, remove the chicken and pat dry with kitchen towel. Combine salt, flour, garlic powder, white pepper, cayenne red pepper powder, mustard, white pepper, and basil in a bowl. Place sour cream in another bowl. Dip the chicken in the flour mixture, then in the sour cream and again in the flour mixture. Heat oil in a skillet over medium heat. Place in the drumsticks and cook for 3-4 minutes until crispy. Serve.

Chicken With White Wine & Lemon Sauce

INGREDIENTS

2 chicken breasts	¼ cup Madeira wine
Salt and freshly ground black pepper, to taste	¼ cup chicken broth
	1 teaspoon mustard
1 lemon, sliced	Chopped fresh parsley, for garnishing
Butter, as required	

DIRECTIONS and Cooking Time: 1 Hour 10 Minutes
Cooking Temperature: 140°f
Attach the sous vide immersion circulator to a Cambro container or pot with water using an adjustable clamp and preheat water to 140°F. Season chicken breasts evenly with salt and black pepper. Place chicken breasts in a cooking pouch with 1-2 lemon slices. Seal pouch tightly after removing the excess air. Place pouch in sous vide bath and set the cooking time for 1 hour. Remove the pouch from the sous vide bath and open carefully, removing chicken wings from pouch. In a medium skillet, melt butter and sear the chicken breasts for 2-3 minutes or until browned on both sides. Transfer chicken to a plate and set aside. Squeeze the juice from ½ of the lemon into the skillet used to sear the chicken breast. Add wine and scrape browned bits from the bottom of the skillet. Cook until wine is reduced by half. Add chicken broth and mustard and cook until sauce reaches desired thickness. Stir in salt and black pepper and remove from heat. Cut chicken breasts into desired slices and divide onto serving plates. Top evenly with the lemon sauce. Garnish with parsley and serve.

Bbq Chicken Breasts

INGREDIENTS

For BBQ Sauce:	¼ cup molasses
3 dried ancho chile peppers, stemmed and seeded	1 tablespoon sea salt
	2 teaspoons ground black pepper
1 dried New Mexico chile pepper, stemmed and seeded	1 teaspoon fresh lemon zest, grated
¼ cup sunflower oil	¼ cup fresh lemon juice
1 small yellow onion,	¼ cup fresh lime juice,
chopped	divided
2 garlic cloves, minced	1 teaspoon fresh lime zest, grated
4½ ounces tomato paste	For Chicken:
½ cup apple cider vinegar	4 skin-on, bone-in chicken breasts
¼ cup brown sugar	Sea salt and freshly ground black pepper, to taste
3 tablespoons cocoa powder	
1½ teaspoons ground cumin	For Garnishing:
	1 orange, cut into 8 wedges
1 teaspoon ground coriander	Fresh cilantro, chopped

DIRECTIONS and Cooking Time: 2 Hours 30 Minutes
Cooking Temperature: 165°f
In a heatproof bowl, add both types of chile peppers. Add enough hot water to cover and set aside for 15 minutes. Drain chile peppers, reserving ½ cup of the soaking water. In a blender, add chile peppers and reserved soaking water and pulse until a smooth paste is formed. Heat oil in a medium pan over medium heat. Add and sauté onion and garlic for 10 minutes. Add chile paste and remaining BBQ sauce ingredients except for 2 tablespoons of lime juice and the lime zest and bring to a boil. Reduce heat to low and simmer for 20-30 minutes. Remove from heat and set aside to cool completely. Stir in remaining lime juice and lime zest. Transfer to a container and refrigerate before using. Attach the sous vide immersion circulator to a Cambro container or pot with water using an adjustable clamp and preheat water to 165°F. Season chicken breasts evenly with salt and black pepper. Divide the chicken breasts into two large pouches. Seal pouches tightly after removing the excess air. Place pouches in sous vide bath and set the cooking time for 2½ hours. Preheat grill to high heat. Grease grill grate. Remove pouches from the sous vide bath and open carefully. Remove chicken breasts and coat each breast with BBQ sauce. Grill chicken breasts for 1 minute per side. Serve with orange wedges and cilantro.

Savory Lettuce Wraps With Ginger-chili Chicken

INGREDIENTS for Servings: 5

½ cup hoisin sauce	Juice of 1 lime
½ cup sweet chili sauce	4 chicken breasts, cubed
3 tbsp soy sauce	Salt and black pepper to taste
2 tbsp grated ginger	
2 tbsp ground ginger	12 lettuce leaves, rinsed
1 tbsp brown sugar	⅛ cup poppy seeds
2 garlic cloves, minced	4 chives

DIRECTIONS and Cooking Time: 1 Hour 45 Minutes

Prepare a water bath and place Sous Vide in it. Set to 141 F. Combine chili sauce, ginger, soy sauce, brown sugar, garlic, and half of lime juice. Heat a saucepan over medium heat and pour in the mixture. Cook for 5 minutes. Set aside. Season the breasts with salt and pepper. Place them in an even layer in a vacuum-sealable bag with the chili sauce mixture. Release air by the water displacement method, seal and submerge the bag in the water bath. Cook for 1 hour and 30 minutes. Once the timer has stopped, remove the chicken and pat dry with kitchen towel. Discard cooking juices. Combine the hoisin sauce with the chicken cubes and mix well. Make piles of 6 lettuce leaves. Share chicken among lettuce leaves and top with the poppy seeds and chives before wrapping.

Classic Chicken Cordon Bleu

INGREDIENTS for Servings: 4

½ cup butter	4 garlic cloves, minced
4 boneless, skinless chicken breasts	8 slices ham
	8 slices Emmental cheese
Salt and black pepper to taste	
1 tsp cayenne pepper	

DIRECTIONS and Cooking Time: 1 Hour 50 Minutes + Cooling Time
Prepare a water bath and place the Sous Vide in it. Set to 141 F. Season the chicken with salt and pepper. Cover with plastic wrap and rolled. Set aside and allow to chill. Heat a saucepan over medium heat and add some black pepper, cayenne pepper, 1/4 cup of butter, and garlic. Cook until the butter melts. Transfer to a bowl. Rub the chicken on one side with the butter mixture. Then place 2 slices of ham and 2 slices of cheese and cover it. Roll each breast with plastic wrap and transfer to the fridge for 2-3 hours or in the freezer for 20-30 minutes. Place the breast in two vacuum-sealable bags. Release air by the water displacement method, seal and submerge the bags in the water bath. Cook for 1 hour and 30 minutes. Once the timer has stopped, remove the breasts and take off the plastic. Heat the remaining butter in a skillet over medium heat and sear the chicken for 1-2 minutes per side.

Chessy Rolled Chicken

INGREDIENTS for Servings: 2

1 chicken breast	¼ cup cream cheese
¼ cup julienned roasted red pepper	6 slices prosciutto
½ cup loosely packed arugula	Salt and black pepper to taste
	1 tbsp oil

DIRECTIONS and Cooking Time: 1 Hour 45 Minutes
Prepare a water bath and place Sous Vide in it. Set to 155 F. Drain the chicken and beat it until getting tiny

thicks. Then cut by half and season with salt and pepper. Spread 2 tbsp of cream cheese and add roasted red pepper and arugula on top. Roll the breasts like sushi and put 3 layers of prosciutto and roll the breasts. Place in a vacuum-sealable bag. Release air by the water displacement method, seal and submerge in water bath. Cook for 90 minutes. Once the timer has stopped, remove the chicken from the bag and sear. Slice tiny and serve.

Chicken Stew With Mushrooms

INGREDIENTS for Servings: 2

2 medium-sized chicken thighs, skinless	1 small carrot, chopped
	1 small onion, chopped
½ cup fire-roasted tomatoes, diced	1 tbsp fresh basil, finely chopped
½ cup chicken stock	
1 tbsp tomato paste	1 garlic clove, crushed
½ cup button mushrooms, chopped	Salt and black pepper to taste
1 medium-sized celery stalk	

DIRECTIONS and Cooking Time: 1 Hour 5 Minutes
Make a water bath, place Sous Vide in it, and set to 129 F. Rub the thighs with salt and pepper. Set aside. Chop the celery stalk into half-inch long pieces. Now, place the meat in a large vacuum-sealable bag along with onion, carrot, mushrooms, celery stalk, and fire roasted tomatoes. Submerge the sealed bag in the water bath and set the timer for 45 minutes. Once the timer has stopped, remove the bag from the water bath and open it. The meat should be falling off the bone easily, so remove the bones. Heat up some oil in a medium-sized saucepan and add garlic. Briefly fry for about 3 minutes, stirring constantly. Add the contents of the bag, chicken stock, and tomato paste. Bring it to a boil and reduce the heat to medium. Cook for 5 more minutes, stirring occasionally. Serve sprinkled with the basil.

Chicken Thighs With Mustard Wine Sauce

INGREDIENTS

4 bone-in, skin-on chicken thighs	1 cup dry white wine
Kosher salt and freshly ground black pepper, to taste	1 tablespoon whole-grain mustard
	2 tablespoons unsalted butter
4 thyme or rosemary sprigs	1 tablespoon fresh parsley leaves, minced
1 tablespoon canola oil	½ teaspoon fresh lemon juice
1 small shallot, minced	

DIRECTIONS and Cooking Time: 4 Hours Cooking Temperature: 165°f

Attach the sous vide immersion circulator to a Cambro container or pot with water using an adjustable clamp and preheat water to 165°F. Season chicken generously with salt and pepper. Place chicken and herbs sprigs in a cooking pouch. Seal pouch tightly after removing the excess air. Place pouch in sous vide bath and set the cooking time for 1-4 hours. Remove pouch from the sous vide bath and open carefully. Take out the chicken thighs, reserving the cooking liquid, and pat dry the chicken thighs with paper towels. Arrange chicken thighs on a cutting board, skin side down. With your hands, press down firmly on each thigh to flatten the skin against the board. In a non-stick skillet, heat oil over medium heat. Place chicken skin side down and cook for 8 minutes. Flip chicken and cook for another 2 minutes then transfer to a paper towel-lined plate. In the same skillet, add the shallot over medium-high heat and sauté for 30 seconds. Add wine and cook for another 2 minutes. Stir in reserved cooking liquid and mustard then remove the skillet from heat. Immediately add butter, parsley, lemon juice, salt, and black pepper and beat until well combined. Serve the chicken with the wine sauce.

Artichoke Stuffed Chicken

INGREDIENTS for Servings: 6

2 pounds chicken breast fillets, butterfly cut	8 garlic cloves, crushed
½ cup chopped baby spinach	Salt and white pepper to taste
10 artichoke hearts	4 tbsp olive oil

DIRECTIONS and Cooking Time: 3hours 15 Minutes

Combine artichoke, pepper, and garlic in a food processor. Blend until completely smooth. Pulse again and gradually add oil until well incorporated. Stuff each breast with equal amounts of artichoke mixture and chopped baby spinach. Fold the breast fillet back together and secure the edge with a wooden skewer. Season with salt and white pepper and transfer to a separate vacuum-sealable bags. Seal the bags and cook en Sous Vide for 3 hours at 149 F.

Turkey Breast With Cloves

INGREDIENTS for Servings: 6

2 pounds turkey breast, sliced	2 tbsp lemon juice
2 garlic cloves, minced	1 tsp fresh rosemary, finely chopped
1 cup olive oil	1 tsp cloves, minced
2 tbsp Dijon mustard	Salt and black pepper to taste

DIRECTIONS and Cooking Time: 1 Hour 45 Minutes

In a large bowl, combine olive oil, with mustard, lemon juice, garlic, rosemary, cloves, salt, and pepper. Mix until well incorporated and add turkey slices. Soak and refrigerate for 30 minutes before cooking. Remove from the refrigerator and transfer to 2 vacuum-sealable bags. Seal the bags and cook en Sous Vide for one hour at 149 F. Remove from the water bath and serve.

Lemon Chicken With Mint

INGREDIENTS for Servings: 3

1 pound chicken thighs, boneless and skinless	¼ cup oil
	1 tsp ginger
	½ tsp cayenne pepper
1 tbsp freshly squeezed lemon juice	1 tsp fresh mint, finely chopped
2 garlic cloves, crushed	½ tsp salt

DIRECTIONS and Cooking Time: 2 Hours 40 Minutes

In a small bowl, combine olive oil with lemon juice, garlic, ground ginger, mint, cayenne pepper, and salt. Generously brush each thigh with this mixture and refrigerate for at least 30 minutes. Remove thighs from the refrigerator. Place in a large vacuum-sealable bag and cook for 2 hours at 149 F. Remove from the vacuum-sealable bag and serve immediately with spring onions.

Lemon Grass Chicken Dish

INGREDIENTS for Servings: 3

1 lb. chicken breast	2 tablespoons coconut sugar
1 stalk of fresh lemon grass, chopped	½ teaspoon salt
2 tablespoons fish sauce	1 tablespoon chili garlic sauce

DIRECTIONS and Cooking Time: 45 Minutes

Prepare your water bath using your Sous Vide immersion circulator and raise the temperature to 150-degrees Fahrenheit   Cut the chicken into bite size portions and put them in a bowl   Chop the lemon grass and place in a blender   Add the fish sauce, sugar, and salt and blend well   Pour the marinade over your chicken and mix well   Insert skewers into the chicken   Keep repeating until all the chicken has been used   Place the skewered chicken in a heavy-duty, resealable bag, seal them using the immersion method and submerge and cook for 45 minutes   Remove the bag transfer it to a water bath to chill   Remove the chicken from the bag and slice it up even more if you prefer   Brush with chili-garlic sauce   Sear the chicken on a skillet over medium heat and then serve

Nutrition Info:Per serving:Calories: 304 ;Carbohydrate: 34g ;Protein: 22g ;Fat: 9g ;Sugar: 7g ;Sodium: 529mg

Cheesy Chicken Balls

INGREDIENTS for Servings: 6

1 pound ground chicken	32 small, diced cubes of mozzarella cheese
2 tbsp onion, finely chopped	1 tbsp butter
¼ tsp garlic powder	3 tbsp panko
Salt and black pepper to taste	½ cup tomato sauce
2 tbsp breadcrumbs	½ oz grated Pecorino Romano cheese
1 egg	Chopped parsley

DIRECTIONS and Cooking Time: 1 Hour 15 Minutes
Prepare a water bath and place the Sous Vide in it. Set to 146 F. In a bowl, mix the chicken, onion, salt, garlic powder, pepper, and seasoned breadcrumbs. Add in egg and combine well. Form 32 medium-size balls and fill with a cube of cheese, make sure the mix covers the cheese well. Place the balls in a vacuum-sealable bag and let chill for 20 minutes. Then, release air by the water displacement method, seal and submerge the bag in the water bath. Cook for 45 minutes. Once the timer has stopped, remove the balls. Melt butter in a skillet over high heat and add panko. Cook until toast. As well cook the tomato sauce. In a serving dish, place the balls and glaze with the tomato sauce. Top with the panko and cheese. Garnish with parsley.

Chicken Thighs With Garlic Mustard Sauce

INGREDIENTS

1½ pound skin-on chicken thighs	1 teaspoon champagne or white wine vinegar
Salt and freshly ground black pepper, to taste	1 large garlic clove, mashed into a paste
2 tablespoons canola oil	1 teaspoon whole-grain Dijon mustard
1 tablespoon butter	

DIRECTIONS and Cooking Time: 4 Hours 10 Minutes
Cooking Temperature: 165°f
Attach the sous vide immersion circulator to a Cambro container or pot with water using an adjustable clamp and preheat water to 165°F. Season chicken generously with salt and pepper. Place chicken in a cooking pouch and seal pouch tightly after removing the excess air. Place pouch in sous vide bath and set the cooking time for 1-4 hours. Remove pouch from the sous vide bath and open carefully. Transfer chicken to a plate, reserving the cooking liquid from the pouch. In a large non-stick skillet, heat oil over high heat. Place chicken skin side down and cook for

2-3 minutes. Transfer chicken to a plate and set aside. Wipe out skillet with paper towels then melt butter over low heat. Add reserved cooking liquid and remaining ingredients and simmer until sauce becomes thick. Place sauce over chicken and serve.

Chicken Parmesan Balls

INGREDIENTS for Servings: 6

1 lb. ground chicken	32 small, diced cubes of mozzarella cheese
2 tablespoons onion, finely chopped	1 tablespoon butter
¼ teaspoon garlic powder	3 tablespoons panko
Salt and pepper as needed	½ cup tomato sauce
2 tablespoons seasoned breadcrumbs	½ oz. grated parmesan cheese
1 egg	Chopped parsley for garnishing

DIRECTIONS and Cooking Time: 45 Minutes
Prepare your Sous Vide water bath using your immersion circulator, and raise the temperature to 145-degrees Fahrenheit Mix the chicken with onion, salt, garlic powder, pepper and seasoned bread crumbs in a bowl Add the egg and mix well Scoop out 32 balls Top each ball with 1 cube of cheese and press the meat around the cheese Put the balls in a zip bag and chill for 20 minutes Seal the bag using the immersion method and cook for 45 minutes Remove the balls from the bag Melt butter over a medium-high heat and add the panko Cook until golden brown. Warm the tomato sauce Transfer the balls in a serving dish and top with tomato sauce, panko and cheese Garnish with chopped parsley and serve by piercing them with a toothpick

Nutrition Info:Calories: 277 Carbohydrate: 15g Protein: 16g Fat: 17g Sugar: 2g Sodium: 414mg

Easiest No-sear Chicken Breast

INGREDIENTS for Servings: 3

1 lb chicken breasts, boneless	Salt and black pepper to taste
1 tsp garlic powder	

DIRECTIONS and Cooking Time: 75 Minutes
Make a water bath, place Sous Vide in it, and set it to 150 F. Pat dry the chicken breasts and season with salt, garlic powder, and pepper. Put the chicken in a vacuum-sealable bag, release air by the water displacement method and seal it. Place in the water and set the timer to cook for 1 hour. Once the timer has stopped, remove and unseal the bag. Remove the chicken and let chill for later use.

Whole Chicken(1)

INGREDIENTS for Servings: 6

1 medium whole chicken 3 garlic cloves 3 ounces chopped celery stalk	3 tbsp mustard Salt and black pepper to taste 1 tbsp butter

DIRECTIONS and Cooking Time: 6 Hours 40 Minutes
Prepare a water bath and place the Sous Vide in it. Set to 150 F. Combine all the ingredients in a vacuum-sealable bag.Release air by the water displacement method, seal and submerge the bag in bath.Set the timer for 6 hours and 30 minutes. Once done, leave chicken to cool lightly before carving.

Sticky Duck Wings

INGREDIENTS for Servings: 6

3lb. duck wings 1 tablespoon mustard ½ cup honey 1 tablespoon soy sauce 1 tablespoon hot sauce	¼ cup ketchup 2 tablespoons Cajun spice blend ¼ cup butter Salt and pepper, to taste

DIRECTIONS and Cooking Time: 2 Hours
Preheat Sous Vide cooker to 150F.   Cut the wings into portions and rub with Cajun blend. Season with some salt and pepper.   Transfer the wings into cooking bags and add butter.   Vacuum seal the wings and submerge in water.   Cook the wings 2 hours. Finishing steps: Preheat your broiler.   Combine remaining ingredients in a bowl.   Remove the wings from the cooker and toss with prepared sauce. Arrange the wings on baking sheet and broil 10 minutes, basting with any remaining sauce during that time.   Serve warm.

Nutrition Info: Calories 305 Total Fat 11g Total Carb 27g Dietary Fiber 7g Protein 18g

Honey Garlic Chicken Wings

INGREDIENTS

For Sauce: 1 ½-inch piece fresh ginger, chopped 3 garlic cloves, chopped 2 tablespoons honey Salt and freshly ground black pepper, to taste	1 tablespoon soy sauce For Wings: 40 split chicken wings Salt and freshly ground black pepper, to taste

DIRECTIONS and Cooking Time: 4 Hours 15 Minutes
Cooking Temperature: 160°f

Attach the sous vide immersion circulator to a Cambro container or pot with water using an adjustable clamp and preheat water to 160°F.   For sauce: in a bowl, add all sauce ingredients and mix until well combined. Reserve 1 tablespoon of sauce in a separate bowl. Season chicken wings lightly with salt and black pepper.   Place chicken wings and all but the 1 tablespoon reserved sauce into a cooking pouch. Seal pouch tightly after removing the excess air. Place pouch in sous vide bath and set the cooking time for 4 hours.   Preheat the oven broiler to high. Line a baking sheet with parchment paper.   Remove pouch from the sous vide bath and open carefully, removing chicken wings from pouch.   Arrange chicken wings onto prepared baking sheet in a single layer. Broil for 10-15 minutes, flipping once halfway through the cooking time.   Remove from oven and transfer into bowl of reserved sauce. Toss to coat well and serve immediately.

Honey Dredged Duck Breast

INGREDIENTS for Servings: 3

1 x 6 oz. boneless duck breast ¼ teaspoon cinnamon ¼ teaspoon smoked paprika	¼ teaspoon cayenne pepper 1 teaspoon honey Salt and pepper as needed

DIRECTIONS and Cooking Time: 3½ Hours
Prepare your water bath using your Sous Vide immersion circulator and raise the temperature to 134.9-degrees Fahrenheit   Remove the duck breast from the packaging and pat dry using a kitchen towel   Score the skin of the duck breast using a crosshatch pattern - do not cut the flesh, sprinkle some salt over   Take a medium sized frying pan/skillet and place it on your stove over medium-high heat   Put the breast in the pan and cook for 3-4 minutes, making sure the skin side is facing down   Remove the breast from your pan and set it on a surface   Add the paprika, cayenne pepper and cinnamon in a small bowl and mix everything well   Spread the mixture over the duck breast and season, add some additional salt and pepper   Now put the breast in a heavy-duty, resealable bag with a teaspoon of honey and seal the bag using the immersion method and submerge it underwater   Cook for about 3½ hours and take it out once done   Pat dry and place in a frying pan over high heat to sear for about 2 minutes, make sure you keep the skin side facing down   Flip it and sear for another 30 seconds, allow to rest and serve!

Nutrition Info: Per serving:Calories: 304 ;Carbohydrate: 25g ;Protein: 18g ;Fat: 15g ;Sugar: 19g ;Sodium: 612mg

Waldorf Chicken Salad

INGREDIENTS for Servings: 4

2 skinless chicken breasts, boneless ½ teaspoon ground black pepper 1 tablespoon corn oil 1 Granny Smith apple, cored and diced 1 teaspoon lime juice ½ cup red grapes, cut in half 1 stick rib celery, diced	1/3 cup mayonnaise 2 teaspoons Chardonnay wine 1 teaspoon Dijon mustard 1 tablespoon kosher salt 1 Romaine lettuce head ½ cup walnuts, toasted and chopped

DIRECTIONS and Cooking Time: 120 Minutes
Prepare your water bath using your Sous Vide immersion circulator, and increase the temperature to 145-degrees Fahrenheit   Take the chicken and season it with black pepper and salt. Put the seasoned chicken breast and corn oil in a large, resealable bag and seal using the immersion method   Cook for 2 hours and then remove the bag   Put the apple slices in a large-sized bowl, add the lime juice, and toss them well.   Add the celery and red grapes and stir well   Put the mayonnaise, Dijon mustard, and Chardonnay wine in a small bowl and mix well   Pour the whole mixture over the fruits and give them a nice toss   Remove the chicken breast from the plastic bag and discard the liquid   Dice the breast and place in a medium-sized bowl   Add some kosher salt and toss well   Put the seasoned chicken in with the rest of the salad and toss well   Dived your romaine lettuce amongst the salad bowls, spoon the salad on top of the lettuce, and garnish with some walnuts   Serve!

Nutrition Info:Per serving:Calories: 304 ;Carbohydrate: 34g ;Protein: 22g ;Fat: 9g ;Sugar: 7g ;Sodium: 529mg

Vegetable Chicken With Soy Sauce
INGREDIENTS for Servings: 4

1 whole bone-in chicken, trussed 1-quart low sodium chicken stock 2 tbsp soy sauce 5 sprigs fresh sage	2 dried bay leaves 2 cups sliced carrots 2 cups sliced celery ½ oz dried mushrooms 3 tbsp butter

DIRECTIONS and Cooking Time: 6 Hours 25 Minutes
Prepare a water bath and place the Sous Vide in it. Set to 149 F.   Combine the soy sauce, chicken stock, herbs, veggies, and chicken. Place in a vacuum-sealable bag. Release air by the water displacement method, seal and submerge the bag in the water bath. Cook for 6 hours.   Once the timer has stopped, remove the chicken and drain the veggies. Dry with a baking sheet. Season with olive oil, salt and pepper. Heat the oven to 450 F. and roast for 10 minutes. In a saucepan, stir the cooking juices. Remove from the heat and mix with butter. Slice the chicken without the

skin and season with kosher salt and ground black pepper. Serve in a platter. Top with the sauce.

Chicken Tikka
INGREDIENTS

4 boneless, skinless chicken breasts Salt and freshly ground black pepper, to taste 2 tablespoons butter 2 cups half-and-half 2 cups canned crushed tomatoes 4 garlic cloves, peeled 1 (1-inch) piece fresh ginger, cut into chunks	1½ tablespoons honey 1 tablespoon ground turmeric 1 tablespoon paprika 1 tablespoon ground cumin 2 teaspoons ground coriander ½ teaspoons salt 2 cups cooked rice Chopped fresh cilantro, for garnishing

DIRECTIONS and Cooking Time: 2 Hours Cooking Temperature: 146°f
Attach the sous vide immersion circulator to a Cambro container or pot with water using an adjustable clamp and preheat water to 146°F.   Season chicken breasts evenly with salt and black pepper.   In a food processor, add half-and-half, tomatoes, garlic, ginger, honey, and spices and pulse until smooth.   Divide chicken and butter into two cooking pouches with two chicken breasts and one tablespoon butter in each pouch. Add mixture from food processor into a third, large pouch. Seal pouches tightly after removing the excess air. Place all pouches in the sous vide bath and set the cooking time for 2 hours.   Remove the pouches from the sous vide bath and open carefully. Remove chicken breasts from pouches and cut into slices of the desired size.   Divide cooked rice onto serving plates. Top with chicken slices and drizzle with sauce. Garnish with cilantro and serve.

Crispy Chicken Bacon Wrap
INGREDIENTS for Servings: 2

1 chicken breast 2 strips pancetta 2 tbsp Dijon mustard	1 tbsp grated Pecorino Romano cheese

DIRECTIONS and Cooking Time: 3 Hours 15 Minutes
Prepare a water bath and place the Sous Vide in it. Set to 146 F. Combine the chicken with salt. Marinade with Dijon mustard on both sides. Top with Pecorino Romano Cheese and wrap the pancetta around the chicken.   Place in a vacuum-sealable bag. Release air by the water displacement method, seal and submerge the bag in the water bath. Cook for 3 hours. Once the timer has stopped, remove the chicken and pat dry. Heat a skillet over medium heat and sear until crispy.

Bacon Wrapped Chicken

INGREDIENTS for Servings: 2

2 chicken breasts 2 strips bacon 2 tablespoons Dijon mustard	1 tablespoon grated parmesan cheese ½ teaspoon salt

DIRECTIONS and Cooking Time: 3 Hours

Prepare your water bath using your Sous Vide immersion circulator, and raise the temperature to 145-degrees Fahrenheit   Season the chicken with salt and spread Dijon mustard on both sides   Sprinkle with parmesan cheese   Wrap the bacon around the chicken breast and place in a zip bag   Cook for 3 hours   Remove the chicken and pat dry   Sear until crispy   Serve!

Nutrition Info: Calories: 284 Carbohydrate: 5g Protein: 18g Fat: 21g Sugar: 2g Sodium: 563mg

Honey Flavored Chicken Wings

INGREDIENTS for Servings: 2

¾ tsp soy sauce ¾ tsp rice wine ¾ tsp honey ¼ tsp five-spice 6 chicken wings ½ inch fresh ginger	½ inch ground mace 1 clove garlic, minced Sliced scallions for serving

DIRECTIONS and Cooking Time: 135 Minutes

Prepare a water bath and place the Sous Vide in it. Set to 160 F.   In a bowl, combine the soy sauce, rice wine, honey, and five-spice. Place the chicken wings and garlic in a vacuum-sealable bag. Release air by the water displacement method, seal and submerge the bag in the water bath. Cook for 2 hours.   Once the timer has stopped, remove the wings and transfer to a baking tray. Bake in the oven for 5 minutes at 380 F. Serve on a platter and garnish with sliced scallions.

Pepper Chicken Salad

INGREDIENTS for Servings: 4

4 chicken breasts, boneless and skinless ¼ cup vegetable oil plus three tbsp for salad 1 medium-sized onion, peeled and finely chopped	6 cherry tomatoes, halved Salt and black pepper to taste 1 cup lettuce, finely chopped 2 tbsp of freshly squeezed lemon juice

DIRECTIONS and Cooking Time: 1 Hour 15 Minutes

Make a water bath, place Sous Vide in it, and set to 149 F.   Thoroughly rinse the meat under the cold water and pat dry using a kitchen paper. Cut the meat into bite-sized pieces and place in a vacuum-sealable bag along with ¼ cup of oil and seal. Submerge the bag in the water bath. Once the timer has stopped, remove the chicken from the bag, pat dry and chill to a room temperature.   In a large bowl mix the onion, tomatoes, and lettuce. Finally, add the chicken breasts and season with three tablespoons of oil, lemon juice, and some salt to taste. Top with Greek yogurt and olives. However, it's optional. Serve cold.

Buffalo Chicken Wings

INGREDIENTS for Servings: 6

3 lb chicken wings 3 tsp salt 2 tsp grounded garlic 2 tbsp smoked paprika 1 tsp sugar	½ cup hot sauce 5 tbsp butter 2 ½ cups almond flour Olive oil for frying

DIRECTIONS and Cooking Time: 1 Hour And 20 Minutes

Make a water bath, place Sous Vide in it, and set to 144 F.   Combine the wings, garlic, salt, sugar and smoked paprika. Coat the chicken evenly. Place in a sizable vacuum-sealable bag, release air by the water displacement method and seal the bag.   Submerge in the water. Set the timer to cook for 1 hour. Once the timer has stopped, remove and unseal the bag. Pour flour into a large bowl, add in chicken and toss to coat. Heat oil in a pan over medium heat, fry the chicken until golden brown. Remove and set aside. In another pan, melt butter and add the hot sauce. Coat the wings with butter and hot sauce. Serve as an appetizer

Avocado Chicken Salad

INGREDIENTS for Servings: 2

1 boneless, skinless chicken breast 1 ripe but firm avocado, cut into ½-inch cubes 1 celery stalk, finely diced Juice of 1 lime ½ tablespoon fresh chives, minced ½ tablespoon fresh parsley, minced	¼ cup red onion, finely diced 2 tablespoons plain Greek yogurt 1 tablespoon mayonnaise, or more to taste 1 teaspoon salt 1 teaspoon pepper Bread or crackers for serving

DIRECTIONS and Cooking Time: 2 Hours

Preheat the water bath to 150°F.   Season chicken with salt and pepper. Seal into a bag. Place in water bath and cook 2 hours. Place in refrigerator and cool completely.   When chicken is cool, cut into ½-inch cubes. Toss with avocado, celery, lime juice, chive, parsley, onion, mayonnaise, yogurt, and salt and pepper to taste. Serve with bread or crackers.

Nutrition Info: Calories 375 Total Fat 242g Total Carb 179g Dietary Fiber 6g Protein 267g

Dill & Rosemary Turkey Breast

INGREDIENTS for Servings: 2

1 pound boneless turkey breasts Salt and black pepper to taste	3 fresh dill sprigs 1 fresh rosemary sprig, chopped 1 bay leaf

DIRECTIONS and Cooking Time: 1 Hour 50 Minutes
Prepare a water bath and place the Sous Vide in it. Set to 146 F. Heat a skillet over medium heat, Put the turkey and sear for 5 minutes. Reserve the fat. Season the turkey with salt and pepper. Place the turkey, dill, rosemary, bay leaf and reserved fat in a vacuum-sealable bag. Release air by the water displacement method, seal and submerge the bag in the water bath. Cook for 1 hour and 30 minutes. Heat a skillet over high heat. Once the timer has stopped, remove the turkey and transfer into the skillet. Sear for 5 minutes.

Hawaiian Chicken

INGREDIENTS

For Glaze:	For Chicken:
2 cups chicken broth 1½ cups soy sauce ¾ cup light brown sugar ½ cup plus 1 tablespoon water, divided ½ cup mirin 1 tablespoon fish sauce 3 tablespoons cornstarch 1 tablespoon water	6 pounds boneless, skinless chicken thighs 1 (3-inch) piece fresh ginger, peeled and cut into three pieces 6 large garlic cloves, minced For Garnishing: 1 cup scallions, thinly sliced

DIRECTIONS and Cooking Time: 3 Hours 5 Minutes
Cooking Temperature: 147°f
Attach the sous vide immersion circulator to a Cambro container or pot with water using an adjustable clamp and preheat water to 147°F. In a large bowl, add chicken broth, soy sauce, brown sugar, ½ cup water,

mirin, and fish sauce and beat until well combined for the glaze. Divide the glaze, chicken, ginger, and garlic into three cooking pouches. Seal the pouches tightly after removing the excess air. Place pouches in sous vide bath and set the cooking time for 3 hours. Remove the pouches from the sous vide bath and open carefully. Strain half of the cooking liquid into a pan. Transfer all chicken into a new cooking pouch and seal it. Return pouch to sous vide bath with the sous vide turned off. Place pan of reserved cooking liquid on stove and bring to a boil. In a small bowl, dissolve cornstarch into 1 tablespoon of water. Add the cornstarch mixture to the cooking liquid, stirring continuously. Cook until the glaze becomes thick. Place chicken on a platter and top with glaze. Garnish with scallions and serve.

Spicy Adobo Chicken

INGREDIENTS for Servings: 2

2 chicken leg quarters 2 garlic cloves, crushed ¼ teaspoon whole black peppercorns ½ tablespoon molasses ¼ cup dark soy sauce	Salt as needed 1 tablespoon canola oil ½ Worcestershire sauce 1 bay leaf ¼ cup white vinegar

DIRECTIONS and Cooking Time: 120 Minutes
Mix the soy sauce, Worcestershire, peppercorns, molasses, garlic, bay leaf and salt. Add the chicken legs in a Sous Vide bag with the marinade and refrigerate for 12 hours or overnight. Prepare your Sous Vide water bath, using your immersion circulator, and raise the temperature to 165-degrees Fahrenheit Submerge the chicken and cook for 2 hours Remove the chicken legs from the bag and air dry for 10-15 minutes. Sear over medium heat in a nonstick pan with canola oil Add the sauce from the bag to the pan and keep cooking until you have reached the desired consistency Serve the chicken with sauce!

Nutrition Info: Calories: 320 Carbohydrate: 33g Protein: 16g Fat: 14g Sugar: 3g Sodium: 255mg

BEEF,PORK & LAMB RECIPES

Bbq Ribs With Spiced Rub
INGREDIENTS

1 tablespoon dried oregano, crushed	1 tablespoon kosher salt
1 tablespoon ground cumin	1 tablespoon freshly ground black pepper
1 tablespoon paprika	2 pork rib racks, trimmed and each cut into 3-4 bone sections
1 tablespoon red chili powder	2 cups barbecue sauce (of your choice)
1 tablespoon onion powder	
1 tablespoon garlic powder	

DIRECTIONS and Cooking Time: 48 Hours Cooking Temperature: 138°f

Attach the sous vide immersion circulator to a Cambro container or pot with water using an adjustable clamp and preheat water to 138°F. In a bowl, mix together oregano, spices, salt, and black pepper. Rub ribs with spice mixture. Place each rib section into a cooking pouch. Seal pouches tightly after removing the excess air. Place pouches in sous vide bath and set the cooking time for 24-48 hours. Cover the sous vide bath with plastic wrap to minimize water evaporation. Add water intermittently to keep the water level up. Preheat the oven broiler. Remove pouches from the sous vide bath and open carefully. Remove rib sections from pouches and pat dry with paper towels. Coat each rib section with BBQ sauce and broil for 1-2 minutes on each side. Serve immediately.

Beef Bourguignon
INGREDIENTS

For Beef:	1 bay leaf
Vegetable oil, as required	Sugar, to taste
¼ cup small bacon, cubed	½ tablespoon all-purpose flour
2 pounds beef, cubed	½ tablespoon cold water
1 bottle nice burgundy wine	Salt and freshly ground black pepper, to taste
1 tablespoon butter, divided	1 rosemary sprig
1 pound mushrooms, chopped roughly	Chopped fresh parsley, for garnishing
20 pearl onions	For Mashed Potatoes:
2 celery stalks, finely chopped	2 russet potatoes, peeled and cubed
2 carrots, peeled and finely chopped	3 tablespoons heavy cream
1 white onion, finely chopped	Butter, as required
	Salt, to taste
2 garlic cloves, mashed	

DIRECTIONS and Cooking Time: 25 Hours Cooking Temperature: 180°f

In a wide cast iron pan, heat enough vegetable oil to cover the bottom of the pan and cook bacon cubes until just browning. Add beef and sear until browned completely. Transfer beef and bacon to a bowl, reserving fat in a separate small bowl. Add some wine and scrape the brown bits from bottom and sides of the pan. Cook until a thick glaze is formed. Move glaze to a small bowl and set aside to cool. In the same pan as used for glaze, melt ½ tablespoon of butter over medium-high heat. Add mushrooms and cook for 5 minutes. Cover and cook for 1-2 minutes. Transfer mushrooms to a bowl. Add more wine to the now-empty pan and scrape the brown bits from bottom and sides of the pan. Cook until a thick glaze is formed. Add glaze to the bowl of reserved glaze and set aside to cool. Melt remaining ½ tablespoon of butter over medium-high heat in the same pan. Add pearl onions and cook for 5 minutes. Transfer the onions into the bowl of mushrooms. Add some wine to the pan and scrape the brown bits from bottom and sides. Cook until a thick glaze is formed. Transfer glaze into the bowl of reserved glaze and set aside to cool. For wine reduction: In the same pan, cook reserved bacon fat over medium-high heat and add celery, carrot, and white onion for 7-10 minutes. Add 3¼ cups of wine, garlic, bay leaf, some cooked bacon, and reserved glaze and cook for 30 minutes, stirring occasionally. Strain wine reduction through a fine strainer. Return strained sauce to the pan and bring to a gentle boil. In a small bowl, dissolve flour into cold water. Add flour mixture to strained wine reduction and cook for 3 minutes. Remove from heat and stir in sugar, salt, and black pepper. Set aside to cool. Attach the sous vide immersion circulator to a Cambro container or pot with water using an adjustable clamp and preheat water to 180°F. Place beef, bacon, mushrooms, pearl onions, rosemary sprigs, and wine reduction in a large cooking pouch. Seal pouch tightly after removing the excess air. Place pouch in sous vide bath and set the cooking time for 24 hours. Cover the sous vide bath with plastic wrap to minimize water evaporation. Add water intermittently to keep the water level up. For mashed potatoes: cook potatoes in a pan of boiling water for 10 minutes. Remove from heat and drain potatoes. Return potatoes to the pan. Add heavy cream and some butter and mash until well combined. Season with salt. Remove pouch from the sous vide bath and open carefully. Remove beef, mushrooms, and pearl onions from pouch, reserving the cooking liquid in a pan. Discard rosemary sprigs. Place pan with reserved liquid over stove and cook for 5-10 minutes or until desired thickness of sauce is reached. Remove from heat and stir in beef, mushrooms, and pearl onions. Serve with mashed potatoes.

Bacon Strips & Eggs

INGREDIENTS for Servings: 2

2 slices British-style bacon rashers cut up into ½ inch by 3-inch slices	4 egg yolks 4 slices crisp toasted bread

DIRECTIONS and Cooking Time: 60 Minutes
Prepare the Sous Vide water bath using your immersion circulator and raise the temperature to 143-degrees Fahrenheit. Gently place each of your egg yolks in the resealable zipper bag and seal it using the immersion method. Submerge it underwater and cook for about 1 hour. In the meantime, fry your bacon slices until they are crisp. Drain them on a kitchen towel. Once the eggs are cooked, serve by carefully removing the yolks from the zip bag and placing it on top of the toast. Top with the slices of bacon and serve!

Nutrition Info: Per serving: Calories: 385 ;Carbohydrate: 49g ;Protein: 16g ;Fat: 16g ;Sugar: 4g ;Sodium: 514mg

Pork Roast With Milk Gravy

INGREDIENTS

For Pork Roast:	For Milk Gravy:
¼ cup olive oil	½ cup butter
½ teaspoon dried parsley, crushed	⅓ cup flour
½ teaspoon dried oregano, crushed	3 cups milk, either 2% or whole
Onion powder, to taste	Cooking liquid from pork roast
Garlic salt, to taste	½ teaspoon beef "better than bouillon" stock (optional)
Salt and freshly ground black pepper, to taste	Salt and freshly ground black pepper, to taste
1½-2-pound pork sirloin roast	

DIRECTIONS and Cooking Time: 6 Hours Cooking Temperature: 150°f
Attach the sous vide immersion circulator to a Cambro container or pot with water using an adjustable clamp and preheat water to 150°F. For pork roast: in a small bowl, mix together all ingredients for pork roast except for the roast. Rub the oil mixture generously over the pork roast. Place pork roast in a cooking pouch. Seal pouch tightly after removing the excess air. Place pouch in sous vide bath and set the cooking time for 4-6 hours. Remove pouch from the sous vide bath and open carefully. Remove pork roast from pouch, reserving cooking liquid into a large bowl. For milk gravy: melt butter over medium-low heat in a medium pan. Slowly add flour, beating continuously. Cook for 2-3 minutes, continuing to beat. While beating, slowly add milk and reserved cooking liquid. Increase heat to medium and cook until gravy becomes thick, stirring continuously. Stir in bouillon, salt, and black pepper and remove from heat. Heat a cast iron grill pan over high heat and sear pork roast for 2-3 minutes or until completely golden brown and serve with gravy. Beef

Spiced Beef Brisket

INGREDIENTS for Servings: 4

2lb. beef brisket	½ tablespoon beef demi-glace
Salt and pepper, to taste	1 teaspoon chopped thyme
2 tablespoons olive oil	1 cup beef stock
½ tablespoon tomato paste	½ cup red wine
4 cloves garlic, minced	2 tablespoons honey
1 tablespoon smoked paprika	¾ lb. carrots, peeled, cut into matchsticks

DIRECTIONS and Cooking Time: 32 Hours
Preheat your Sous Vide cooker to 155F. Season the brisket with salt and pepper. Place the brisket into Sous Vide cooking bag. Place aside. Heat ½ tablespoon olive oil in a saucepan. Add tomato paste, garlic, smoked paprika, demi-glace, thyme, stock, and wine. Simmer 5 minutes. Stir in the honey and season to taste. Simmer 1 minute. Pour the mixture into the bag with beef and vacuum seal the bag. Carefully place the bag into the cooker and cook 32 hours. Finishing steps: 25 minutes before the beef is done, toss the carrots with 1 tablespoon olive oil. Roast the carrots 20-25 minutes at 450F. Remove the bag from cooker and open carefully. Strain the sauce into a small saucepot. Simmer 3 minutes over medium heat. Heat the remaining olive oil in a large skillet. Sear the beef 3 minutes per side. Serve the beef with roasted carrots and prepared sauce.

Nutrition Info: Calories 309 Total Fat 14g Total Carb 24g Dietary Fiber 3g Protein 13g

Savory Harissa Lamb Kabobs

INGREDIENTS for Servings: 10

3 tbsp olive oil	Salt to taste
4 tsp red wine vinegar	1½ pounds boneless lamb shoulder, cubed
2 tbsp chili paste	1 cucumber, peeled and chopped
2 garlic cloves, minced	
1½ tsp ground cumin	Zest and juice of ½ lemon
1½ tsp ground coriander	1 cup Greek-style yogurt
1 tsp hot paprika	

DIRECTIONS and Cooking Time: 2 Hours 30 Minutes

Prepare a water bath and place the Sous Vide in it. Set to 134 F. Combine 2 tbsp of olive oil, vinegar, chili, garlic, cumin, coriander, paprika, and salt. Place the lamb and sauce in a vacuum-sealable bag. Release air by water displacement method, seal and submerge the bag in the bath. Cook for 2 hours. Once the timer has stopped, remove the lamb and pat dry with kitchen towel. Discard cooking juices. Mix the cucumber, lemon zest and juice, yogurt, and pressed garlic in a small bowl. Set aside. Fill the skewer with the lamb and roll it. Heat the oil in a skillet over high heat and cook the skewer for 1-2 minutes per side. Top with the lemon-garlic sauce and serve.

Cheesy Ham Frittatas

INGREDIENTS for Servings: 8

1 small onion /finely chopped	1 tablespoon butter
2 garlic cloves /minced	4 tablespoons milk
12 eggs /lightly beaten	Salt and freshly ground black pepper, to taste
1 package /3 ounces cream cheese /softened	4 slices fully-cooked ham /diced
	4 ounces shredded Colby cheese

DIRECTIONS and Cooking Time: 60 Minutes
Preheat water to 180°F in a sous vide cooker or with an immersion circulator. In a medium skillet, melt butter over medium heat and sauté onion until softened, 3-4 minutes, stirring frequently. Add garlic and sauté about 1 minute more. Remove onion mixture from heat and set aside. Spray eight 8-ounce jars with cooking spray. Place eggs, cream cheese and milk in a blender container and add salt and pepper to taste. Process egg mixture until thoroughly combined. Pour egg mixture into jars, add ham and stir gently. Close jars fingertip tight, submerge in water and cook for 1 hour. Remove jars from water and remove lids. Slide a thin knife around the inside of the jars and invert jars on serving dishes to remove frittatas. Sprinkle cheese over frittatas and serve immediately. Enjoy!

Nutrition Info: Calories: 242; Total Fat: 17g Saturated Fat: 9g; Protein: 18g; Carbs: 5g; Fiber: 0g; Sugar: 1g

Bbq Pork Ribs

INGREDIENTS for Servings: 4

1 lb pork ribs	1 tsp garlic powder
Salt and black pepper to taste	1 cup BBQ sauce

DIRECTIONS and Cooking Time: 1 Hour 10 Minutes
Make a water bath, place Sous Vide in it, and set to 140 F. Rub salt and pepper on the pork ribs, place in a vacuum-sealable bag, release air and seal it. Put in the water and set the timer to 1 hour. Once the timer has stopped, remove and unseal the bag. Remove ribs and coat with BBQ sauce. Set aside. Preheat a grill. Once it is hot, sear the ribs all around for 5 minutes. Serve with a dip of choice.

Oxtail Over Vegetable Mash

INGREDIENTS

For Oxtail:	2 tablespoons butter
8 medium whole onions, unpeeled	2 celery sticks, finely chopped
1 full garlic bulb, unpeeled	1 medium leek, thinly sliced
1 cup white wine	10 closed cup mushrooms, thinly sliced
½ cup Demerara sugar	
⅛ teaspoon ground cloves	2 teaspoons English mustard
pinch of cayenne pepper	3 cups cooking liquid from oxtail
salt and freshly cracked black pepper, to taste	4 tablespoons onion puree from oxtail
4 pounds oxtail pieces	pinch of cayenne pepper
For Sauce:	salt and freshly cracked black pepper, to taste
4 medium carrots, peeled and cut into half-moons	

DIRECTIONS and Cooking Time: 21 Hours 15 Mins
Cooking Temperature: 180°f
Preheat oven to 392°F and line a baking sheet with a piece of foil. Arrange onions and garlic bulb onto prepared baking sheet. Roast for 50 minutes. After 15 minutes, remove garlic bulb from oven and keep aside. Remove onions from oven and keep aside with garlic to cool completely. After cooling, squeeze onion pulp and garlic pulp from the skins and retain. Into a small pan, add wine, sugar, cloves, cayenne pepper, salt, black pepper, onion and garlic pulp and bring to a boil. Simmer for 10-15 minutes. With an immersion blender, blend the onion mixture into a thick paste. Remove from heat and keep aside cool completely. Attach the sous vide immersion circulator using an adjustable clamp to a Cambro container or pot filled with water and preheat to 180°F. Into a cooking pouch, add oxtail pieces and onion puree and freeze for 15 minutes. Remove from freezer and seal pouch tightly after squeezing out the excess air. Place pouch in sous vide bath and set the cooking time for 20 hours. Remove pouch from sous vide bath and carefully open it. Remove oxtail pieces from pouch. Through a sieve, strain cooking liquid into a bowl and refrigerate to cool. (Reserve 4 tablespoons of this onion puree separately for the sauce.) After cooling, remove solid fat from top. Remove meat from bones and, using 2 forks, shred. Remove any large chunks of fat. For sauce:

in a large pan, melt butter and sauté carrots, celery and leek until tender. Add oxtail meat, mustard, cooking liquid, and onion puree, and bring to a boil. Reduce heat and simmer, covered, for 10-15 minutes. Add mushrooms and simmer for 5 minutes. Stir in cayenne pepper, salt and black pepper, and remove from heat. This oxtail mixture is great served over mashed potatoes.

Frog Legs With Risotto
INGREDIENTS

For Frogs Legs:	For Risotto:
4 pounds frog legs	4-6 cups vegetable
½ cup plus 3	broth
tablespoons butter,	15 ounces pure,
divided	unsweetened carrot
5 chicken broth ice	juice
cubes	3 tablespoons
5 fresh thyme sprigs	grapeseed oil
8 garlic cloves, minced	1½ cups Vialone Nano
2 lemon slices	risotto
1 bay leaf	1 medium onion,
½ teaspoon red	minced
pepper flakes, crushed	1 cup chardonnay
kosher salt and freshly	white wine
ground black pepper,	1 cup bagged frozen
to taste	carrot/pea mix
3 tablespoons grape	½ cup mascarpone
seed oil	cheese

DIRECTIONS and Cooking Time: 45 Mins Cooking Temperature: 135°f
Attach the sous vide immersion circulator using an adjustable clamp to a Cambro container or pot filled with water and preheat to 135°F. With a sharp knife, cut between the doubled frog legs to separate into two. Into a cooking pouch, add frog leg pieces, ½ cup of butter, thyme, garlic, bay leaf, red pepper flakes, salt and black pepper. Seal pouch tightly after squeezing out the excess air. Place pouch in sous vide bath and set the cooking time for 45 minutes. Remove pouch from sous vide bath and carefully open it. Remove frog pieces from pouch. With paper towels, pat frog pieces completely dry. In a large sauté pan, heat oil and remaining butter over medium-high heat, and sear frog pieces until browned slightly. Meanwhile for risotto: in a pan, add broth and carrot juice and bring to a boil. Reduce heat to low and allow to simmer. In a large heavy-bottomed pan, heat oil over medium heat and sauté risotto rice and onion for 2 minutes. Add wine and cook until absorbed, stirring continuously. Add hot broth mixture ½ cup at a time, and cook until absorbed, stirring continuously. (This process will take 15 minutes.) Add carrots/peas and cook for 3 minutes, stirring continuously. Remove from heat and stir in mascarpone cheese, salt and black pepper. Divide risotto onto serving plates. Top with frog meat and serve immediately.

Tomato Pork Chops With Potato Puree
INGREDIENTS for Servings: 4

1 pound skinless pork chops	1 stalk celery, cut up into 1-inch dice
Salt and black pepper to taste	1 quartered shallot
	3 sprigs fresh thyme
1 cup beef stock	1 oz red mashed
½ cup tomato sauce	potatoes

DIRECTIONS and Cooking Time: 5 Hours 40 Minutes
Prepare a water bath and place the Sous Vide in it. Set to 182 F. Sprinkle the chops with salt and pepper, then place in a vacuum-sealable bag. Add in stock, tomato sauce, shallot, whiskey, celery, and thyme. Release air by the water displacement method, seal and submerge the bag in the water bath. Cook for 5 hours. Once the timer has stopped, remove the chops and transfer to a plate. Reserve the cooking liquids. Heat a saucepan over high heat and pour the drained juices; let simmer. Reduce the heat and stir for 20 minutes. Then add in chops and cook for 2-3 more minutes. Serve with potato puree.

Perfect Leg Of Lamb
INGREDIENTS for Servings: 6-8

¾ cup dry mustard powder	1 whole leg of lamb
2 handfuls mint, chopped	2 cups balsamic vinegar
2 handfuls rosemary, chopped	Salt and pepper, to taste

DIRECTIONS and Cooking Time: 24 Hours
Heat water bath to 131F. Remove the rump and release the meat from the bone. Score the lamb, creating a diamond pattern. Generously season the lamb with salt and pepper. Rub in mustard powder. Sprinkle the lamb with herbs and vacuum seal in the bag. Cook the lamb 24 hours. Finishing steps: Remove the lamb from the bag. Place onto baking sheet. Pour cooking juices into a saucepan. Add balsamic vinegar and cook until reduced by half. Preheat oven to 450F. Brush the lamb with balsamic glaze and pop in the oven 10-15 minutes. Serve.

Nutrition Info: Calories 209 Total Fat 7g Total Carb 8g Dietary Fiber 2g Protein 22g

Glazed Lamb Leg
INGREDIENTS for Servings: 4

1 lamb leg	4 garlic cloves
2 tbsp tomato paste	4 thyme sprigs
2 cups balsamic vinegar	Salt and pepper to taste

DIRECTIONS and Cooking Time: 24 Hours

Preheat your Sous Vide machine to 167ºF. Combine the vinegar and tomato paste in a medium pan and reduce the mixture until thick over the medium heat. Rub salt and pepper into the leg, pour the sauce over it. Put the leg into the vacuum bag. Add thyme and garlic cloves Seal the bag and set the timer for 24 hours. When the time is up, carefully open the bag, remove the leg and pour the cooking juices into a pan. Reduce the liquid over medium heat until thick, mixing it carefully with a spoon and making sure it does not burn. Pour the sauce over the leg and serve.

Nutrition Info: Per serving:Calories 315, Carbohydrates 10 g, Fats 23 g, Protein 17 g

Beef Tri-tip With Bbq Sauce

INGREDIENTS for Servings: 6

2 ½ lb. beef tri-tip	½ cup barbecue sauce, divided
2 teaspoons kosher salt	2 teaspoons light brown sugar
1 teaspoon freshly ground black pepper	

DIRECTIONS and Cooking Time: 6 Hours

Set the Sous Vide cooker to 130F. Season beef with 1 teaspoon salt and ½ teaspoon black pepper. Transfer meat to zip-lock bag and add ¼ cup barbecue sauce. Seal the bag using water immersion technique and place in water bath for 6 hours. When the timer goes off, remove the bag from the water bath. Finishing steps: Take out the meat and pat dry with kitchen towels. Preheat broiler to medium heat and place the meat on the foil-lined broiler-safe baking sheet. Brush the meat with remaining sauce and sprinkle with sugar, remaining salt and pepper. Broil for 5 minutes or until caramelized. Place the meat on serving platter and let it rest for 10 minutes. Slice before serving.

Nutrition Info: Calories 163 Total Fat 6g Total Carb 8g Dietary Fiber 2g Protein 12g

Red Wine Beef Ribs

INGREDIENTS for Servings: 3

1 pound beef short ribs	¼ cup apple cider vinegar
¼ cup red wine	1 garlic clove, minced
1 tsp honey	1 tsp Paprika
½ cup tomato paste	Salt and black pepper to taste
2 tbsp olive oil	
½ cup beef stock	

DIRECTIONS and Cooking Time: 6 Hours 15 Minutes

Prepare a water bath and place the Sous Vide in it. Set to 140 F. Rinse and drain the ribs. Season with salt, pepper, and paprika. Place in a vacuum-sealable bag in a single layer along with wine, tomato paste, beef broth, honey, and apple cider. Release air by the water displacement method, seal and submerge the bag in the water bath. Set the timer for 6 hours. Pat the ribs dry. Discard cooking liquids. In a large skillet, heat up the olive oil over medium heat. Add garlic and stir-fry until translucent. Put in ribs and brown for 5 minutes per side.

Cumin & Garlic Pork Kabobs

INGREDIENTS for Servings: 4

1 pound boneless pork shoulder, cubed	1 tsp coriander
Salt to taste	1 tsp garlic powder
1 tbsp ground nutmeg	1 tsp brown sugar
1 tbsp minced garlic	1 tsp fresh ground black pepper
1 tsp cumin	1 tbsp olive oil

DIRECTIONS and Cooking Time: 4 Hours 20 Minutes

Prepare a water bath and place the Sous Vide in it. Set to 149 F. Brush the pork with salt, garlic, nutmeg, cumin, coriander, pepper, and brown sugar and place in a vacuum-sealable bag. Release air by the water displacement method, seal and submerge the bag in the water bath. Cook for 4 hours. Heat a grill over high heat. Once the timer has stopped, remove the pork and transfer to the grill. Sear for 3 minutes until browned.

Beer Braised Pork Ribs

INGREDIENTS for Servings: 4

2 pounds pork ribs, chopped into bone sections	12 ounce can light beer
1 big onion, finely chopped	Salt and pepper to taste
	1 tbsp butter

DIRECTIONS and Cooking Time: 18 Hours 10 Minutes

Rub the pork ribs with salt and pepper. Put the ribs into the vacuum bag, add chopped onion and beer. Preheat your sous vide machine to 176ºF. Set the cooking time for 18 hours. When the time is up, carefully dry the ribs with the paper towels. Sear the ribs in 1 tbsp butter on both sides for about 40 seconds until crusty. Serve with mashed potatoes, cole slaw or white rice.

Nutrition Info: Per serving:Calories 283, Carbohydrates 17 g, Fats 15 g, Protein 20 g

Chipotle Baby Back Ribs

INGREDIENTS

For BBQ Sauce:	2 teaspoons ground
3 dried ancho chiles, stemmed and seeded	black pepper
	1 teaspoon fresh
1 dried New Mexico chile, stemmed and seeded	lemon zest, grated
	¼ cup fresh lemon juice
¼ cup sunflower oil	¼ cup fresh lime juice, divided
1 small yellow onion, chopped	
	1 teaspoon fresh lime zest, grated
2 garlic cloves, minced	
4½ ounces tomato paste	For Ribs:
	2 racks baby back pork ribs, each rack cut in half
½ cup apple cider vinegar	
	Sea salt and freshly ground black pepper, to taste
¼ cup brown sugar	
¼ cup molasses	
3 tablespoons cocoa powder	For Garnishing:
	1-2 limes, cut into wedges
1½ teaspoons ground cumin	
	Scallions, chopped
1 teaspoon ground coriander	Fresh cilantro, chopped
1 tablespoon sea salt	

DIRECTIONS and Cooking Time: 48 Hours Cooking Temperature: 143°f
Add chiles to a heatproof bowl. Add enough hot water to cover and set aside for 15 minutes. Drain chiles, reserving ½ cup of soaking water. Add chiles and reserved soaking water to a blender and pulse until a smooth paste is formed. In a medium pan, heat oil over medium heat and sauté onion and garlic for 10 minutes. Add tomato paste and remaining BBQ sauce ingredients except lime zest and 2 tablespoons of lime juice and bring to a boil. Reduce heat to low and simmer for 20-30 minutes. Remove from heat and set aside to cool completely. Once cool, stir in remaining lime juice and the lime zest. Transfer to a container and refrigerate before use. For ribs: Attach the sous vide immersion circulator to a Cambro container or pot with water using an adjustable clamp and preheat water to 143°F. Season rib racks with salt and black pepper. Divide rib racks into 2 cooking pouches. Seal pouches tightly after removing the excess air. Place pouches in sous vide bath and set the cooking time for 12-48 hours. Cover the sous vide bath with plastic wrap to minimize water evaporation. Add water intermittently to keep the water level up. Preheat grill to high heat and grease grill grate. Remove pouches from the sous vide bath and open carefully. Remove ribs from pouches. Coat each rib rack with BBQ sauce. Grill for 1 minute per side. Serve, garnishing with lime wedges, scallions, and cilantro.

Awesome Pork Chops With Balsamic Glaze

INGREDIENTS for Servings: 2

2 pork chops	4 tbsp balsamic vinegar
Salt and black pepper to taste	
	2 tsp fresh rosemary, chopped
1 tbsp olive oil	

DIRECTIONS and Cooking Time: 3 Hours 20 Minutes
Prepare a water bath and place the Sous Vide in it. Set to 146 F. Combine the pork with salt and pepper and place in a vacuum-sealable bag. Release air by the water displacement method, seal and submerge in the water bath. Cook for 3 hours. Once the timer has stopped, remove the pork and dry it. Heat olive oil in a frying pan and sauté the chops for 5 minutes until browned. Add in balsamic vinegar and simmer. Repeat the process for 1 minute. Plate and garnish with rosemary and balsamic sauce.

Authentic Italian Sausage
INGREDIENTS for Servings: 4

2 and a ½ cups, seedless red grapes with their stems removed	4 sweet Italian sausage
	2 tablespoons, balsamic vinegar
1 tablespoon, chopped fresh rosemary	Salt
2 tablespoons, butter	Ground black pepper

DIRECTIONS and Cooking Time: 1 Hour 3 Minutes
Prepare your Sous Vide water bath by dipping your immersion circulator and raising the temperature to 160ºF Take a heavy-duty zip bag and add butter, grapes, rosemary, sausages in a single layer Seal using immersion method and cook for 1 hour underwater Remove the sausages and transfer to plate Take a small sized saucepan and add grapes alongside the liquid Add balsamic vinegar and simmer for about 3 minutes over medium-high heat Sear the sausages in the same saucepan for 3 minutes and serve with the grapes Enjoy!

Nutrition Info: Per serving: Calories 995, Carbohydrates 10 g, Fats 51 g, Protein 33 g

Short Ribs Provençale
INGREDIENTS for Servings: 4

2 lbs. beef short ribs	1 tablespoon olive oil
1 teaspoon salt	1 tablespoon flour
1 teaspoon pepper	2 cups red wine
3 cloves garlic	2 cups beef stock
2 sprigs fresh thyme	1 tablespoon tomato paste
1 sprig fresh rosemary	
2 bay leaves	Crusty bread for serving
1 tablespoon butter	

DIRECTIONS and Cooking Time: 48hrs. 30min
Preheat the water bath to 140 degrees F. Season the beef liberally with salt and pepper. Place in bag with garlic, thyme, rosemary, and bay leaves. Seal and place

in water bath. Cook 48 hours. 48 hours later, prepare the sauce. Remove the beef from the bag and pat dry. In a Dutch oven or heavy-bottomed pan, melt butter with olive oil. Add beef and sear until brown on all sides. Remove beef to a plate. Stir flour into the pan and cook 30 seconds, then deglaze with wine, stirring rapidly and scraping the bottom. Stir in beef stock, tomato paste, and any liquid that collected in the sous vide bag. Reduce sauce to your desired consistency. Serve over short ribs.

Nutrition Info: Calories: 551 Protein: 473gCarbs: 87gFat: 282g

Simple Corned Beef

INGREDIENTS for Servings: 4

15 ounces beef brisket	1 cup beer
1 tbsp salt	2 onions, sliced
¼ cup beef stock	½ tsp oregano
1 tsp paprika	1 tsp cayenne pepper

DIRECTIONS and Cooking Time: 5 Hours 10 Minutes
Prepare a water bath and place Sous Vide in it. Set to 138 F. Cut the beef into 4 pieces. Place in separate vacuum-sealable bags. Whisk beer, stock and spices in a bowl. Stir in the onions. Divide the mixture between the bags. Release air by the water displacement method, seal and submerge the bag in water bath. Set the timer for 5 hours. Once the timer has stopped, remove the bag and tranfer to a plate.

Pork & Zucchini Ribbons

INGREDIENTS for Servings: 2

2 (6-ounce) bone-in pork loin chops	2 teaspoons red wine vinegar
Salt and black pepper as needed	2 teaspoons honey
3 tablespoons extra-virgin olive oil	2 tablespoons rice bran oil
1 tablespoon freshly squeezed lemon juice	2 medium zucchini, sliced into ribbons
	2 tablespoons pine nuts, toasted up

DIRECTIONS and Cooking Time: 3 Hours
Prepare the Sous Vide water bath using your immersion circulator and raise the temperature to 140-degrees Fahrenheit. Take the pork chops and season it with salt and pepper, transfer to a heavy duty zip bag and add 1 tablespoon of oil . Seal using the immersion method and cook for 3 hours. Prepare the dressing by whisking lemon juice, honey, vinegar, 2 tablespoons of olive oil and season with salt and pepper. Once cooked, remove the bag from the water bath and discard the liquid. Heat up rice bran oil in a large skillet over high heat and add the pork chops, sear until browned (1 minute per side) Once done, transfer it to a cutting board and allow to rest for 5 minutes. Take a medium bowl and add the zucchini ribbons with dressing   Thinly slice the pork chops and discard the bone.   Place the pork on top of the zucchini.   Top with pine nuts and serve!

Nutrition Info: Per serving:Calories: 174 ;Carbohydrate: 4g ;Protein: 19g ;Fat: 9g ;Sugar: 2g ;Sodium: 302mg

Perfect Roast Steak

INGREDIENTS for Servings: 4

4 tbsp sesame oil	1 tsp onion powder
4 chuck tender roast steaks	1 tsp dried parsley
	Salt and black pepper
1 tsp garlic powder	to taste

DIRECTIONS and Cooking Time: 20 Hours 20 Minutes
Prepare a water bath and place the Sous Vide in it. Set to 130 F. Heat the sesame oil in a skillet over high heat and sear the steaks for 1 minute per side. Set aside and allow to cool. Combine the garlic powder, onion powder, parsley, salt and pepper. Rub the steaks with the mixture and place into a vacuum-sealable bag. Release air by the water displacement method, seal and submerge the bag in the water bath. Cook for 20 hours. Once the timer has stopped, remove the steaks and pat dry with kitchen towel. Discard the cooking juices.

Herbed Rack Of Lamb

INGREDIENTS for Servings: 4

2 racks of lamb, Frenched	1 clove garlic, minced
	1 teaspoon minced thyme
2 teaspoons Herbs de Provence	2 teaspoons fresh mint
Salt and pepper to taste	½ teaspoon onion powder
Sauce:	
2 tablespoons butter	

DIRECTIONS and Cooking Time: 2 ½ Hours
Fill the Sous Vide cooker with water and heat to 134F. Season the rack generously with salt and pepper. Sprinkle with Herbs de Provence and place the racks into Sous Vide cooking bags. Vacuum seal the racks and submerge in water. Cook the lamb 2 ½ hours. Finishing steps: Remove the racks from the bag. Place aside and pat dry. Melt butter in a saucepan over medium heat. Stir in garlic, thyme, mint, and onion powder. Brush the lamb with butter and sear in a heated skillet over medium-high heat. Serve warm, but before serving slice into racks.

Nutrition Info: Calories 434 Total Fat 28g Total Carb 8g Dietary Fiber 2g Protein 42g

Brined Bbq Ribs

INGREDIENTS

For Brine: 3-4 pounds Pork spare ribs 6 cups water 1/2 cup brown sugar 1/2 cup salt For Spice Rub: 3 teaspoons dried basil 2 teaspoons brown sugar 2 teaspoons white sugar	3 teaspoons garlic powder 3 teaspoons paprika 3 teaspoons ancho chiles 2 teaspoons salt 1 teaspoon cumin seeds Freshly ground black pepper, to taste For Serving: BBQ sauce (of your choice)

DIRECTIONS and Cooking Time: 24 Hours Cooking Temperature: 155°f

Cut each rib into 3-4 rib portions. For brine: add water, sugar, and salt to a large bowl and stir until sugar and salt dissolve completely. Add pork ribs, cover, and refrigerate for 24 hours. Attach the sous vide immersion circulator to a Cambro container or pot with water using an adjustable clamp and preheat water to 155°F. For spice rub: mix all spice rub ingredients together in a bowl. Drain ribs and rinse under cold running water then pat dry ribs with paper towels. Season all ribs generously with spice rub. Place each rib portion into a cooking pouch. Seal pouches tightly after removing the excess air. Place pouches in sous vide bath and set the cooking time for 24 hours. During cooking, cover the sous vide bath with plastic wrap to minimize water evaporation. Add water intermittently to keep the water level up. Remove pouches from the sous vide bath and open carefully. Remove rib portions from pouches and pat dry ribs completely with paper towels. Preheat grill to high heat. Grill each rib portion until browned on both sides. Serve immediately with your favorite BBQ sauce.

Ribeye With Pepper Sauce

INGREDIENTS

For Steak: 4-pounds bone-in ribeye steaks Dry spice rub of your choice Kosher salt, to taste Sunflower oil, as required ½ teaspoon Sichuan peppercorns	For Sauce: 1 tablespoon butter 1 tablespoon plain flour 2 tablespoons Brandy 5 tablespoons heavy cream Milk, as required Salt, to taste

DIRECTIONS and Cooking Time: 7 Hours Cooking Temperature: 131°f

Attach the sous vide immersion circulator to a Cambro container or pot with water using an adjustable clamp and preheat water to 131°F. Season steak generously with dry rub and salt. Place steak in a large cooking pouch. Seal pouch tightly after removing the excess air. Place pouch in sous vide bath and set the cooking time for 7 hours. For sauce: in a pestle and mortar, crush peppercorns lightly. Heat a dry frying pan and toast crushed peppercorns until fragrant. In the same frying pan, melt butter and stir in the flour. Add brandy and stir until a paste is formed. Add cream and stir until smooth to remove any lumps. Stir in a little milk and cook until desired thickness of sauce is reached. Stir in salt and remove from heat. Remove pouch from the sous vide bath and open carefully. Remove steak from pouch and pat dry with paper towels. Lightly grease a cast iron frying pan with oil and heat. Add steak and cook for 1 minute on each side. Remove from heat and transfer onto a cutting board. Cut steak into slices, going against the grain of the meat. Serve immediately with sauce.

Loin Pork With Almonds

INGREDIENTS for Servings: 2

3 tbsp olive oil 3 tbsp mustard 2 tbsp honey Salt and black pepper to taste 2 bone-in pork loin chops 2 tsp red wine vinegar	1 tbsp lemon juice 2 tbsp canola oil 2 cups mixed baby lettuce 2 tbsp thinly sliced sundried tomatoes 2 tsp almonds, toasted

DIRECTIONS and Cooking Time: 3 Hours 20 Minutes

Prepare a water bath and place the Sous Vide in it. Set to 138 F. Combine 1 tbsp of olive oil, 1 tbsp of honey, and 1 tbsp of mustard and season with salt and pepper. Brush the loin with the mixture. Place in a vacuum-sealable bag. Release air by the water displacement method, seal and submerge the bag in the water bath. Cook for 3 hours. Meanwhile, prepare the dressing mixing the lemon juice, vinegar, 2 tbsp of olive oil, 2 tbsp of mustard, and the remaining honey. Season with salt and pepper. Once the timer has stopped, remove the loin. Discard cooking juices. Heat canola oil in a skillet over high heat and sear the loin for 30 seconds per side. Allow resting for 5 minutes. For the salad, combine in a bowl the lettuce, sun-dried tomatoes and almonds. Mix in 3/4 of the dressing Top loin with the dressing and serve with the salad.

Overnight Breakfast Ham

INGREDIENTS for Servings: 8

8 thick slices ham or Canadian bacon 1 tablespoon butter /melted	1 tablespoon vegetable oil

DIRECTIONS and Cooking Time: 6 To 12 Hours

Preheat water to 145°F in a sous vide cooker or with an immersion circulator. Vacuum-seal ham slices and butter in a sous vide bag or use a plastic zip-top freezer bag /remove as much air as possible from the bag before sealing. Submerge bag in water and cook overnight /6 to 12 hours. Remove ham slices from cooking bag and pat dry. Heat oil in a large nonstick skillet and sear ham slices until lightly crisped and browned on one side only, about 1 minute. Arrange slices browned-sides up on a platter and serve immediately. Enjoy!

Nutrition Info: Calories: 240; Total Fat: 6g; Saturated Fat: 2g; Protein: 42g; Carbs: 2g; Fiber: 0g; Sugar: 0g

Amazing Prime Rib

INGREDIENTS for Servings: 12

Kosher salt 1 tablespoon, black peppercorn coarsely ground 1 tablespoon, green peppercorn coarsely ground 1 tablespoon, pink peppercorn coarsely ground	3-pound, bone-in beef Ribeye roast 1 tablespoon, dried celery seeds 2 tablespoon, dried garlic powder 4 sprigs, rosemary 1 quart, beef stock 2 egg whites

DIRECTIONS and Cooking Time: 6 Hours
Season the beef with kosher salt and chill for 12 hours Prepare the Sous Vide water bath by dipping the immersion cooker and waiting until the temperature has been raised to 132ºF   Transfer beef to zip bag and seal using immersion method   Cook for 6 hours Preheat your oven to 425ºF and remove the beef, pat it dry   Take a bowl and whisk together peppercorn, celery seeds, garlic powder and rosemary   Brush the top of your cooked roast with egg white and season with the mixture and salt   Place the roast on a baking rack and roast for 10-15 minutes. Allow it to rest 10-15 minutes and carve   Take a large saucepan and add the cooking liquid from the bag, bring to a boil and simmer until half.   Carve the roast and serve with the juice

Nutrition Info: Per serving: Calories 532, Carbohydrates 10 g, Fats 40 g, Protein 33 g

Tomato Pork Shanks With Carrots

INGREDIENTS for Servings: 4

2 pork shanks 1 (14.5-ounce) can diced tomatoes with juice 1 cup beef stock 1 cup finely diced onion	½ cup finely diced fennel bulb ½ cup finely diced carrots Salt to taste ½ cup red wine 1 bay leaf

DIRECTIONS and Cooking Time: 48 Hours 30 Minutes
Prepare a water bath and place the Sous Vide in it. Set to 149 F. Remove the belly fat from the shanks and place it in a vacuum-sealable bag. Add the remaining ingredients Release air by the water displacement method, seal and submerge the bag in the water bath. Cook for 48 hours.   Once the timer has stopped, remove the shank and discard bay leaf. Reserve the cooking juices. Put the shank in a baking sheet and grill for 5 minutes until browned. Heat a saucepan over medium heat and stir in cooking juices. Cook for 10 minutes until thickens. Drizzle the pork with the sauce and serve.

Popular South African Lamb & Cherry Kebabs

INGREDIENTS for Servings: 6

¾ cup white wine vinegar ½ cup dry red wine 2 onions, chopped 4 garlic cloves, minced Zest of 2 lemons 6 tbsp brown sugar 2 tbsp caraway seeds, crushed 1 tbsp cherry jam 1 tbsp cornflour 1 tbsp curry powder	1 tbsp grated ginger 2 tsp salt 1 tsp allspice 1 tsp ground cinnamon 4½ pounds lamb shoulder, cubed 1 tbsp butter 6 pearl onions, peeled and halved 12 dried cherries, halved 2 tbsp olive oi

DIRECTIONS and Cooking Time: 8 Hours 40 Minutes
Prepare a water bath and place the Sous Vide in it. Set to 141 F.   Combine well the vinegar, red wine, onions, garlic, lemon zest, brown sugar, caraway seeds, cherry jam, corn flour, curry powder, ginger, salt, allspice, and cinnamon.   Place the lamb in a large vacuum-sealable bag. Release air by the water displacement method, seal and submerge the bag in the water bath. Cook for 8 hours. Before 20 minutes to the end, heat the butter in a saucepan and sauté the pearl onions for 8 minutes until softened. Set aside and allow to cool. Once the timer has stopped, remove the lamb and pat dry with kitchen towel. Reserve the cooking juices and transfer into a saucepan over medium heat and cook for 10 minutes until reduced by half. Fill the skewer with all kebab ingredients and roll them. Heat olive oil in a grill over high heat and cook the kebabs for 45 seconds per side.

Hamburger Patties

INGREDIENTS

2 pounds fresh ground beef Kosher salt and	1 tablespoon vegetable oil 4 soft hamburger

freshly ground black pepper, to taste 4 cheese slices	buns, toasted lightly Hamburger toppings, as desired

DIRECTIONS and Cooking Time: 4 Hours Cooking Temperature: 138°f

Attach the sous vide immersion circulator to a Cambro container or pot with water using an adjustable clamp and preheat water to 138°F. Divide beef into 4 equal-sized portions. Make patties that are slightly wider than the buns from each portion. Season each patty generously with salt and black pepper. Divide patties into four cooking pouches. Seal pouches tightly after removing the excess air. Place pouches in sous vide bath and set the cooking time for 40 minutes-4 hours. Remove pouches from the sous vide bath and open carefully. Remove patties from pouches and pat dry with paper towels. Season each patty with salt and black pepper and set aside at room temperature for 10 minutes. In a large cast iron skillet, heat oil over high heat and cook patties for 1 minute. Flip patties and place a cheese slice over each patty. Cook for 45-60 seconds. Place 1 patty over each prepared bun. Top with desired topping and serve immediately.

Tasty Short Ribs With Bbq Sauce

INGREDIENTS for Servings: 6

2 tbsp butter 1½ pounds beef short ribs Salt and black pepper to taste 3 tbsp toasted sesame oil 1½ cups barbecue sauce	10 garlic cloves, smashed 3 tbsp champagne vinegar 2 tbsp minced fresh ginger ⅛ cup chopped scallions ⅛ cup sesame seeds

DIRECTIONS and Cooking Time: 12 Hours 15 Minutes

Prepare a water bath and place the Sous Vide in it. Set to 186 F. Season the ribs with salt and pepper. Heat sesame oil in a skillet over high heat and sear each rib for 1 minute per side. Combine the BBQ sauce, garlic, vinegar, and ginger. Place three ribs in each vacuum-sealable bag with the BBQ sauce. Release air by the water displacement method, seal and submerge the bag in the water bath. Cook for 12 hours. Once the timer has stopped, remove the ribs and pat dry with kitchen towel. Heat a saucepan over medium heat and pour the cooking juices. Cook for 4-5 minutes until sticky. Heat the butter in a skillet over high heat and sear the ribs for 1 minute per side. Top with the BBQ sauce. Garnish with scallions and sesame seeds.

Beef Carnitas

INGREDIENTS

For Carnitas: 1 teaspoon dried oregano 2 teaspoons garlic powder 1 teaspoon onion powder 1 teaspoon ground cumin ¼ teaspoon ground cloves ¼ teaspoon ground allspice Salt and freshly ground black pepper, to taste	2-pound chuck roast For Sauce: 2 tangerines, seeded and chopped 2-3 chipotle peppers in adobo sauce 1 tablespoon honey 1 tablespoon oregano leaves ½ cup cooking liquid from chuck rust For Serving: Corn tortillas Avocado, peeled, pitted, and cut into slices

DIRECTIONS and Cooking Time: 24 Hours Cooking Temperature: 156°f

Attach the sous vide immersion circulator to a Cambro container or pot with water using an adjustable clamp and preheat water to 156°F. For carnitas: in a small bowl, combine oregano and spices. Season roast with salt and pepper lightly and then coat with spice mixture. Place roast in a cooking pouch. Seal pouch tightly after removing the excess air. Place pouch in sous vide bath and set the cooking time for 18-24 hours. Cover the sous vide bath with plastic wrap to minimize water evaporation. Add water intermittently to keep the water level up. Remove pouch from the sous vide bath and open carefully. Remove roast legs from pouch, reserving ½ cup of cooking liquid. For sauce: in a pan, add all sauce ingredients except cooking liquid and bring to a gentle boil. Cook for 10 minutes, stirring occasionally. Remove from heat and stir in reserved cooking liquid. Shred beef with two forks and set aside. Arrange tortillas on serving plates. Place shredded beef on each tortilla. Top with sauce and avocados and serve.

Maple Tenderloin With Sautéed Apple

INGREDIENTS for Servings: 4

1 pound pork tenderloin 1 tbsp fresh rosemary, chopped 1 tbsp maple syrup 1 tsp black pepper Salt to taste	1 tbsp olive oil 1 apple, diced 1 thinly sliced small shallot ¼ cup vegetable broth ½ tsp apple cider

DIRECTIONS and Cooking Time: 2 Hours 20 Minutes

Prepare a water bath and place the Sous Vide in it. Set to 135 F. Remove the skin from the tenderloin and cut by the half. Combine the rosemary, maple syrup, ground pepper, and 1 tbsp of salt. Sprinkle over the tenderloin. Place in a vacuum-sealable bag. Release air by the water displacement method, seal and submerge the bag in the water bath. Cook for 2 hours. Once the timer has stopped, remove the bag and dry it. Reserve the cooking juices. Heat olive oil in a skillet over medium heat and sear the tenderloin for 5 minutes. Set aside. Low the heat and put in apple, rosemary springs, and shallot. Season with salt and sauté for 2-3 minutes until golden. Add in vinegar, broth, and cooking juices. Simmer for 3-5 minutes more. Cut the tenderloin into medallions and serve with the apple mix.

Pancetta & Lamb Stew

INGREDIENTS for Servings: 6

2 pounds boneless lamb shoulder, cubed	3 cloves garlic, smashed
4 oz pancetta, cut into strips	1 pound fingerling potatoes, cut lengthwise
1 cup red wine	4 oz dried Portobello mushrooms
2 tbsp tomato paste	
1 cup beef stock	3 sprigs fresh rosemary
4 large shallots, quartered	3 sprigs fresh thyme
4 baby carrots, chopped	Salt and black pepper to taste
4 stalks celery, chopped	

DIRECTIONS and Cooking Time: 24 Hours 25 Minutes

Prepare a water bath and place the Sous Vide in it. Set to 146 F. Heat a skillet over high heat and cook the pancetta until browned. Set aside. Season the lamb with salt and pepper and sear in the same skillet; set aside. Pour in wine and stock, and cook for 5 minutes. Place wine mix, lamb, pancetta, searing juices, veggies and herbs in a vacuum-sealable bag. Release air by the water displacement method, seal and submerge the bag in the water bath. Cook for 24 hours. Once the timer has stopped, remove the bag and transfer cooking juices to a hot saucepan over medium heat and cook for 15 minutes Stir in the lamb to sear for a few minutes and serve.

Jalapeño Lamb Roast

INGREDIENTS for Servings: 6

1 ½ tbsp canola oil	½ cup cilantro leaves, chopped
1 tbsp black mustard seeds	1 shallot, minced
1 tsp cumin seeds	1 clove garlic, minced
Salt and black pepper to taste	2 red jalapenos, minced
4 lb butterflied lamb leg	1 tbsp red wine vinegar
½ cup mint leaves, chopped	1 ½ tbsp olive oil

DIRECTIONS and Cooking Time: 3 Hours

Place a skillet over low heat on a stove top. Add ½ tablespoon of olive oil; once it has heated, add in cumin and mustard seeds and cook for 1 minute. Turn off heat and transfer seeds to a bowl. Sprinkle with salt and black pepper. Mix. Spread half of the spice mixture inside the lamb leg and roll it. Secure with a butcher's twine at 1- inch intervals. Season with salt and pepper and massage. Spread half of the spice mixture evenly over of lamb leg, then carefully roll it back up. Make a water bath and place Sous Vide in it. Set to 145 F. Place the lamb leg in vacuum-sealable bag, release air by the water displacement method, seal and submerge it in the water bath. Set the timer for 2 hours 45 minutes and cook. Make the sauce; add to the cumin mustard mixture shallot, cilantro, garlic, red wine vinegar, mint, and red chili. Mix and season with salt and pepper. Set aside. Once the timer has stopped, remove and unseal the bag. Remove the lamb and pat dry using a paper towel. Add canola oil to a cast iron, preheat over high heat for 10 minutes. Place in lamb and sear to brown on both sides. Remove twine and slice lamb. Serve with sauce.

Meatloaf With Chipotle Glaze

INGREDIENTS

For Meatloaf:	½ teaspoon freshly ground black pepper
2 tablespoons olive oil	1 pound ground beef
1 red bell pepper, seeded and chopped	½ pound Italian sausage, casing removed
½ yellow onion, chopped	1 tablespoon canola oil
2 eggs	For Glaze:
¼ cup heavy cream	½ cup honey
¼ cup breadcrumbs	2 tablespoons canola oil
1 tablespoon soy sauce	
½ teaspoon paprika	1 tablespoon Dijon mustard
pinch of cayenne pepper	1 tablespoon chipotle in adobo sauce, pureed
¼ teaspoon garlic powder	
1 teaspoon kosher salt	1 teaspoon kosher salt

DIRECTIONS and Cooking Time: 2-6 Hours Cooking Temperature: 140°f

Attach the sous vide immersion circulator using an adjustable clamp to a Cambro container or pot filled with water and preheat to 140°F. For the meatloaf: in a skillet, heat the olive oil over a medium heat. Add bell pepper and onion, and sauté for 4-5 minutes. Remove from heat and keep aside to cool completely. Into a large bowl, add the cooled onion mixture, egg, cream, breadcrumbs, soy sauce, spices, salt and black pepper, and mix until well-combined. Add the beef and sausage and, using your hands, knead until well-combined, then shape beef mixture into a loaf. Place the meatloaf into a cooking pouch, and seal tightly after squeezing out the excess air.   Place pouch in sous vide bath and set the cooking time for 2-4 hours. While the meatloaf is cooking: For the glaze: in a bowl, add all glaze ingredients and beat until well-combined.   Just before the end of the sous vide cooking period: Preheat broiler to a high setting and place a rack into the top position of the oven. Remove pouch from sous vide bath and carefully open it. Remove meatloaf from pouch. With paper towels, pat meatloaf completely dry.   In a cast iron skillet, heat the canola oil over a high heat.   Add the meatloaf and cook for 1-2 minutes per side, or until browned completely.   Remove from heat and coat the top of the meatloaf evenly with the glaze.   Broil for 1-2 minutes.

Pulled Pork

INGREDIENTS for Servings: 6

2lb. pork shoulder, trimmed	2 tablespoons maple syrup
1 tablespoon ketchup	2 tablespoons soy sauce
4 tablespoons Dijon mustard	

DIRECTIONS and Cooking Time: 24 Hours
Preheat your Sous Vide cooker to 158ºF.   In a bowl, combine ketchup, mustard, maple syrup, and soy sauce.   Place the pork with prepared sauce into Sous Vide bag.   Vacuum seal the bag and submerge in water.   Cook the pork 24 hours.   Open the bag and remove pork.   Strain cooking juices into a saucepan. Torch the pork to create a crust.   Simmer the cooking juices in a saucepan until thickened.   Pull pork before serving.   Serve with thickened sauce.

Nutrition Info: Per serving:Calories 504, Carbohydrates 16.1 g, Fats 32.8 g, Protein 36 g

Sweet Pork Chops With Pear & Carrots

INGREDIENTS for Servings: 2

2 boneless pork chops	1 pear, shredded
Salt and black pepper to taste	1 tsp olive oil
10 sage leaves	1 tsp honey
2 cups shredded carrots	Juice of ½ lemon
1 tbsp apple cider vinegar	2 tbsp chopped fresh parsley
	1 tbsp butter

DIRECTIONS and Cooking Time: 4 Hours 15 Minutes
Season the chops with salt and pepper. Put sage leaves over the chops and allow resting. Prepare a water bath and place Sous Vide in it. Set to 134 F. Place the chops in a vacuum-sealable bag. Release air by the water displacement method, seal and submerge the bag in water bath. Cook for 2 hours.   Meanwhile, in a bowl

mix well the carrots, pear, vinegar, olive oil, honey, and lemon juice.Season with salt and pepper. Top with parsley and allow chilling for 1 hour and 30 minutes. Heat the butter in a skillet over medium heat until melt.   Once the timer has stopped, remove the chops and dry it. Transfer to the skillet and sear for 1 minute per side. Serve with the carrot mix and garnish with sage.

Beef Bone Marrow

INGREDIENTS for Servings: 4

2 pieces' large beef bone marrow, split lengthwise	Kosher salt as needed Ground black pepper as needed

DIRECTIONS and Cooking Time: 60 Minutes
Prepare the Sous Vide water bath using your immersion circulator and increase the temperature to 155-degrees Fahrenheit   Add the bones in a zip bag and seal using the immersion method   Submerge underwater and cook for 1 hour   Once done, remove the cooked bone marrow from the bag and transfer it to a baking sheet (make sure to keep the marrow side facing up)   Season with salt and pepper   Broil the bones for about 2 minutes until the marrow is golden brown   Serve!

Nutrition Info: Per serving:Calories: 815 ;Carbohydrate: 18g ;Protein: 67g ;Fat: 48g ;Sugar: 67g ;Sodium: 436mg

Shredded Bbq Roast

INGREDIENTS for Servings: 3

1 pound beef chuck roast	2 tbsp BBQ seasoning

DIRECTIONS and Cooking Time: 14 Hours 20 Minutes
Make a water bath, place the Sous Vide in it, and set to 165 F.   Preheat a grill. Pat dry the meat using a paper towel and rub with BBQ seasoning. Set aside for 15 minutes. Place meat in vacuum-sealable bag, release air by water displacement method and seal bag. Submerge in the water bath. Set the timer for 14 hours and cook. Once the timer has stopped, remove the bag and unseal it. Remove the meat and shred it. Serve.

Smoked Sausage & Cabbage Potatoes

INGREDIENTS for Servings: 4

½ head green cabbage, cored and thinly sliced	2 tablespoons cider vinegar
1 Granny smith apple, peeled and cored, cut	2 tablespoons packed brown sugar
	Salt and black pepper,

up into small dices	as needed
24 oz. red potatoes cut up into quarters and into ¼ inch thick wedges	1 pound precooked smoked pork sausage sliced up into 4 portions with each portion sliced into half lengthwise
1 small onion thinly sliced	½ cup chicken broth
¼ teaspoon celery salt	2 tablespoons unsalted butter

DIRECTIONS and Cooking Time: 2 Hours
Prepare the Sous Vide water bath using your immersion circulator and raise the temperature to 185-degrees Fahrenheit. Take a large bowl and add the cabbage, potatoes, onion, apple, cider vinegar, brown sugar, and celery salt. Season with salt and pepper Divide the mixture and sausage among 2 resealable zip bags and add ¼ cup of chicken broth to each bags. Seal using the immersion method and cook for 2 hours. Take a skillet and place it over medium-high heat and add 1 tablespoon of butter, heat it up and add the bag contents to the skillet. Bring it to a boil and reduce the heat, cook until the liquid evaporates. It should take about 5-6 minutes for the onion, potatoes, cabbage to be browned. Transfer to a serving platter and repeat the process with the remaining cabbage- sausage mix. Serve!

Nutrition Info: Per serving:Calories: 510 ;Carbohydrate: 39g ;Protein: 18g ;Fat: 32g ;Sugar: 10g ;Sodium: 496mg

Pork Chop With Corn, Peppers, & Tomatoes

INGREDIENTS

2 bone-in pork chop	1 handful cherry tomatoes
½ teaspoon ground ginger	1 bell pepper, peeled, seeded, and sliced into strips
Salt and freshly ground black pepper, to taste	1 garlic clove, minced
1 ear of corn, kernels removed and cob discarded	2 tablespoons sesame oil

DIRECTIONS and Cooking Time: 1 Hour Cooking Temperature: 144°f
Attach the sous vide immersion circulator to a Cambro container or pot with water using an adjustable clamp and preheat water to 144°F. Season pork chops generously with ground ginger, salt, and pepper. Place pork chops and remaining ingredients in a large cooking pouch. Seal pouch tightly after removing the excess air. Place pouch in sous vide bath and set the cooking time for 1 hour. Remove pouch from the sous vide bath and open carefully. Transfer the pork chops to a serving plate, reserving the vegetables. Heat a cast iron skillet and sear reserved vegetables

for 1 minute. Transfer vegetables onto plate with pork chops and serve.

Prime Rib With Celery Herb Crust

INGREDIENTS for Servings: 3

1 ½ lb rib eye steak, bone in	½ tsp pink pepper
Salt and black pepper to taste	1 tbsp garlic powder
½ tbsp celery seeds, dried	2 sprigs rosemary, minced
	2 cups beef stock
	1 egg white

DIRECTIONS and Cooking Time: 5 Hours 15 Minutes
Rub salt on the meat and marinate for 1 hour. Make a water bath, place Sous Vide in it, and set to 130 F. Place beef in a vacuum-sealable bag, release air by the water displacement method and seal the bag. Submerge the bag in the water bath. Set the timer for 4 hours and cook. Once ready, remove the beef and pat dry; set aside. Mix the black pepper powder, pink pepper powder, celery seeds, garlic powder, and rosemary. Brush the beef with the egg white. Dip the beef in the celery seed mixture to coat graciously. Place in a baking sheet and bake in an oven for 15 minutes. Remove and allow to cool on a cutting board. Gently slice the beef, cutting against the bone. Pour liquid in a vacuum bag and beef broth in a pan and bring to boil over medium heat. Discard floating fat or solids. Place beef slices on a plate and drizzle sauce over it. Serve with a side of steamed green vegetables.

Garlic Burgers

INGREDIENTS for Servings: 4

1 pound lean ground beef	4 tomato slices
3 garlic cloves, crushed	¼ cup lentils, soaked
2 tbsp breadcrumbs	¼ cup oil, divided in half
3 eggs, beaten	1 tbsp cilantro, finely chopped
4 burger buns	Salt and black pepper to taste
4 crisphead lettuce leaves	

DIRECTIONS and Cooking Time: 70 Minutes
Prepare a water bath, place Sous Vide in it, and set to 139 F. Meanwhile, in a bowl, combine lentils with beef, garlic, cilantro, breadcrumbs, eggs, and three tablespoons of oil. Season with salt and black pepper. Using your hands, shape burgers and lay on a lightly floured working surface. Gently place each burger in a vacuum-sealable bag and seal. Submerge in the water bath and cook for 1 hour. Once the timer has stopped, carefully remove the burgers from the bag and pat them dry with paper towel. Set aside. Heat up the remaining oil in a large skillet. Brown burgers for 2-3 minutes on each side for extra crispiness. Drizzle burgers with your favorite sauce and transfer to buns.

Garnish as with lettuce and tomato and serve immediately.

White Wine Veal & Mushroom Chops

INGREDIENTS for Servings: 4

4 cups button mushrooms, sliced	1 pound lean veal cuts, chopped into bite-sized pieces
3 large carrots, sliced	
1 cup celery root, finely chopped	1 tbsp cayenne pepper
2 tbsp butter, softened	Salt and black pepper to taste
1 tbsp extra-virgin olive oil	¼ cup white wine
	A handful fresh celery leaves, chopped

DIRECTIONS and Cooking Time: 3 Hours 20 Minutes
Prepare a water bath, place Sous Vide in it, and set to 144 F. In a large bowl, combine meat with mushrooms, sliced carrots, celery root, olive oil, cayenne pepper, salt, and black pepper. Stir well and transfer to a large vacuum-sealable bag. Submerge the sealed bag in the water bath and cook for 3 hours. Once done, remove the meat from the bag and pat dry. Reserve the cooking liquids. Melt the butter in a large saucepan. Simmer cooking liquids until slightly thickened. Pour in white wine and bring it to a boil for 1 minute. Sprinkle with finely chopped celery leaves and serve warm with the sauce on the side.

Tasty Tenderloin With Avocado Dip

INGREDIENTS for Servings: 3

1 pork tenderloin	Salt and black pepper to taste
1 jar avocado butter	
Fresh rosemary sprigs	

DIRECTIONS and Cooking Time: 2 Hours 10 Minutes
Prepare a water bath and place Sous Vide in it. Set to 146 F. Season the tenderloin with salt and pepper. Brush with some avocado butter and place in a vacuum-sealable bag. Add rosemary springs. Release air by the water displacement method, seal and submerge the bag in water bath. Cook for 2 hours. Once the timer has stopped, remove the tenderloin and dry it. Season with salt and pepper, add more avocado butter and sear on a hot skillet. Cut in slices and serve.

Lamb Chops & Mint Pistachio

INGREDIENTS for Servings: 4

2 full racks lamb sliced into chops	½ cup unsalted pistachio nuts, shelled
Kosher salt and black	3 tablespoons lemon
pepper as needed	juice
1 cup packed fresh mint leaves	2 cloves garlic, minced
½ cup packed fresh parsley	6 tablespoons extra-virgin olive oil
½ cup scallion, sliced	

DIRECTIONS and Cooking Time: 120 Minutes
Prepare the Sous Vide water bath using your immersion circulator and raise the temperature to 125-degrees Fahrenheit Season the lamb with salt and pepper Put in a zip bag and seal using the immersion method. Cook for 2 hours After 20 minutes, take the lamb out and set the grill to high Add the mint, parsley, pistachios, scallions, garlic, and lemon juice in a food processor and form a paste Drizzle 4 tablespoons of olive oil as you process, and keep going until you have a smooth paste Season with salt and pepper Brush your cooked lamb with 2 tablespoons of olive oil and grill for 1 minute per side Serve the chops with pesto

Nutrition Info: Per serving:Calories: 474 ;Carbohydrate: 0g ;Protein: 18g ;Fat: 44g ;Sugar: 0g ;Sodium: 368mg

Italian Sausage & Autumn Grape

INGREDIENTS for Servings: 4

2 ½ cups seedless purple grapes with stem removed	4 whole sweet Italian sausages
1 tablespoon chopped fresh rosemary	2 tablespoons balsamic vinegar
2 tablespoons butter	Salt and ground black pepper, as needed

DIRECTIONS and Cooking Time: 60 Minutes
Prepare the Sous Vide water bath using your immersion circulator and raise the temperature to 160-degrees Fahrenheit. Take a plastic bag and add the grapes, rosemary, butter, and sausage in one layer. Seal using the immersion method. Cook for 1 hour. Remove the sausage to serving platter and pour the grapes and liquid in a saucepan. Add the balsamic vinegar and simmer for 3 minutes over medium-high heat and season the mixture with salt and pepper. Grill the sausage on medium-high heat for 3-4 minutes and serve with the grapes.

Nutrition Info: Per serving:Calories: 341 ;Carbohydrate: 11g ;Protein: 28g ;Fat: 21g ;Sugar: 6g ;Sodium: 602mg

Party Beef Hot Dogs

INGREDIENTS for Servings: 4

8 hot dogs	Mustard
8 hot dog buns	Ketchup

DIRECTIONS and Cooking Time: 1 Hour

Prepare the Sous Vide water bath by dipping the immersion cooker and waiting until the temperature has been raised to 140ºF   Add the hot dogs to your zip bag and seal using immersion method   Submerge and cook for 60 minutes   Serve by adding the hot dogs in the bun and dressing with a bit of mustard and ketchup   Enjoy!

Nutrition Info: Per serving: Calories 150, Carbohydrates 9 g, Fats 10 g, Protein 6 g

Sage & Cider Chops

INGREDIENTS for Servings: 2

1 sprig chopped rosemary	2 pork chops
	1 cup hard cider,
Salt and black pepper	divided
to taste	1 teaspoon sage
1 chopped garlic clove	1 tbsp vegetable oil
	1 tbsp sugar

DIRECTIONS and Cooking Time: 70 Minutes
Prepare a water bath and place the Sous Vide in it. Set to 138 F. In a bowl, combine salt, pepper, sage, rosemary, and garlic. Rub the chops with this mixture and place in a vacuum-sealable bag. Add 1/4 cup of hard cider. Release air by the water displacement method, seal and submerge the bag in the water bath. Cook for 45 minutes.   Once done, remove the bag. Heat oil in a skillet over medium heat and cook the veggies. Add in the chops and sear until golden. Allow resting for 5 minutes. Pour cooking juices into the skillet along with with 1 cup of cider and sugar. Keep stirring until melted. To serve, top the chops with the sauce.

Ground Beef Stew

INGREDIENTS for Servings: 3

4 medium-sized eggplants, halved	¼ cup extra virgin olive oil
½ cup lean ground beef	1 tbsp fresh celery leaves, finely chopped
2 medium-size tomatoes, chopped	Salt and black pepper to taste
2 tbsp toasted almonds, finely chopped	1 tsp thyme

DIRECTIONS and Cooking Time: 60 Minutes
Prepare a water bath and place the Sous Vide in it. Set to 180 F. Slice eggplants in half, lengthwise. Scoop the flesh and transfer to a bowl. Generously sprinkle with salt and let sit for ten minutes.   Heat up 3 tablespoons of oil over medium heat. Briefly fry the eggplants, for 3 minutes on each side and remove from the frying pan. Use some kitchen paper to soak up the excess oil. Set aside.   Put ground beef to the same frying pan. Stir-fry for 5 minutes, stir in tomatoes and simmer until the tomatoes have

softened. Add in eggplants, almonds and celery leaves and cook for 5 minutes. Turn off heat and stir in thyme. Transfer everything to a large vacuum-sealable bag. Release air by the water displacement method, seal and submerge the bag in the water bath. Set the timer for 40 minutes.   Once the timer has stopped, remove the bag and pour the contents over a large bowl. Taste and adjust the seasonings. Serve garnished with parsley, if desired.

Pork Cutlets

INGREDIENTS for Servings: 6

2 pounds ground pork	Salt and black pepper to taste
½ cup breadcrumbs	
1 egg	1 tbsp flour
1 tsp paprika	2 tbsp butter

DIRECTIONS and Cooking Time: 75 Minutes
Prepare a water bath and place the Sous Vide in it. Set to 140 F. Combine the pork, egg, paprika, flour, and salt. Shape into cutlets and place each in a small vacuum-sealable bag. Release air by the water displacement method, seal and submerge the bag in water bath. Set the timer for 60 minutes.   Once the timer has stopped, remove the bag. Melt the butter in a pan over medium heat. Coat the cutlets with the bradcrumbs and cook until golden on all sides. Serve and enjoy.

Pork Belly

INGREDIENTS

2 pounds pork belly	1 teaspoon ground white pepper
1 teaspoon Chinese five-spice powder	3 tablespoons white vinegar
2 teaspoons salt	

DIRECTIONS and Cooking Time: 8 Hours 15 Minutes
Cooking Temperature: 158°f
Attach the sous vide immersion circulator to a Cambro container or pot with water using an adjustable clamp and preheat water to 158°F.   Using a sharp paring knife, slide cuts through the pork belly skin 1 inch apart horizontally. Be careful to only cut through the skin and not too deep into the underlying fatty layer. Insert 2 skewers, crisscrossed, into the pork belly.   In a small bowl, mix together Chinese five-spice powder, salt, and white pepper. Rub the underside of the pork belly generously with half of the salt mixture.   Place pork belly in a large cooking pouch. Seal pouch tightly after removing the excess air. Place pouch in sous vide bath and set the cooking time for 6-8 hours.   Preheat the oven broiler to high. Arrange a rack on a baking sheet.   Remove pouch from the sous vide bath and open carefully. Remove pork belly from pouch and pat dry pork belly with paper towels.   Generously sprinkle underside of pork belly with remaining salt mixture. Flip the belly over and coat with a very thin

layer of vinegar. Place pork belly on the rack that is on the baking sheet. Broil for 10-15 minutes, rotating baking sheet occasionally. Transfer pork belly to a cutting board and cut into bite-sized pieces with a large knife. Serve immediately.

Bbq Beef Brisket

INGREDIENTS for Servings: 8

1 ½ pound beef brisket	Salt and black pepper to taste
1 tbsp olive oil	1 tbsp garlic powder

DIRECTIONS and Cooking Time: 48 Hours 15 Minutes

Prepare a water bath and place the Sous Vide in it. Set to 150 F. Rub the salt, pepper and garlic powder over the meat and place it in a vacuum-sealable bag. Release air by the water displacement method, seal and submerge in the water bath. Set the timer for 48 hours. After 2 days, heat the olive oil in a pan over medium heat. Remove the beef from the bag and sear all sides.

Siu-style Chinese Baby Back Ribs

INGREDIENTS for Servings: 6

1/3 cup hoisin sauce	1-inch piece fresh grated ginger
1/3 cup dark soy sauce	1 ½ teaspoon five spice powder
1/3 cup granulated sugar	½ teaspoon salt
3 tablespoons honey	½ teaspoon white pepper
3 tablespoons sherry vinegar	½ teaspoon fresh ground black pepper
1 tablespoon fermented bean paste	3 lbs. baby back ribs with the membrane removed
2 teaspoons sesame oil	
2 crushed garlic cloves	Cilantro leaves for garnishing

DIRECTIONS and Cooking Time: 4 Hours

Prepare the Sous Vide water bath using your immersion circulator and raise the temperature to 167-degrees Fahrenheit. Take a large bowl and add the hoisin sauce, dark soy sauce, sugar, sherry vinegar, honey, bean paste, sesame oil, garlic, five spice powder, salt, ginger, white pepper, and black pepper. Take a small-sized bowl and add 1/3 cup of the marinade, chill for later use. Add the ribs to the remaining marinade and mix well to coat the ribs. Divide the mixture among 3 large resealable bags and seal using the immersion method. Cook for 4 hours. Heat up the grill to 400-degrees Fahrenheit and transfer the ribs to the grill, brush with the reserved marinade and cook for 3 minutes. Flip them up and brush with more marinade, cook for another 3 minutes. Transfer the dish to the cutting board and

allow it to rest for 5 minutes, slice the rack into ribs and garnish with cilantro leaves. Serve!

Nutrition Info: Per serving:Calories: 1041 ;Carbohydrate: 33g ;Protein: 52g ;Fat: 77g ;Sugar: 26g ;Sodium: 567mg

Delicious Basil & Lemon Pork Chops

INGREDIENTS for Servings: 4

4 boneless pork rib chops	4 tbsp butter
Salt and black pepper to taste	2 garlic cloves, smashed
Zest and juice of 1 lemon	2 bay leaves
	1 fresh basil sprig

DIRECTIONS and Cooking Time: 1 Hour 15 Minutes

Prepare a water bath and place the Sous Vide in it. Set to 141 F Season the chops with salt and pepper. Place the chops with the lemon zest and juice, garlic, bay leaves, basil, and 2 tbsp of butter in a vacuum-sealable bag. Release air by the water displacement method, seal and submerge the bag in the water bath. Cook for 1 hour. Once the timer has stopped, remove the chops and pat dry with kitchen towel. Reserve the herbs. Heat the remaining butter in a skillet over medium heat and sear for 1-2 minutes per side.

Marinated Tri-tip

INGREDIENTS

3 tablespoons low-sodium soy sauce	1 tablespoon red miso
1 tablespoon honey	1 teaspoon garlic powder
1-2 teaspoons chili paste with fermented soy bean	1 teaspoon ginger powder
1 teaspoon onion powder	1 teaspoon sesame oil (optional)
	3-pound tri-tip roast

DIRECTIONS and Cooking Time: 4 Hours Cooking Temperature: 135°f

Attach the sous vide immersion circulator to a Cambro container or pot with water using an adjustable clamp and preheat water to 135°F. Mix all ingredients in a large bowl except tri-tip. Add tri-tip and coat generously with mixture. Place tri-tip in a cooking pouch. Seal pouch tightly after removing the excess air. Place pouch in sous vide bath and set the cooking time for 4 hours. Preheat grill to high heat. Remove pouch from the sous vide bath and open carefully. Remove tri-tip from pouch and pat dry with paper towels. Grill tri-tip for 1 minute on each side. Remove from grill and cut into desired slices. Serve immediately.

Divine Sirloin With Sweet Potato Purée

INGREDIENTS for Servings: 4

4 sirloin steaks 2 pounds sweet potatoes, cubed Salt and black pepper to taste	¼ cup steak seasoning 4 tbsp butter Canola oil for searing

DIRECTIONS and Cooking Time: 1 Hour 20 Minutes
Prepare a water bath and place the Sous Vide in it. Set to 129 F. Place the seasoned steaks in a vacuum-sealable bag. Release air by the water displacement method, seal and submerge the bag in the water bath. Cook for 1 hour. Boil the potatoes for 15 minutes. Drain it and transfer to a bowl with butter. Mash and season with salt and pepper. Once the timer has stopped, remove the steaks and pat dry. Heat the oil in a pot over medium heat. Sear for 1 minute. Serve with the potato puree.

Sirloin Steaks With Mushroom Cream Sauce

INGREDIENTS for Servings: 3

3 (6-oz) boneless sirloin steaks Salt and black pepper to taste 4 tsp unsalted butter 6 oz white mushrooms, quartered 2 large shallots, minced	1 tbsp olive oil 2 cloves garlic, minced ½ cup beef stock ½ cup heavy cream 2 tsp mustard sauce Thinly sliced scallions for garnishing

DIRECTIONS and Cooking Time: 1 Hour 20 Minutes
Prepare a water bath, place Sous Vide in it, and set to 135 ºF. Season the beef with pepper and salt and place them in a 3 separate vacuum-sealable bag. Add 1 teaspoon of butter to each bag. Release air by the water displacement method, seal and submerge the bag in the water bath. Set to 45 minutes. Ten minutes before the timer stops, heat oil and the remaining butter in a skillet over medium heat. Once the timer has stopped, remove and unseal the bag. Remove the beef, pat dry, and place in the skillet. Reserve the juices in the bags. Sear on each side for 1 minute and transfer to cutting board. Slice and set aside. In the same skillet, add the shallots and mushrooms. Cook for 10 minutes and add the garlic. Cook for 1 minute. Add the stock and reserved juices. Simmer for 3 minutes. Add in heavy cream, bring to a boil on high heat and reduce to lower heat after 5 minutes. Turn the heat off and stir in the mustard sauce. Place the steak on a plate, top with mushroom sauce and garnish with scallions.

Lamb Chops With Basil Chimichurri

INGREDIENTS for Servings: 4

Lamb Chops:	Basil Chimichurri:
3 lamb racks, frenched 3 cloves garlic, crushed Salt and black pepper to taste 1 ½ cups fresh basil, finely chopped 2 banana shallots, diced	3 cloves garlic, minced 1 tsp red pepper flakes ½ cup olive oil 3 tbsp red wine vinegar Salt and black pepper to taste

DIRECTIONS and Cooking Time: 3 Hours 40 Minutes
Prepare a water bath and place the Sous Vide in it. Set to 140 F. Pat dry the racks with a kitchen towel and rub with pepper and salt. Place meat and garlic in a vacuum-sealable bag, release air by water displacement method and seal the bag. Submerge the bag in the water bath. Set the timer for 2 hours and cook. Make the basil chimichurri: mix all the listed ingredients in a bowl. Cover with cling film and refrigerate for 1 hour 30 minutes. Once the timer has stopped, remove the bag and open it. Remove the lamb and pat dry using a paper towel. Sear with a torch to golden brown. Pour the basil chimichurri on the lamb. Serve with a side of steamed greens.

Indian Style Pork

INGREDIENTS for Servings: 4

5lb. pork tenderloin, sliced 2 cups yogurt 2 tablespoons tandoori paste 1 tablespoon curry paste	1 cup sour cream 1-inch ginger, minced 2 cloves garlic, minced Salt and pepper, to taste

DIRECTIONS and Cooking Time: 2 Hrs.
In a large bowl, combine yogurt, sour cream, tandoori paste, curry paste, garlic, and ginger. Add sliced pork. Cover and marinate 20 minutes in a fridge. Preheat your Sous Vide cooker to 135 degrees F. Remove the pork from marinade and place into Sous Vide bag. Vacuum seal the bag. Submerge pork in the water bath and cook 2 hours. Remove the bag from water and open carefully. Heat 1 tablespoon olive oil in a large skillet. Sear the pork 3 minutes per side. Serve warm.

Nutrition Info: Calories: 363 Protein: 174gCarbs: 11gFat: 15g

Tzatziki Sauce & Meatball

INGREDIENTS for Servings: 2

1 oz. ground lamb meat	¼ teaspoon ground cinnamon
¼ cup fresh parsley, chopped	1 cup whole milk yogurt
¼ cup onion, minced	½ cup diced cucumber
¼ cup toasted pine nuts, finely chopped	3 tablespoons fresh mint, chopped
2 garlic cloves, minced	1 teaspoon lemon juice
Kosher salt as needed	¼ teaspoon cayenne pepper
2 teaspoons ground coriander	Pitta bread

DIRECTIONS and Cooking Time: 120 Minutes
Prepare the Sous Vide water bath using your immersion circulator and raise the temperature to 134-degrees Fahrenheit Add the lamb, onion, pine nuts, 2 teaspoons of salt, garlic, cinnamon and coriander in a medium-sized bowl and mix well using your hand Roll the lamb mix into 20 balls and divide them into two large, heavy-duty resealable zip bags Seal them using the immersion method. Submerge underwater and cook for about 2 hours. While they are cooking, put the yogurt, mint, cucumber, cayenne, lemon juice and 1 teaspoon of salt in a medium-sized bowl to prepare the Tzatziki sauce Once done, remove the balls and broil them for 3-5 minutes over a foil-lined, broiler-safe baking sheet (with broiler set to high) Serve the balls with your Tzatziki sauce along with some pitta bread

Nutrition Info: Per serving:Calories: 251 ;Carbohydrate: 20g ;Protein: 17g ;Fat: 12g ;Sugar: 3g ;Sodium: 545mg

Persian Tofu

INGREDIENTS

1 x 15-ounce package firm tofu, drained, pressed and sliced into ½-inch-thick planks	1 teaspoon ground turmeric
	1 teaspoon kosher salt
	2 teaspoons freshly ground black pepper
4 garlic cloves, roughly minced	2 limes, cut into wedges
2 tablespoons extra-virgin olive oil	Sumac, for serving

DIRECTIONS and Cooking Time: 2 Hours Cooking Temperature: 180°f
Attach the sous vide immersion circulator using an adjustable clamp to a Cambro container or pot filled with water and preheat to 180°F. Into a small bowl, add garlic, olive oil, turmeric, salt and black pepper. Rub tofu evenly with the mixture. Into a cooking pouch, add tofu patties. Seal pouch tightly after squeezing out the excess air. Place pouch in sous vide bath and set the cooking time for 2 hours. Preheat broiler to high. Line a baking sheet with a piece of foil. Remove pouch from sous vide bath and carefully open it. Remove tofu from pouch. Arrange tofu slices onto prepared baking sheet in a single layer and drizzle with any remaining oil from pouch. Broil for 2-3 minutes per side. Transfer tofu slices onto a serving plate. Squeeze lime juice from wedges over tofu. Sprinkle with sumac and serve immediately.

Spicy Masala Lamb Racks

INGREDIENTS for Servings: 4

1-1.5 lbs. frenched baby lamb racks	2 teaspoons Garam Masala spice blend
½ teaspoon salt	½ teaspoon pepper

DIRECTIONS and Cooking Time: 90 Minutes
Prepare the Sous Vide water bath using your immersion circulator and raise the temperature to 135-degrees Fahrenheit Season the lamb rack with pepper and salt on all sides Rub the rack with Garam Masala Place the rack in a heavy-duty resealable zip bag, making sure the bone side is facing up Seal the bag using the immersion method, and cook for 90 minutes Remove the meat and pat dry using kitchen towel Sear with a blow torch Slice the rack into lollipop shape and serve!

Nutrition Info: Per serving:Calories: 335 ;Carbohydrate: 3g ;Protein: 21g ;Fat: 26g ;Sugar: 0g ;Sodium: 2mg

Tasty Mediterranean Meatballs

INGREDIENTS for Servings: 4

1 pound ground beef	1 garlic clove, minced
½ cup bread crumbs	1 tsp salt
¼ cup milk	½ tsp dried basil
1 egg, beaten	1 tbsp sesame oil
2 tbsp chopped fresh basil	

DIRECTIONS and Cooking Time: 1 Hour 55 Minutes
Prepare a water bath and place the Sous Vide in it. Set to 141 F. Combine beef, bread crumbs, milk, egg, basil, garlic, salt, and basil and shape into 14-16 meatballs. Place 6 meatballs in each vacuum-sealable bag. Release air by the water displacement method, seal and submerge the bags in the water bath. Cook for 90 minutes. Heat the oil in a skillet over medium heat. Once the timer has stopped, remove the meatballs and transfer to the skillet and sear for 4-5 minutes. Discard the cooking juices. Serve.

Pulled Pork(1)

INGREDIENTS for Servings: 12

1/3 cup packed brown sugar /divided	1/2 teaspoon liquid smoke

3 tablespoons plus 1 teaspoon kosher salt /divided 3 tablespoons paprika 1 tablespoon garlic powder 1 tablespoon ground mustard 1 boneless pork shoulder /about 6 pounds	1 cup cider vinegar 3/4 cup brown mustard 1/3 cup ketchup 1 teaspoon garlic powder 1 teaspoon cayenne pepper, plus more to taste 1/2 teaspoon freshly ground black pepper, plus more to taste

DIRECTIONS and Cooking Time: 20 To 26 Hours
Preheat water to 165°F in a sous vide cooker or with an immersion circulator. For the rub, mix 1 tablespoon brown sugar and 3 tablespoons kosher salt with paprika, garlic powder and ground mustard until thoroughly combined. Rub about half of the spice mixture into the pork shoulder, pressing firmly. Vacuum-seal pork shoulder and liquid smoke in a sous vide bag or use a plastic zip-top freezer bag /remove as much air as possible from the bag before sealing. Submerge bag in water and cook for 18 to 24 hours. Preheat oven to 300°F. Remove pork shoulder from cooking bag, reserving the cooking juices. Pat pork shoulder dry with paper towels and rub with remaining spice mixture. Set pork shoulder on a wire rack on a rimmed baking sheet and roast until surface is crisp and dark, about 1 1/2 hours. Meanwhile, for the sauce, mix cider vinegar, brown mustard, ketchup, brown sugar, garlic powder, cayenne pepper, black pepper with remaining brown sugar and kosher salt in a medium saucepan. Add 1 cup juices from cooking bag, heat to a boil and reduce heat to a simmer. Simmer sauce until sugar is dissolved and sauce is reduced to desired consistency, stirring occasionally, about 10 minutes. Set pork shoulder on a large cutting board and shred into bite-size pieces with two forks. Season pulled pork to taste with salt and serve immediately with the sauce. Enjoy!

Nutrition Info: Calories: 380; Total Fat: 11g; Saturated Fat: 4g; Protein: 61g; Carbs: 6g; Fiber: 0g; Sugar: 6g Wisconsin Beer Brats

Sunday Roast

INGREDIENTS for Servings: 6

3lbs. chuck roast 2 tablespoons coarse salt 1 tablespoon coarse pepper	1 large sprig fresh rosemary 1 tablespoon olive oil

DIRECTIONS and Cooking Time: 24hr. 20min
Preheat the water bath to 140 degrees F. Season the beef with salt and pepper. Seal it into a bag with the rosemary. Place in water bath and cook 24 hours.

After 24 hours, remove beef from bag and pat dry. Sear in olive oil in a hot pan until brown on all sides.

Nutrition Info: Calories: 305 Protein: 475gCarbs: 74gFat: 101g

Red Pepper Salad & Pork Chop

INGREDIENTS for Servings: 4

4 pork chops 1 small red bell pepper, diced 1 small yellow onion, diced 2 cups frozen corn kernels	¼ cup cilantro, chopped Salt and pepper as needed Vegetable oil as needed

DIRECTIONS and Cooking Time: 1 Hour
Prepare the Sous Vide water bath using your immersion circulator and raise the temperature to 140-degrees Fahrenheit. Season the pork carefully with salt Transfer the pork to a resealable zip bag and seal using the immersion method. Submerge underwater and cook for 1 hour Take a pan and put it over medium heat and add the oil, allow it to heat up Add the onion, red pepper, corn and sauté for a while until they are slightly browned Season with salt and pepper Finish the corn mix with a garnish of chopped cilantro, keep it aside Remove the pan from heat and wipe the oil Place it back to medium-high heat Put the oil and allow it to heat up Transfer the cooked pork chops to the pan and sear each side for 1 minute Serve the pork chops with the salad!

Nutrition Info: Per serving:Calories: 657 ;Carbohydrate: 49g ;Protein: 25g ;Fat: 41g ;Sugar: 25g ;Sodium: 489mg

Pleasing Pork In Salsa Verde

INGREDIENTS for Servings: 8

2 pounds boneless pork shoulder, cubed Salt to taste 1 tbsp ground cumin 1 tsp fresh ground black pepper 1 tbsp olive oil 1 pound tomatillos 3 poblano pepper, finely seeded and diced	½ white onion finely diced 1 serrano seeded and diced 3 crushed garlic cloves 1 bunch roughly chopped cilantro 1 cup chicken broth ½ cup lime juice 1 tbsp oregano

DIRECTIONS and Cooking Time: 24 Hours 25 Minutes
Prepare a water bath and place the Sous Vide in it. Set to 149 F. Season the pork with salt, cumin and pepper. Heat oil in a skillet over high heat and sear the pork for 5-7 minutes. Set aside. In the same skillet, cook tomatillos, poblano, onion, serrano, and garlic for 5 minutes. Transfer to a food processor and add in

cilantro, lime juice, chicken broth, and oregano. Blend for 1 minute. Place the pork and sauce in a vacuum-sealable bag. Release air by the water displacement method, seal and submerge the bag in the water bath. Cook for 24 hours. Once the timer has stopped, remove the bag and transfer into serving bowls. Sprinkle with salt and pepper. Serve with rice.

Goat Cheese Lamb Ribs

INGREDIENTS for Servings: 2

Ribs:	1 tbsp fennel pollen
2 half racks lamb ribs	½ tsp cayenne pepper
2 tbsp vegetable oil	To Garnish:
1 clove garlic, minced	8 oz goat cheese,
2 tbsp rosemary	crumbled
leaves, chopped	2 oz roasted walnuts,
Salt and black pepper	chopped
to taste	3 tbsp parsley,
	chopped

DIRECTIONS and Cooking Time: 4 Hours 10 Minutes
Make a water bath, place the Sous Vide in it, and set to 134 F. Mix the listed lamb ingredients except for the lamb. Pat dry the lamb using a kitchen towel and rub with the spice mixture. Place the meat in a vacuum-sealable bag, release air by the water displacement method, seal and submerge the bag in the water bath. Set the timer for 4 hours. Once the timer has stopped, remove the lamb. Preheat a grill over high heat and add in oil. Sear the lamb until golden brown. Cut the ribs between the bones. Garnish with goat cheese, walnuts and parsley. Serve with a hot sauce dip.

Cream Poached Pork Loin

INGREDIENTS

3-pound boneless	2 onions, thinly sliced
pork loin roast	¼ cup cognac
Kosher salt and	1 cup heavy cream
freshly ground black	1 cup whole milk
pepper, to taste	

DIRECTIONS and Cooking Time: 4 Hours 10 Minutes
Cooking Temperature: 145°f
Attach the sous vide immersion circulator to a Cambro container or pot with water using an adjustable clamp and preheat water to 145°F. Season pork roast evenly with salt and black pepper. Heat a large cast iron skillet over medium-high heat and sear pork roast for 15 minutes or until golden brown on both sides. Transfer pork roast to a platter, leaving grease in the pan. In the same pan, add onions and sauté. After 5 minutes, add cognac and bring to a boil. Reduce heat and simmer for 1 minute. Remove from heat and set aside to cool for at least 10 minutes. Place pork, onions, cream, and milk in a cooking pouch. Seal pouch tightly after removing the excess air. Place pouch in sous vide bath and set the cooking time for 4

hours. Remove pouch from the sous vide bath and open carefully. Remove pork roast from pouch and transfer to a cutting board, reserving cooking liquid. Cover pork roast with a piece of foil to keep warm. Place cream mixture from pouch in a large skillet over medium heat and bring to a boil. Cook for 10 minutes, stirring occasionally. Stir in salt and black pepper and remove from heat. Cut pork roast into slices of the desired size and serve alongside cream sauce.

Rolled Beef

INGREDIENTS for Servings: 8

Beef:	4oz. peas
8 4oz. sliced beef	1 sprig thyme
Salt and pepper, to	1 pinch sugar
taste	4oz. carrots, chopped
¼ cup vegetable oil, to	8 teaspoon Dijon
fry	mustard
Filling:	16 slices bacon

DIRECTIONS and Cooking Time: 37 Hrs.
Preheat Sous Vide cooker to 176 degrees F. Place the peas in a Sous Vide bag. Add the carrots, a pinch of sugar and salt to taste. Vacuum seal the bag and place in a water bath. Cook the veggies 30 minutes. Remove from the bag. Cover the beef slices with parchment paper. Pound with a meat tenderizer to make the beef this. Spread the mustard over meat, and top each slice with two pieces bacon. Roll the meat into roulade, then roll the meat over veggies and secure the roulades with a kitchen twine. Season with salt and pepper. Heat the oil in a skillet and sear the roulades on all sides. Cool the roulades and transfer in a Sous Vide bag. Vacuum seal the beef and cook 37 hours at 153 degrees F. Remove the meat from the cooker. Allow cooling completely before removing from the bag. Remove the kitchen twine and slice before serving.

Nutrition Info: Calories: 287 Protein: 12gCarbs: 4gFat: 23g

Cream-poached Pork Loin

INGREDIENTS for Servings: 4

1 – 3 lbs. boneless	2 thinly sliced onion
pork loin roast	¼ cup cognac
Kosher salt and	1 cup whole milk
pepper as needed	1 cup heavy cream

DIRECTIONS and Cooking Time: 4 Hours
Prepare the Sous Vide water bath using your immersion circulator and raise the temperature to 145-degrees Fahrenheit. Season the pork with pepper and salt, take a large iron skillet and place it over medium-heat for 5 minutes. Add the pork and sear for 15 minutes until all sides are browned. Transfer to a platter, add the onion to the rendered fat

(in the skillet) and cook for 5 minutes. Add the cognac and bring to a simmer. Allow it to cool for 10 minutes. Add the pork, onion, milk, and cream to a resealable zipper bag and seal using the immersion method. Submerge underwater and cook for 4 hours. Once cooked, remove the bag from the water and take the pork out, transfer the pork to cutting board and cover it to keep it warm. Pour the bag contents to a skillet and bring the mixture to a simmer over medium heat, keep cooking for 10 minutes and season with salt and pepper. Slice the pork and serve with the cream sauce.

Nutrition Info: Per serving:Calories: 1809 ;Carbohydrate: 23g ;Protein: 109g ;Fat: 140g ;Sugar: 19g ;Sodium: 621mg

Tamari Steak With Scramble Eggs

INGREDIENTS for Servings: 4

¼ cup milk	1 tsp onion powder
1 cup Tamari sauce	Salt and black pepper
½ cup brown sugar	to taste
⅓ cup olive oil	2 ½ pounds skirt
4 garlic cloves, chopped	steak
	4 eggs

DIRECTIONS and Cooking Time: 1 Hour 55 Minutes
Prepare a water bath and place the Sous Vide in it. Set to 130 F. Combine the Tamari sauce, brown sugar, olive oil, onion powder, garlic, sea salt and pepper. Place the steak in a vacuum-sealable bag with the mixture. Release air by the water displacement method, seal and submerge the bag in the water bath. Cook for 1 hour and 30 minutes. In a bowl, combine eggs, milk, and salt. Stir well. Scramble the eggs in a skillet over medium heat . Set aside. Once the timer has stopped, remove the steak and pat it dry. Heat a skillet over high heat and sear the steak for 30 seconds per side. Cut into tiny strips. Serve with the scrambled eggs.

Bacon Wrapped Filet With Horseradish Cream

INGREDIENTS

6-8 pound beef tenderloin	For Beef Tenderloin:
Transglutaminase, as required	1 cup heavy cream
	¼ cup prepared horseradish, drained well
Thin bacon strips, as required	2 tablespoons coarse grain mustard
Fresh thyme sprigs, as required	1 tablespoon Dijon mustard
Vegetable oil, as required	Salt and freshly

For Horseradish Cream:	ground black pepper, to taste

DIRECTIONS and Cooking Time: 6 Hours Cooking Temperature: 131°f
Attach the sous vide immersion circulator to a Cambro container or pot with water using an adjustable clamp and preheat water to 131°F. Carefully remove silver skin from tenderloin then remove all fats. Cut tenderloin into steaks of the desired size. Arrange a parchment paper on a cutting board. Place bacon strips on parchment paper and dust with the transglutaminase. Arrange 1 tenderloin filet over dusted side of 1 bacon strip. Roll the bacon strip over the filet to wrap and press firmly to adhere. Repeat with remaining fillets. Arrange 1 thyme sprig over each wrapped fillet and sprinkle with salt. Place each filet in an individual cooking pouch. Seal pouches tightly after removing the excess air. Place pouches in sous vide bath and set the cooking time for 2-6 hours. For horseradish cream: in a bowl, add heavy cream and beat with a mixer until thick but not too stiff. Fold in remaining horseradish cream ingredients. Remove pouches from the sous vide bath and open carefully. Remove fillets from pouches and pat dry with paper towels. Heat a cast iron skillet over high heat and sear each fillet until browned on both sides. Serve immediately alongside horseradish cream.

Teriyaki Beef Cubes

INGREDIENTS for Servings: 2

2 fillet mignon steaks	1½ tablespoons sesame seeds, toasted
½ cup teriyaki sauce (extra 6 tablespoons)	Rice noodles
2 tablespoons soy sauce	2 tablespoons sesame oil
2 teaspoons fresh chilis, chopped	1 tablespoon scallion for garnishing, finely chopped

DIRECTIONS and Cooking Time: 60 Minutes
Prepare the Sous Vide water bath using your immersion circulator and raise the temperature to 134-degrees Fahrenheit Slice the steaks into small portions and put them in a zipper bag Add ½ a cup of teriyaki sauce to the bag. Seal using the immersion method, submerge and cook for 1 hour. Add the soy sauce and chopped chilis in a small bowl Add the sesame seeds in another bowl After 50 minutes of cooking, start cooking the rice noodles according to the package's instructions Once done, drain the noodles and put them on a serving platter Take the bag out from the water and remove the beef. Discard the marinade Take a large skillet and put it over a high heat. Add your sesame oil and allow the oil to

heat up. Add the beef and 6 tablespoons of teriyaki sauce, and cook for 5 seconds Transfer the cooked beef to your serving platter and garnish with toasted sesame seeds and scallions Serve with the prepped chili-soy dip

Nutrition Info: Per serving:Calories: 445 ;Carbohydrate: 15g ;Protein: 38g ;Fat: 26g ;Sugar: 7g ;Sodium: 597mg

Pork Tenderloin

INGREDIENTS for Servings: 3

1 pork tenderloin /about 1 pound 1/4 teaspoon kosher salt, plus more to taste 8 sprigs fresh thyme /divided 2 garlic cloves /sliced, divided	1/4 teaspoon freshly ground black pepper, plus more to taste 2 scallions /sliced, divided 1 tablespoon olive oil 1 tablespoon butter

DIRECTIONS and Cooking Time: 1 Hour
Preheat water to 140°F in a sous vide cooker or with an immersion circulator.   Generously season tenderloin with salt and pepper and vacuum-seal in a sous vide bag with about half of the thyme, half of the garlic and half of the scallions /or use a plastic zip-top freezer bag, removing as much air as possible from the bag before sealing. Submerge bag in water and cook for 1 hour.   Remove tenderloin from cooking bag and pat dry with paper towel. Heat oil in a large nonstick skillet over medium-high heat. Season tenderloin to taste with salt and pepper and sear until lightly browned on all sides, about 2 minutes. Add butter to skillet with remaining thyme, garlic and scallions and baste tenderloin until browned, about 1 minute more. Remove tenderloin to a rimmed platter and drizzle with the butter mixture from the skillet. Let tenderloin stand for about 5 minutes before slicing as desired to serve. Enjoy!

Nutrition Info: Calories: 296; Total Fat: 14g; Saturated Fat: 5g; Protein: 40g; Carbs: 1g; Fiber: 0g; Sugar: 0g

Crusted Prime Rib Roast

INGREDIENTS

For Rib Roast: ½ tablespoon garlic powder ¼ tablespoon ancho Chile powder 3-4-pound prime rib roast Salt and freshly ground black pepper,	2 fresh rosemary sprigs For Crust: 8 garlic cloves, peeled and root cut off 4 fresh thyme sprigs 4 fresh rosemary sprigs
to taste 4 fresh thyme sprigs	2-4 tablespoons olive oil

DIRECTIONS and Cooking Time: 5-10 Hours Cooking Temperature: 131°f
Attach the sous vide immersion circulator to a Cambro container or pot with water using an adjustable clamp and preheat water to 131°F.   In a small bowl, mix together garlic powder, ancho Chile powder, salt, and black pepper. Coat prime rib roast generously with spice mixture.   Place roast and herb sprigs in a cooking pouch. Seal pouch tightly after removing the excess air. Place pouch in sous vide bath and set the cooking time for a minimum of 5 and no more than10 hours. Longer cooking times will be required for for more tender results.   Preheat oven to 400°F.   For crust: place garlic cloves and herb sprigs on a square of tinfoil and drizzle with olive oil. Fold the tin foil around the garlic mixture to make a sealed pouch. Bake for 30 minutes.   Remove from oven and mash roasted garlic into a paste with a fork. Set aside. Preheat oven to 450°F.   Remove pouch from the sous vide bath and open carefully. Remove roast from pouch and pat dry with paper towels.   Coat roast evenly with garlic paste. Arrange roast in a roasting pan and bake for 5 minutes, then serve.

Jerk Pork Ribs

INGREDIENTS for Servings: 6

5 lb (2) baby back pork ribs, full racks	½ cup jerk seasoning mix

DIRECTIONS and Cooking Time: 20 Hours 10 Minutes
Make a water bath, place Sous Vide in it, and set to 145 F. Cut the racks into halves and season them with half of jerk seasoning. Place the racks in separate vacuum-sealable racks. Release air by the water displacement method, seal and submerge the bags in the water bath. Set the timer to 20 hours.   Cover the water bath with a bag to reduce evaporation and add water every 3 hours to avoid the water drying out. Once the timer has stopped, remove and unseal the bag. Transfer the ribs to a foiled baking sheet and preheat a broiler to high. Rub the ribs with the remaining jerk seasoning and place them in the broiler. Broil for 5 minutes. Slice into single ribs.

Mesmerizing Beef Burgers

INGREDIENTS for Servings: 4

10-ounce, ground beef 2 hamburger buns 2 slices, American cheese	Salt Pepper Condiments, topping Butter, toasting

DIRECTIONS and Cooking Time: 1 Hour
Prepare the Sous Vide water bath by dipping the immersion cooker and waiting until the temperature has been raised to 137ºF Shape the beef into patties and season them with salt and pepper Transfer to zip bag and seal using immersion method, cook for 1 hour Toast the buns in butter warm cast iron pan Once the burgers are cooked, transfer them to the pan and sear for 30 seconds per side Place cheese on top and allow to melt Assemble burger with topping and condiments Serve!

Nutrition Info: Per serving: Calories 288, Carbohydrates 34 g, Fats 12 g, Protein 11 g

Venison Burgers

INGREDIENTS

1½ pound ground venison	cooking oil, as required
½ pound high quality ground smoked bacon	4 artisan hamburger buns, as required
6 ounces beer	toppings and condiments of your choice
salt and freshly ground black pepper, to taste	

DIRECTIONS and Cooking Time: 4 Hours Cooking Temperature: 140°f
Attach the sous vide immersion circulator using an adjustable clamp to a Cambro container or pot filled with water and preheat to 140°F. Into a large bowl, add ground venison, ground bacon, beer, salt and black pepper, and gently mix until well-combined. Make 4 patties, using ½ pound of mixture each time. In cooking pouches, gently place the patties. Seal pouch tightly after squeezing out the excess air. Place pouch in sous vide bath and set the cooking time for 1-4 hours, depending on how well done you prefer burgers. Remove pouches from sous vide bath and carefully open them. Remove patties from pouches. With paper towels, pat patties completely dry. Season patties with a little salt and black pepper. In a cast iron skillet, heat oil over high heat, and sear burgers for 45 seconds per side. Place 1 patty in each burger and serve with your desired topping and condiments.

Lamb Sweetbreads

INGREDIENTS

4 cups milk, divided	3 ½ ounces soft flour
10 ounces lamb sweetbreads	salt and freshly ground black pepper, to taste
1 ounce dried rosemary, crushed	oil, as required

DIRECTIONS and Cooking Time: 45 Mins Cooking Temperature: 144°f
Into a large bowl, add 2 cups of milk and the lamb sweetbreads, and allow to soak for 8 hours. Attach the sous vide immersion circulator using an adjustable clamp to a Cambro container or pot filled with water and preheat to 144°F. Drain lamb sweetbreads. Into a large pan, add 4 cups of water and bring to a boil. Add lamb sweetbreads and cook for 10 seconds. Remove lamb sweetbreads from boiling water and immediately plunge into a large bowl of ice water to cool. After cooling, peel off any excess sinew. Into a cooking pouch, add lamb sweetbreads and the remaining 2 cups of milk. Seal pouch tightly after squeezing out the excess air. Place pouch in sous vide bath and set the cooking time for 40 minutes. Remove pouch from sous vide bath and carefully open it. Remove lamb sweetbreads from pouch. With paper towels, pat lamb sweetbreads completely dry. In a bowl, mix together the flour, rosemary, salt and black pepper. Roll lamb sweetbreads evenly with flour mixture. In a cast iron pan, heat some oil and fry and pan fry lamb sweetbreads until crisp. Serve immediately.

Tofu With Caramelized Onions

INGREDIENTS

1 x 14-ounce package firm or extra-firm tofu, drained, pressed and cut into 6 planks	⅓ cup barbecue sauce
	1 tablespoon unsalted butter
1 tablespoon extra-virgin olive oil	1 large yellow onion, thinly sliced
	salt and freshly ground black pepper, to taste

DIRECTIONS and Cooking Time: 2 Hours Cooking Temperature: 180°f
Attach the sous vide immersion circulator using an adjustable clamp to a Cambro container or pot filled with water and preheat to 180°F. Into a cooking pouch, add tofu in a single layer. Add barbecue sauce and seal pouch tightly after squeezing out the excess air. Place pouch in sous vide bath and set the cooking time for 2 hours. Meanwhile, for caramelized onions: in a sauté pan, heat olive oil and butter over medium heat and cook onion for 20 minutes, stirring occasionally. Season with salt and black pepper. Preheat broiler to high. Remove pouch from sous vide bath and carefully open it. Remove tofu from pouch, reserving cooking liquid. Arrange tofu onto a baking sheet and broil for 4 minutes. Arrange caramelized onion in the center of a serving plate and

top with tofu.   Drizzle with some reserved cooking liquid and serve.

Pork Sausage
INGREDIENTS

3 pounds raw, natural casing sausages	2-6 teaspoons kosher salt
6-ounces beer	1 tablespoon butter

DIRECTIONS and Cooking Time: 4 Hours Cooking Temperature: 171°f

Attach the sous vide immersion circulator to a Cambro container or pot with water using an adjustable clamp and preheat water to 171°F.   Place sausages in a single layer in cooking pouches. Add a few tablespoons of beer and 2 teaspoons of salt to each pouch. Seal pouches tightly after removing the excess air. Place pouches in sous vide bath and set the cooking time for 4 hours.   Remove pouches from the sous vide bath and open carefully. Remove sausages from pouch and pat dry with paper towels.   In a skillet, melt butter over medium heat and cook sausages for 3 minutes, flipping occasionally.   Serve immediately.

FISH & SEAFOOD RECIPES

Herb Butter Lemon Cod

INGREDIENTS for Servings: 6

8 tbsp butter	½ tbsp minced fresh
6 cod fillets	chives
Salt and black pepper	½ tbsp minced fresh
to taste	basil
Zest of ½ lemon	½ tbsp minced fresh
1 tbsp minced fresh	sage
dill	

DIRECTIONS and Cooking Time: 37 Minutes
Prepare a water bath and place the Sous Vide in it. Set to 134 F. Season the cod with salt and pepper. Place the cod and lemon zest in a vacuum-sealable bag. In a separate vacuum-sealable bag, place the butter, half of dill, chives, basil, and sage. Release air by the water displacement method, seal and submerge both bags in the water bath. Cook for 30 minutes. Once the timer has stopped, remove the cod and pat dry with kitchen towel. Discard the cooking juices. Remove the butter from the other bag and pour over the cod. Garnish with the remaining dill.

Tuna Confit

INGREDIENTS for Servings: 4

1 1/2 teaspoons kosher salt	1 pound tuna steak /cut into 1" cubes
1/2 teaspoon freshly ground black pepper	1 lemon /thinly peel zest with vegetable
1/4 teaspoon red pepper flakes	peeler
Pinch of sugar	1 garlic clove /peeled, thinly sliced
2 sprigs fresh herbs /such as thyme, parsley or tarragon	1/2 cup vegetable oil

DIRECTIONS and Cooking Time: 1 Hour
In a large bowl, mix salt, pepper, red pepper flakes and sugar until thoroughly combined. Add tuna and toss to coat. Add herbs, lemon peel and garlic to tuna. Cover bowl and refrigerate for at least 4 hours. Preheat water to 125°F in a sous vide cooker or with an immersion circulator. Pour tuna with marinade into a sous vide bag, add oil and vacuum-seal /or use a plastic zip-top freezer bag, removing as much air as possible from the bag before sealing. Submerge bag in water and cook for 1 hour. Strain tuna and serve as desired. Enjoy!

Nutrition Info: Calories: 329; Total Fat: 21g; Saturated Fat: 5g; Protein: 34g; Carbs: 0g; Fiber: 0g; Sugar: 0g

Spicy Fish Tortillas

INGREDIENTS for Servings: 6

⅓ cup whipping cream	½ sweet onion, chopped
4 halibut fillets, skinned	6 tortillas
1 tsp chopped fresh cilantro	Shredded iceberg lettuce
¼ tsp red pepper flakes	1 large tomato, sliced
	Guacamole for garnish
Salt and black pepper to taste	1 lime, quartered
1 tbsp cider vinegar	

DIRECTIONS and Cooking Time: 35 Minutes
Prepare a water bath and place the Sous Vide in it. Set to 134 F. Combine fillets with the cilantro, red pepper flakes, salt, and pepper. Place in a vacuum-sealable bag. Release air by the water displacement method, submerge the bag in the bath. Cook for 25 minutes. Meantime, mix the cider vinegar, onion, salt, and pepper. Set aside. Once the timer has stopped, remove the fillets and pat dry with kitchen towel. Using a blowtorch and sear the fillets. Chop into chunks. Put the fish over the tortilla, add lettuce, tomato, cream, onion mixture and guacamole. Garnish with lime.

Mustardy Swordfish

INGREDIENTS for Servings: 4

2 tbsp olive oil	½ tsp Coleman's
2 swordfish steaks	mustard
Salt and black pepper to taste	2 tsp sesame oil

DIRECTIONS and Cooking Time: 55 Minutes
Prepare a water bath and place Sous Vide in it. Set to 104 F. Season swordfish with salt and pepper. Mix well the olive oil and mustard. Place the swordfish in a vacuum-sealable bag with the mustard mix. Release air by the water displacement method. Allow to rest in the fridge for 15 minutes. Seal and submerge the bag in the water bath. Cook for 30 minutes. Heat sesame oil in a skillet over high heat. Once the timer has stopped, remove the swordfish and pat dry with kitchen towel. Discard cooking juices. Transfer into the skillet and sear for 30 seconds per side. Cut the swordfish into slices and serve.

Sous Vide Lobster With Tarragon

INGREDIENTS for Servings: 4

1lb. lobster tail, cleaned ¾ cup butter, cubed 2 sprigs tarragon	1 lime, cut into wedges Salt, to taste

DIRECTIONS and Cooking Time: 1 Hour
Preheat Sous Vide cooker to 134F.   In a Sous Vide bag, combine lobster tail, cubed butter, tarragon, and salt. Vacuum seal the bag.   Submerge the bag in a water bath and cook 1 hour.   Finishing steps: Remove the bag from the water bath.   Open carefully, and transfer the lobster onto a plate.   Drizzle the lobster tail with cooking/butter sauce.   Serve with lime wedges.

Nutrition Info: Calories 412 Total Fat 35g Total Carb 2g Dietary Fiber 5g Protein 21g

Smoked Prawn
INGREDIENTS for Servings: 2

24 pieces of de-shelled small prawns Smoked salt	4 tablespoons extra-virgin olive oil Pepper as needed

DIRECTIONS and Cooking Time: 15 Minutes
Take a large-sized pot of water and heat to a temperature of 149-degrees Fahrenheit using your Sous Vide immersion circulator   Add the prawns, olive oil, pepper and smoked salt in a heavy-duty plastic zipper bag   Seal it using the immersion method, and cook for 15 minutes   Once cooked, place the prawns in a hot pan and sear until they turn golden brown   Add some extra smoked salt to enhance the flavors.   Serve!

Nutrition Info: Calories: 560 Carbohydrate: 86g Protein: 25g Fat: 12g Sugar: 11g Sodium: 390mg

Shrimp Scampi
INGREDIENTS for Servings: 4

4 tablespoons unsalted butter	½ teaspoon freshly ground black pepper
2 tablespoons freshly squeeze lemon juice	1 lb. jumbo shrimps, peeled and de-veined
2 cloves fresh garlic, minced	½ cup of panko bread crumbs
1 teaspoon fresh lemon zest	1 tablespoon fresh parsley, minced
1 teaspoon kosher salt	

DIRECTIONS and Cooking Time: 30 Minutes
Prepare your Sous-vide water bath to a temperature of 135-degrees Fahrenheit   Place a large-sized skillet over medium heat   Add 3 tablespoons of butter and melt in the skillet   Add the lemon juice, salt, pepper and zest along with the garlic   Remove the heat immediately and allow it to cool for about 5 minutes   Add the shrimps in a large-sized, resealable bag and add the butter mixture   Seal the bag using the

immersion method, submerge underwater and cook for 30 minutes   In the meantime, melt more butter /1 tablespoon into the pan and place it over a medium heat again   Add the bread crumbs when the butter stops foaming and toss them well. Remove from the heat   After cooking the shrimps for 25 minutes, prepare your broiler by heating it to high   When the timer goes off, divide the shrimps along with the cooking liquid, into 4 broiler-safe ramekins/dishes   Top up with crumbs   Broil for 2 minutes until a golden brown   Sprinkle with some parsley and Serve!

Nutrition Info: Calories: 293 Carbohydrate: 4g Protein: 16g Fat: 24g Sugar: 0g Sodium: 513mg

Salmon With Yogurt Dill Sauce
INGREDIENTS for Servings: 2

2 salmon fillets ½ teaspoon salt ½ teaspoon pepper 2-4 sprigs fresh dill 1 cup plain Greek yogurt	For sauce: 1 tablespoon fresh dill, minced Juice of 1 lemon ½ teaspoon salt ½ teaspoon pepper

DIRECTIONS and Cooking Time: 20min
Season salmon with salt and pepper. Seal into the bag with dill. Refrigerate ½ hour. Preheat the water bath to 140 degrees F. Place salmon into the water bath and cook 20 minutes. Meanwhile, prepare the sauce. Combine all sauce ingredients and season to taste. When salmon is cooked, arrange on a plate and top with sauce.

Nutrition Info: Calories: 498Protein: 712gCarbs: 116gFat: 156g

Gourmet Lobster With Mayonnaise
INGREDIENTS for Servings: 2

2 lobster tails 1 tbsp butter 2 sweet onions, chopped 3 tbsp mayonnaise	Salt to taste A pinch of black pepper 2 tsp lemon juice

DIRECTIONS and Cooking Time: 40 Minutes
Prepare a water bath and place the Sous Vide in it. Set to 138 F.   Heat water in a casserole over high heat, until boiling. Open the lobster tails shells and immerse into the water. Cook for 90 seconds. Transfer to an ice-water bath. Allow cooling for 5 minutes. Crack the shells and remove the tails.   Place the tails with butter in a vacuum-sealable bag. Release air by the water displacement method, seal and submerge the bag in the water bath. Cook for 25 minutes.   Once the timer has stopped, remove the tails and pat dry. Seat aside. Allow chilling for 30 minutes. In a bowl, combine the mayonnaise, sweet onions, pepper, and lemon juice. Chop the tails, add to the mayonnaise mixture, and stir well. Serve with toasted bread.

Mahi-mahi Corn Salad

INGREDIENTS for Servings: 4

4 mahi-mahi portions	2 tablespoons fresh
½ teaspoon paprika	basil, chopped
½ teaspoon onion	For dressing
powder	2 tablespoons lime
½ teaspoon garlic	juice
powder	1 teaspoon ancho
¼ teaspoon cayenne	chile powder
pepper	1 tablespoon olive oil
Salt and pepper as	Salt and pepper as
needed	needed
For the Salad	For garnishing
3 cups corn	Lime wedge
½ pint cherry	1 tablespoon fresh
tomatoes, halved	basil
1 red bell pepper,	
diced	

DIRECTIONS and Cooking Time: 15-35 Minutes
Prepare your Sous-vide water bath to a temperature of 122-degrees Fahrenheit   Season the mahi-mahi fillet with salt and pepper and put it in a sous vide zip bag. Whisk together the garlic powder, paprika, onion powder, and cayenne. Sprinkle the spice mix on top of the fish and seal the bag.   Transfer the bag to the water bath and cook for 15-35 minutes   Preheat the oven to 400-degrees Fahrenheit   Add the corn and red pepper on a baking tray. Drizzle the olive oil over the top with salt and pepper. Cook until the corn kernels are soft.   In a bowl, mix the cooked corn, roasted red peppers, tomatoes, and basil and whisk them well. In another bowl mix well the ingredients for the dressing and pour over the corn kernels. Take the Mahi-mahi fillet out of the bag and pat dry. Sear over high-heat in a pan about 2 minutes per side. For serving, take a large spoonful of the corn mix and place on the plates. Add the mahi-mahi fillet on top. Garnish with lime wedge and basil. Serve!

Nutrition Info: Per serving:Calories: 412 ;Carbohydrate: 24g ;Protein: 44g ;Fat: 6g ;Sugar: 18g ;Sodium: 385mg

Dill Mackerel

INGREDIENTS

2 mackerel fillets, pin	fresh lemon rind, as
boned	required
sea salt, to taste	oil, as required

DIRECTIONS and Cooking Time: 25 Mins Cooking Temperature: 122°f
Attach the sous vide immersion circulator using an adjustable clamp to a Cambro container or pot filled with water and preheat to 122°F.   Season mackerel fillets evenly with a little salt.   Into a cooking pouch, add mackerel fillets and lemon zest. Seal pouch tightly after squeezing out the excess air. Place pouch in sous vide bath and set the cooking time for 20 minutes. Remove pouches from sous vide bath and carefully open it. Remove fillets from pouch. With paper towels, pat fillets completely dry.   In a skillet, heat some oil over high heat and cook fillets for 1-2 minutes.   Serve immediately.

Sea Scallops & Sprinkled Sesame

INGREDIENTS for Servings: 4

12 pieces' fresh sea	2 tablespoons sake
scallops, side muscles	1 tablespoon all-
removed	purpose flour
Salt and ground black	1 teaspoon cornstarch
pepper as needed	1 tablespoon sesame
2 tablespoons miso	oil
2 tablespoons	Black and white
unsalted melted	sesame seeds for
butter	garnish

DIRECTIONS and Cooking Time: 30 Minutes
Prepare your Sous-vide water bath to a temperature of 122-degrees Fahrenheit. Season the scallops with pepper and salt   Divide the scallops between two separate resealable zip bags and seal the bags using the immersion method. Submerge the bags and cook for 30 minutes   Add the miso, sake and remaining seasoning of black pepper in a bowl and mix well to prepare the miso seasoning   Once cooked, take the scallops out from the bag and pat dry   In another bowl, mix in melted butter, flour, cornstarch, and salt. Mix well   Brush the mixture all over the scallops   Pour some sesame oil into a large-sized skillet   Place the skillet over a high heat and wait until the oil shimmers. Add the scallops to the oil and sear both sides for 1 minute /30 secs each side   Once done, move it to a serving plate and drizzle the miso dressing over the top. Garnish with the sesame seeds and serve!

Nutrition Info: Calories: 259 Carbohydrate: 17g Protein: 13g Fat: 17g Sugar: 6g Sodium: 478mg

Teriyaki Salmon(1)

INGREDIENTS for Servings: 2

1-inch fresh ginger,	4 oz. egg noodles
peeled and sliced	2 teaspoons soy sauce
10 oz. skinless salmon	2 teaspoons thinly
fillets	sliced scallions
1 tablespoon sesame	4 oz. lettuce, chopped
oil	1/8 small red onion,
½ cup + 1 teaspoon	sliced thinly
teriyaki sauce	1 tablespoon roasted
1 tablespoon sesame	sesame dressing
seeds, toasted	

DIRECTIONS and Cooking Time: 15mins

Add a half of your teriyaki sauce evenly to 2 vacuum pack bags with your salmon, seal, and set to marinate in the refrigerator for about 15 minutes. Set the Sous Vide cooker to preheat to 131F. Add your vacuum bags in the bath and allow to cook for about 15 minutes. Cook egg noodles using the directions on the package Drain well, return to cooking pot and stir in sesame oil and soy sauce, reserving one teaspoon. Divide pasta between serving plates. Combine the other half of teriyaki sauce, ginger, soy sauce, and scallions to a small bowl and stir to combine. Combine onion and lettuce then drizzle with a teaspoon of roasted sesame dressing. When the timer goes off, remove salmon from the water bath, reserving cooking liquid. Top the pasta with salmon fillets and drizzle all with reserved cooking liquid. Garnish salmon with sesame seeds and serve with prepared salad and dipping sauce.

Nutrition Info:Calories: 291 Protein: 33gCarbs: 12gFat: 12g

Shrimp With Creamy Wine Sauce

INGREDIENTS for Servings: 4

1 pound large shrimp /peeled, deveined 2 garlic cloves /sliced 1/4 teaspoon salt 1/4 teaspoon freshly ground black pepper 1 tablespoon olive oil 2 shallots /minced 3/4 cup white wine	2 tablespoons butter /softened 2 tablespoons cream cheese /softened 2 tablespoons chopped fresh parsley leaves 1 tablespoon freshly grated Parmesan cheese 1 teaspoon red pepper flakes

DIRECTIONS and Cooking Time: 30 Minutes
Preheat water to 140°F in a sous vide cooker or with an immersion circulator. Vacuum-seal shrimp, garlic, salt and pepper in a sous vide bag, or use a plastic zip-top freezer bag /remove as much air as possible from the bag before sealing. Arrange shrimp in a single layer in bag, submerge bag in water and cook for 30 minutes. Meanwhile, for the sauce, heat olive oil in a large nonstick skillet over medium heat and sauté shallots for about 3 minutes. Add wine and simmer to reduce, stirring occasionally, 3-4 minutes. Add butter and cream cheese to sauce and whisk until melted and incorporated. Pour shrimp into sauce and stir to coat. Transfer shrimp and sauce to a bowl and sprinkle with parsley, Parmesan cheese and red pepper flakes to serve. Enjoy!

Nutrition Info:Calories: 257; Total Fat: 12g; Saturated Fat: 6g; Protein: 24g; Carbs: 6g; Fiber: 0g; Sugar: 1g

Rosemary Squid

INGREDIENTS for Servings: 3

1 pound fresh squid, whole ½ cup extra virgin olive oil 1 tbsp of pink Himalayan salt	1 tbsp of dried rosemary 3 garlic cloves, crushed 3 cherry tomatoes, halved

DIRECTIONS and Cooking Time: 1 Hour And 15 Minutes
Thoroughly rinse each squid under the running water. Using a sharp paring knife, remove the heads and clean each squid. In a large bowl, combine olive oil with salt, dried rosemary, cherry tomatoes, and crushed garlic. Submerge squid in this mixture and refrigerate for 1 hour. Then remove and drain. Place squid and cherry tomatoes in a large vacuum-sealable bag. Cook en sous vide for one hour at 136 F.

Drunken Mussels

INGREDIENTS for Servings: 2

2 pounds mussels in their shells 2 garlic cloves, chopped	1 cup dry white wine 4 tbsp butter Salt to taste

DIRECTIONS and Cooking Time: 15 Minutes
Preheat your cooking machine to 194ºF. Season the mussels with salt and put into the vacuum bag. Reduce the air in the bag to 30% (70% of vacuum) otherwise the shell won't open. Add dry white wine, garlic cloves and butter Seal the bag, put it into the water bath and set the timer for 15 minutes. Serve sprinkled with lemon juice.

Nutrition Info:Per serving:Calories 369, Carbohydrates 18 g, Fats 25 g, Protein 18 g

Coconut Shrimp

INGREDIENTS

1 package shrimp * ¼ cup bone broth ¼ cup coconut milk 1 x 1-inch piece fresh ginger, finely chopped 3 kaffir lime leaves, sliced	butter, as required 1 tablespoon flavored garlic lovers' seasoning chopped fresh cilantro, for garnishing

DIRECTIONS and Cooking Time: 35 Mins Cooking Temperature: 135°f
Attach the sous vide immersion circulator using an adjustable clamp to a Cambro container or pot filled with water and preheat to 135°F. Into a cooking pouch, add all ingredients except cilantro. Seal pouch tightly after squeezing out the excess air. Place pouch in sous vide bath and set the cooking time for 35

minutes. Remove pouch from sous vide bath and carefully open it. Remove shrimp mixture from pouch and transfer into a serving bowl. Garnish with cilantro and serve immediately.

Cranberry Bbq Salmon

INGREDIENTS

2 tablespoons BBQ sauce 2 tablespoons cranberry sauce 1 tablespoon cranberry juice 1 teaspoon fresh lime juice	1 tablespoon extra-virgin olive oil ⅛ teaspoon salt 2 x 5-ounce boneless salmon fillets fresh cilantro, for garnishing

DIRECTIONS and Cooking Time: 35 Mins Cooking Temperature: 140°f
Into a large bowl, add all ingredients except salmon fillets and cilantro, and mix until well-combined. Set aside 1½ tablespoons of marinade in a small bowl. Add salmon fillets to large bowl of marinade and coat generously. Refrigerate, covered for 1-2 hours. Attach the sous vide immersion circulator using an adjustable clamp to a Cambro container or pot filled with water and preheat to 140°F. Remove the salmon fillets from marinade and place into a cooking pouch. Seal pouch tightly after squeezing out the excess air. Place pouch in sous vide bath and set the cooking time for 25-30 minutes. Preheat broiler to high. Remove pouch from sous vide bath and carefully open it. Remove fillets from pouch. With paper towels, pat fillets completely dry. Coat fillets evenly with reserved marinade. Arrange salmon fillets onto a broiler-safe pan and broil for 1-2 minutes. Garnish with cilantro and serve immediately.

Lemon Butter Sole

INGREDIENTS for Servings: 3

3 sole filets 1 ½ tbsp unsalted butter ¼ cup lemon juice	½ tsp lemon zest Lemon pepper to taste 1 sprig parsley for garnishing

DIRECTIONS and Cooking Time: 45 Minutes
Make a water bath, place Sous Vide in it, and set to 132 F. Pat dry the sole and place in 3 separate vacuum-sealable bag. Release air by the water displacement method and seal the bags. Submerge in the water bath and set the timer for 30 minutes. Place a small pan over medium heat, add in butter. Once it has melted remove from the heat. Add lemon juice and lemon zest and stir. Once the timer has stopped, remove and unseal the bag. Transfer the sole filets to serving plates, drizzle butter sauce over and garnish with parsley. Serve with a side of steam green vegetables.

Seared Tuna Steaks

INGREDIENTS for Servings: 4

1 teaspoon kosher salt 1/4 teaspoon cayenne pepper 3 tablespoons olive oil /divided	2 tuna steaks /1" thick, about 10 ounces each 1 teaspoon butter 1 tablespoon whole peppercorns

DIRECTIONS and Cooking Time: 40 Minutes
Preheat water to 105°F in a sous vide cooker or with an immersion circulator. Season tuna steaks with salt and cayenne pepper and vacuum-seal with 1 tablespoon olive oil in a sous vide bag, or use a plastic zip-top freezer bag /remove as much air as possible from the bag before sealing. Submerge bag in water and cook for 30 minutes. Remove tuna steaks from bag and blot dry with paper towels. Heat remaining 2 tablespoons olive oil and butter in a large nonstick skillet over medium-high heat. Cook peppercorns until softened and beginning to pop, about 5 minutes. Place tuna steaks in skillet and sear until browned, about 1 minute per side. Cut tuna steaks in half and serve with the peppercorns from the skillet. Enjoy!

Nutrition Info: Calories: 359; Total Fat: 20g; Saturated Fat: 4g; Protein: 42g; Carbs: 0g; Fiber: 0g; Sugar: 0g

"smoked" Shrimp

INGREDIENTS for Servings: 4

1 teaspoon smoked coarse sea salt 1 teaspoon Szechuan peppercorns 1 pound jumbo shrimp	1 tablespoon minced ginger 2 tablespoons olive oil /divided 4 scallions /chopped

DIRECTIONS and Cooking Time: 20 Minutes
Preheat water to 150°F in a sous vide cooker or with an immersion circulator. Heat salt and peppercorns in a dry nonstick skillet over medium heat just until fragrant. Finely grind salt mixture with a mortar and pestle. Sprinkle salt mixture and ginger over shrimp, drizzle with 1 tablespoon oil and vacuum-seal in a sous vide bag, or use a plastic zip-top freezer bag /remove as much air as possible from the bag before sealing. Arrange shrimp in a single layer in bag, submerge bag in water and cook for 15 minutes. Heat remaining oil in a large nonstick skillet and sauté shrimp and scallions until shrimp are lightly golden and scallions are wilted, stirring frequently, 2 to 3 minutes. Serve immediately and enjoy!

Nutrition Info: Calories: 200; Total Fat: 9g; Saturated Fat: 2g; Protein: 26g; Carbs: 3g; Fiber: 0g; Sugar: 0g

Coconut Shrimp Soup

INGREDIENTS for Servings: 6

8 large raw shrimp, peeled and de-veined	1 stem of lemongrass, white part only, chopped
1 tbsp butter	1 tsp shrimp paste
Salt and black pepper to taste	1 tsp sugar
For Soup	1½ cups coconut milk
1 pound zucchini	1 tsp tamarind paste
4 tbsp lime juice	1 cup water
2 yellow onions, chopped	½ cup coconut cream
	1 tbsp fish sauce
1-2 small red chilis, finely chopped	2 tbsp fresh basil, chopped

DIRECTIONS and Cooking Time: 55 Minutes
Prepare a water bath and place the Sous Vide in it. Set to 142 F. Place the shrimp and butter in a vacuum-sealable bag. Season with salt and pepper. Release air by the water displacement method, seal and submerge the bag in the water bath. Cook for 15-35 minutes. Meanwhile, peel the zucchini and discard the seeds. Chop in cubes. In a food processor, add the onion, lemongrass, chili, shrimp paste, sugar, and 1/2 cup of coconut milk. Blend until purée. Heat a casserole over lower heat and combine the onion mixture, remaining coconut milk, tamarind paste and water. Add in zucchini and cook for 10 minutes. Once the timer has stopped, remove the shrimp and transfer to the soup. Whisk the coconut cream, lime juice and basil. Serve in soup bowls.

Aromatic Shrimps

INGREDIENTS for Servings: 2

1-pound large shrimps, peeled and deveined	Any aromatics of your choice
1 tsp olive oil	Salt to taste
	2 tbsp lemon juice

DIRECTIONS and Cooking Time: 30 Minutes
Preheat your cooking machine to 125ºF. Season the shrimps with salt and put into the vacuum bag. Add 1 tsp olive oil and aromatics. Seal the bag, put it into the water bath and set the timer for 30 minutes. Serve with any sauce of your choice or sprinkled with lemon juice.

Nutrition Info: Per serving:Calories 153, Carbohydrates 9 g, Fats 1 g, Protein 27 g

Salted Salmon In Hollandaise Sauce

INGREDIENTS for Servings: 4

4 salmon fillets	1 tsp lemon juice
Salt to taste	1 tsp water
Hollandaise Sauce	
4 tbsp butter	½ diced shallot
1 egg yolk	A pinch of paprika

DIRECTIONS and Cooking Time: 1 Hour 50 Minutes
Season the salmon with salt. Allow chilling for 30 minutes. Prepare a water bath and place the Sous Vide in it. Set to 148 F. Place all the sauce ingredients in a vacuum-sealable bag. Release air by the water displacement method, seal and submerge the bag in the water bath. Cook for 45 minutes. Once the timer has stopped, remove the bag. Set aside. Lower the temperature of the Sous Vide to 120 F and place salmon in a vacuum-sealable bag. Release air by the water displacement method, seal and submerge the bag in the water bath. Cook for 30 minutes. Transfer the sauce to a blender and mix until light yellow. Once the timer has stopped, remove the salmon and pat dry. Serve topped with the sauce.

Garlic Squid

INGREDIENTS for Servings: 4

4 small clean squids	2 tbsp olive oil
2 garlic cloves, chopped	Salt and pepper to taste

DIRECTIONS and Cooking Time: 2 Hours
Preheat your cooking machine to 140ºF. Season the squid with salt and put into the vacuum bag. Add olive oil and chopped garlic Seal the bag, put it into the water bath and cook for 2 hours. Serve sprinkled with lemon juice.

Nutrition Info: Per serving:Calories 171, Carbohydrates 8 g, Fats 7 g, Protein 19 g

Leek & Shrimp With Mustard Vinaigrette

INGREDIENTS for Servings: 4

6 leeks	1 tbsp rice vinegar
5 tbsp olive oil	1 tsp Dijon mustard
Salt and black pepper to taste	1/3 pound cooked bay shrimp
1 shallot, minced	Chopped fresh parsley

DIRECTIONS and Cooking Time: 1 Hour 20 Minutes
Prepare a water bath and place the Sous Vide in it. Set to 183 F. Cut the top of the leeks and remove the bottom parts. Wash them in cold water and sprinkle with 1 tbsp of olive oil. Season with salt and pepper. Place in a vacuum-sealable bag. Release air by the water displacement method, seal and submerge the bag in the water bath. Cook for 1 hour. Meanwhile, for the vinaigrette, in a bowl combine the shallot, Dijon mustard, vinegar, and 1/4 cup of olive oil. Season with salt and pepper. Once the timer has stopped, remove the bag and transfer to an ice-water bath. Allow cooling. Put the leeks in 4 plates and

season with salt. Add the shrimp and drizzle with vinaigrette. Garnish with parsley.

Baby Octopus Dish

INGREDIENTS for Servings: 4

1 tablespoon extra-virgin olive oil Kosher salt and black pepper as needed	1 lb. baby octopus 1 tablespoon lemon juice, freshly squeezed

DIRECTIONS and Cooking Time: 50 Minutes
Prepare your Sous-vide water bath to a temperature of 134-degrees Fahrenheit   Add the octopus in a heavy-duty resealable zipper bag   Seal the bag using the immersion method and cook underwater for 50 minutes   Once cooked, remove the octopus and pat it dry   Toss the cooked octopus with some olive oil and lemon juice and season it with salt and pepper   Serve!

Nutrition Info: Calories: 378 Carbohydrate: 4g Protein: 25g Fat: 29g Sugar: 0g Sodium: 392mg
Special Tips If you want a nice crispy chard, grill the cooked and seasoned octopus for 1 minute on each side.

Crabmeat With Lime Butter Sauce

INGREDIENTS for Servings: 4

6 garlic cloves, minced 1 pound crabmeat	Zest and juice from ½ lime 4 tbsp butter

DIRECTIONS and Cooking Time: 70 Minutes
Prepare a water bath and place the Sous Vide in it. Set to 137 F. Combine well the half of garlic, lime zest and half of lime juice. Set aside. Place the crabmeat, butter and lime mixture in a vacuum-sealable bag. Release air by the water displacement method, seal and submerge the bag in the water bath. Cook for 50 minutes. Once the timer has stopped, remove the bag. Discard the cooking juices.   Heat a saucepan over medium-low heat and pour in remaining butter, remaining lime mixture and remaining lime juice. Serve the crab in 4 ramekins, sprinkled with lime butter.

Tom Yum Goong Prawns

INGREDIENTS for Servings: 2

12 large-sized, peeled, tail-on shrimp Kosher salt and pepper as needed 1 stalk of lemon grass with outer leaves removed and lightly smashed into slices of 1 inch	4 oyster mushrooms, halved lengthwise 8 cherry tomatoes ½ white onion, sliced into ½ inch wedges 3 tablespoons fish sauce 1 teaspoon palm sugar 10 tablespoons

5 kaffir lime leaves, torn in half 1 piece of 2-inches galangal, thinly sliced 4 Thai Chilis, stalk removed, and smashed	coconut milk 3 tablespoons freshly squeezed lime juice 3 tablespoons Thai roasted chili paste ¼ cup cilantro, roughly chopped

DIRECTIONS and Cooking Time: 15 Minutes
Prepare your Sous-vide water bath to a temperature of 149-degrees Fahrenheit   Lightly season your shrimps with pepper and salt   Take a heavy-duty resealable bag and put the shrimp in it   Seal the bag using the immersion method and submerge it underwater. Cook for about 15 minutes   Take a pot filled with boiling water and add the lemon grass, galangal, kaffir lime leaves, and the Thai chilis to the pot. Boil for 10 minutes to prepare the soup   Add the mushrooms, onion, and tomatoes, and keep boiling for another 2 minutes   Add the fish sauce alongside the sugar and bring the mixture to a boil, let it boil for 2 minutes   Remove the heat immediately and stir in the lime juice, coconut milk, cilantro and chili paste   Season with some fish sauce, lime juice or palm sugar   Remove the bag out from the water bath and remove the shrimp out, transfer them to your soup pot   Mix them well and serve!

Nutrition Info: Calories: 348 Carbohydrate: 7g Protein: 24g Fat: 2g Sugar: 3g Sodium: 458mg

Sole Fish With Bacon

INGREDIENTS for Servings: 2

2 5oz. sole fish fillets 2 tablespoons olive oil 2 slices bacon	½ tablespoon lemon juice Salt and pepper, to taste

DIRECTIONS and Cooking Time: 25 Minutes
Preheat Sous Vide cooker to 132F.   Cook the bacon in a non-stick skillet and cook bacon until crispy. Remove the bacon and place aside.   Season fish fillets with salt, pepper, and lemon juice. Brush the fish with olive oil.   Place the fish in a Sous Vide bag. Top the fish with the bacon. Vacuum seal the bag.   Submerge in a water bath and cook 25 minutes.   Finishing steps: Remove the fish from the bag.   Serve while warm.

Nutrition Info: Calories 298 Total Fat 29g Total Carb 4g Dietary Fiber 0g Protein 24g

Curry Shrimp With Noodles

INGREDIENTS for Servings: 2

1 pound shrimp, tail-on 8 oz vermicelli noodles, cooked and drained	1 tsp rice wine 1 tsp curry powder 1 tbsp soy sauce 1 green onion, sliced 2 tbsp vegetable oil

DIRECTIONS and Cooking Time: 25 Minutes
Prepare a water bath and place the Sous Vide in it. Set to 149 F. Place the shrimp in a vacuum-sealable bag. Release air by the water displacement method, seal and submerge the bag in the water bath. Cook for 15 minutes. Heat oil in a pan over medium heat and add in rice wine, curry powder and soy sauce. Mix well and combine the noodles. Once the timer has stopped, remove the shrimp and transfer to the noodle mix. Garnish with green onion.

Redfish With Creole Mayo

INGREDIENTS

For fish:	½ teaspoon Creole
red fish fillets *	mustard
Creole seasoning, as	1 small clove garlic,
required	minced
olive oil, as required	pinch of salt
For Mayo:	¼ teaspoon cayenne
1 egg yolk	pepper
½ cup olive oil	chopped fresh parsley,
	as required

DIRECTIONS and Cooking Time: 25 Mins Cooking Temperature: 122°f
Attach the sous vide immersion circulator using an adjustable clamp to a Cambro container or pot filled with water and preheat to 122°F. Season fish fillets with Creole seasoning evenly. Into a large cooking pouch, place fish fillets. Seal pouch tightly after squeezing out the excess air. Place pouch in sous vide bath and set the cooking time for 20 minutes. Meanwhile, for mayo: to a bowl, add egg yolk and beat until smooth. Slowly add oil, beating continuously until a heavy cream like mixture is formed. Add all remaining ingredients except parsley, and beat until well-combined. Keep aside until serving. Preheat broiler to high. Remove pouches from sous vide bath and carefully open them. Remove fillets from pouches. With paper towels, pat fillets completely dry. Arrange fillets onto a broiler-safe pan and drizzle with some oil. Broil until golden brown. Add parsley into mayo and stir to combine. Serve fish with the topping of mayo.

Swordfish & Potato Salad With Kalamata Olives

INGREDIENTS for Servings: 2

Potatoes	Salad
3 tbsp olive oil	1 cup baby spinach
1 pound sweet	leaves
potatoes	1 cup cherry
2 tsp salt	tomatoes, halved
3 fresh thyme sprigs	¼ cup Kalamata
Fish	olives, chopped
1 tbsp olive oil	1 tbsp olive oil

1 swordfish steak	1 tsp Dijon mustard
Salt and black pepper	3 tbsp cider vinegar
to taste	¼ tsp salt
1 tsp canola oil	

DIRECTIONS and Cooking Time: 3 Hours 5 Minutes
To make the potatoes: prepare a water bath and place the Sous Vide in it. Set to 192 F. Place the potatoes, olive oil, sea salt and thyme in a vacuum-sealable bag. Release air by the water displacement method, seal and submerge the bag in the water bath. Cook for 1 hour and 15 minutes. Once the timer has stopped, remove the bag and do not open. Set aside. To make the fish: Make a water bath and place the Sous Vide in it. Set to 104 F. Season the swordfish with salt and pepper. Place in a vacuum-sealable bag with the olive oil. Release air by the water displacement method, seal and submerge the bag in the water bath. Cook for 30 minutes. Heat canola oil in a skillet over high heat. Remove the swordfish and pat pat dry with kitchen towel. Discard the cooking juices. Transfer the swordfish into the skillet and cook for 30 seconds per side. Cut into slices and cover with plastic wrap. Set aside. Finally, make the salad: to a salad bowl, add the cherry tomatoes, olives, olive oil, mustard, cider vinegar, and salt and mix well. Add in baby spinach. Remove the potatoes and cut by the half. Discard cooking juices. Top the salad with potatoes and swordfish to serve.

Butter Shrimps

INGREDIENTS for Servings: 4

16 shrimps, peeled	1 shallot, minced
and deveined	2 tsp thyme
1 tbsp unsalted butter,	1 tsp lemon zest,
melted	grated

DIRECTIONS and Cooking Time: 25 Minutes
Preheat your cooking machine to 125ºF. Put all ingredients in the vacuum bag. Seal the bag, put it into the water bath and set the timer for 25 minutes. Serve immediately as an appetizer or tossed with penne pasta.

Nutrition Info: Per serving:Calories 257, Carbohydrates 23 g, Fats 5 g, Protein 30 g

Scallops With Lemon Meyer Glaze

INGREDIENTS

2 pounds sea scallops,	2 tablespoon scallions,
muscles removed	white and green parts
4 slices Meyer lemon	separated, finely
Salt and freshly	chopped (greens
ground black pepper,	reserved for garnish)
to taste	pinch of red chili
½ cup fresh orange	flakes
juice	4 tablespoons dry
juice and zest of 2	

Meyer lemons	sherry
2 tablespoons butter	2 teaspoons honey

DIRECTIONS and Cooking Time: 40 Mins Cooking Temperature: 122°f

Attach the sous vide immersion circulator using an adjustable clamp to a Cambro container or pot filled with water and preheat to 122°F. Into 2 cooking pouches, divide scallops, salt and black pepper. In each pouch, place 2 lemon slices. Seal pouches tightly after squeezing out the excess air. Place pouches in sous vide bath and set the cooking time for 30 minutes. In a bowl, mix together orange juice and enough lemon juice to get ⅔ cup liquid. Keep aside. Remove pouches from sous vide bath and carefully open them. Remove scallops from the pouches. For the sauce: in a skillet, melt butter over medium-high heat and sauté white part of scallion and chili flakes until soft. With a slotted spoon, transfer scallion into a bowl and keep aside. To the same skillet, add scallops and gently sear for 90 seconds per side. With a slotted spoon, transfer scallops onto a platter. To the same skillet, add sherry and scrape browned pieces from bottom. Add cooked scallion whites, juice mixture, and some of lemon zest and bring to a boil. Cook until desired thickness sauce is achieved. Add honey 1 teaspoon at a time, and stir to combine. Place sauce over scallops evenly. Garnish with scallion greens and some lemon zest, and serve immediately.

Moroccan Red Snapper

INGREDIENTS for Servings: 4

4 pieces cleaned red snapper	3 oranges
2 tablespoons butter	1 yellow onion
Salt and pepper as needed	1 diced zucchini
For Citrus Sauce	1 teaspoon saffron threads
1 lemon	1 teaspoon diced chili pepper
1 grapefruit	1 tablespoon sugar
1 lime	3 cups fish stock
2 tablespoons canola oil	3 tablespoons chopped cilantro

DIRECTIONS and Cooking Time: 30 Minutes

Prepare your Sous-vide water bath to a temperature of 132-degrees Fahrenheit Season the snapper fillets with salt and pepper and transfer them to a heavy-duty Sous Vide zip bag. (use multiple bags if necessary) Divide the butter equally between the bags if more than one bag is used. If not, add the whole amount of butter to the single bag Seal using the immersion method and submerge underwater, cook for 30 minutes While the fish is being cooked, start preparing your sauce by peeling the fruits and dicing up the flesh (make sure to remove the pith) Take a large-sized pan and place it over medium-heat, add the oil and allow it to heat up Add in the onion and

zucchini and sauté for 2-3 minutes Add the saffron, fruits, diced pepper and sugar and cook for 1 more minute Add the fish stock and bring the mix to a boil, lower down the heat to low and simmer for 10 minutes Remove the heat and stir in cilantro, keep it on the side Take the fish out from the bag and transfer them to your serving platter Spoon the fruity-saffron sauce over the top and serve

Nutrition Info: Per serving:Calories: 285 ;Carbohydrate: 21g ;Protein: 32g ;Fat: 5g ;Sugar: 3g ;Sodium: 602mg

Poached Lobster Pasta

INGREDIENTS

For Lobster:	For Sauce:
4-5 frozen lobster tails, thawed and removed from shells, reserving the shells	¼ cup tomato paste
	2 plum tomatoes, chopped
1 teaspoon salt	2 cloves garlic, sliced
½ cup unsalted butter	2 fresh parsley sprigs
1 tablespoon chili paste	2 fresh thyme sprigs
1 clove garlic, crushed	½ cup dry white wine
1-2 fresh parsley sprigs	2 tablespoons white wine vinegar
1-2 fresh thyme sprigs	4-5 cups whipping cream
3 tablespoons olive oil reserved lobster shells	1 pound linguine (or pasta of your choice) salt and freshly ground white pepper, to taste

DIRECTIONS and Cooking Time: 55 Mins Cooking Temperature: 140°f

Attach the sous vide immersion circulator using an adjustable clamp to a Cambro container or pot filled with water and preheat to 140°F. Remove lobster meat from tails and season with a little salt. Into a cooking pouch, add lobster, butter, chili paste, garlic and herbs. Seal pouch tightly after squeezing out the excess air. Place pouch in sous vide bath and set the cooking time for 30 minutes. Remove pouch from sous vide bath and carefully open it. Remove lobster meat from the pouch and cut into small chunks. Meanwhile, for the sauce: in a heavy large pan, heat oil over high heat and cook reserved lobster shells for 4-5 minutes. Reduce heat to low and stir in the tomato paste. Cook for a few minutes. Add tomatoes, garlic, herbs, wine and vinegar, and stir to combine. Add cream and bring to a boil, then reduce heat to medium-low and simmer for 20 minutes, stirring occasionally. Meanwhile, prepare pasta according to package's directions, then drain. With a metal strainer, strain sauce into large bowl, pressing on solids to extract as much liquid as possible. Transfer liquid into another pan over low heat. Add cooked pasta, lobster meat, salt and white pepper and toss to coat well. Serve immediately.

Egg Bites With Salmon & Asparagus

INGREDIENTS for Servings: 6

6 whole eggs	½ oz minced shallot
¼ cup crème fraiche	2 tsp chopped, fresh
¼ cup goat cheese	dill
4 spears asparagus	Salt and black pepper
2 oz smoked salmon	to taste
2 oz chèvre cheese	

DIRECTIONS and Cooking Time: 70 Minutes
Prepare a water bath and place the Sous Vide in it. Set to 172 F. Blend the eggs, crème fraiche, goat cheese and salt. Diced the asparagus and add to the mix with the shallots. Cut salmon and add to the bowl as well. Add the dill. Combine well. Add the egg and salmon mixture into 6 jars. Add 1/6 chevre into the jars, seal and submerge the jars in the water bath. Cook for 60 minutes. Once the timer has stopped, remove the jars and top with salt.

Citrus Fish With Coconut Sauce

INGREDIENTS for Servings: 6

2 tbsp vegetable oil	1 tsp cumin powder
4 tomatoes, peeled and chopped	1 tsp cayenne pepper
	½ tsp salt
2 red bell peppers, diced	6 cod fillets, skin removed, cubed
1 yellow onion, diced	14 ounces coconut
½ cup orange juice	milk
¼ cup lime juice	¼ cup shredded
4 garlic cloves, minced	coconut
1 tsp caraway seeds, crushed	3 tbsp chopped fresh cilantro

DIRECTIONS and Cooking Time: 1 Hour 57 Minutes
Prepare a water bath and place the Sous Vide in it. Set to 137 F. Combine in a bowl, the orange juice, lime juice, garlic, caraway seeds, cumin, cayenne pepper, and salt. Brush the fillets with the lime mixture. Cover and allow to chill in the fridge for 1 hour. Meantime, heat oil in a saucepan over medium heat and put in tomatoes, bell peppers, onion, and salt. Cook for 4-5 minutes until softened. Pour the coconut milk over the tomato mixture and cook for 10 minutes. Set aside and allow to cool. Take out the fillets from the fridge and place in 2 vacuum-sealable bags with the coconut mixture. Release air by the water displacement method, seal and submerge the bags in the water bath. Cook for 40 minutes. Once the timer has stopped, remove the bags and transfer the contents into a serving bowl. Garnish with the shredded coconut and cilantro. Serve with rice.

Poached Salmon

INGREDIENTS for Servings: 2

2 skinless, center-cut salmon fillets	Kosher salt and black pepper as needed
1 large-sized shallot, sliced into thin rings	¾ cup extra virgin olive oil
12 whole Thai basil leaves, lightly bruised	1 teaspoon ginger, minced
	3 Oz mixed greens* - optional
	1 lemon

DIRECTIONS and Cooking Time: 25 Minutes
Prepare your Sous-vide water bath to a temperature of 128-degrees Fahrenheit Season the salmon with salt and pepper and add the fillets in a heavy-duty zipper bag. Add in the shallot slices, olive oil, ginger, mixed greens and basil leaves Whisk well and seal the bag using the immersion method Submerge the bag underwater and cook for about 25 minutes Once done, transfer the greens from the bag to a serving platter Take the salmon fillets and put them on top of your serving platter Pass the rest of the mixture through a metal mesh and into a medium-sized bowl Add some lemon juice to your olive oil Mix well and drizzle the mixture on top of your salmon Serve!

Nutrition Info: Per serving:Calories: 298 ;Carbohydrate: 0g ;Protein: 27g ;Fat: 18g ;Sugar: 0g ;Sodium: 425mg

Smoky Salmon

INGREDIENTS for Servings: 3

3 salmon filets, skinless	2 tsp smoked paprika
1 tbsp sugar	1 tsp mustard powder

DIRECTIONS and Cooking Time: 1 Hour 20 Minutes
Prepare a water bath, place Sous Vide in it, and set it to 115 F. Season the salmon with 1 teaspoon of salt and place in a zipper bag. Refrigerate for 30 minutes. In a bowl, mix the sugar, smoked salt, remaining salt, and mustard powder and mix to combine. Remove the salmon from the fridge and rub with the monk powder mixture. Place salmon in a vacuum-sealable bag, release air by the water displacement method and seal the bag. Submerge in the water bath and set the timer for 45 minutes. Once the timer has stopped, remove the bag and unseal it. Remove the salmon and pat dry using a kitchen towel. Place a non – stick skillet over medium heat, add the salmon and sear it for 30 seconds. Serve with a side of steamed greens.

Singaporean Prawn Noodle

INGREDIENTS for Servings: 2

20 pieces small, tail-on shrimp	2 nests vermicelli noodle, cooked and

1 teaspoon Chinese white wine 1 teaspoon curry powder 1 tablespoon light soy sauce	drained 1 green onion, thinly sliced 2 tablespoons vegetable oil

DIRECTIONS and Cooking Time: 15 Minutes
Prepare your Sous-vide water bath to a temperature of 149-degrees Fahrenheit   Put the prawns in a resealable zip bag and seal using the immersion method   Cook for 15 minutes   Place a skillet over a medium heat   Add the vegetable oil, Chinese white wine, curry powder and soy sauce   Whisk well and add the noodles. Cook until everything is mixed   Add the prawns and toss   Top it up with some green onions. Serve!

Nutrition Info: Calories: 239 Carbohydrate: 2g Protein: 16g Fat: 7g Sugar: 0g Sodium: 443mg

Parsley Prawns With Lemon

INGREDIENTS for Servings: 4

12 large prawns, peeled and deveined 1 tsp salt 1 tsp sugar 3 tsp olive oil	1 bay leaf 1 sprig parsley, chopped 2 tbsp lemon zest 1 tbsp lemon juice

DIRECTIONS and Cooking Time: 35 Minutes
Make a water bath, place Sous Vide in it, and set to 156 F. In a bowl, add prawns, salt, and sugar, mix and let it sit for 15 minutes. Place prawns, bay leaf, olive oil, and lemon zest in a vacuum-sealable bag. Release air by the water displacement method and seal. Submerge in bath and cook for 10 minutes.Once the timer has stopped, remove and unseal the bag. Dish prawns and drizzle with lemon juice.

Monkfish Medallions

INGREDIENTS for Servings: 2

1 monkfish steak Kosher salt as needed Ground black pepper as needed	4 tablespoons unsalted butter 1 tablespoon chopped fresh parsley

DIRECTIONS and Cooking Time: 30 Minutes
Prepare your Sous-vide water bath to a temperature of 130-degrees Fahrenheit   Season the fish with pepper and salt   Add the fish in a large-sized resealable bag and seal it using the immersion method. Submerge underwater and cook for about 30 minutes   Once done, take the bag out and transfer the steak to a cutting board   Slice it into ½ inch thick medallions   Place a large-sized skillet over medium high heat   Add the butter and let it melt   Add the monkfish medallions and brown them for about 5 minutes until they turn golden brown   Remove the heat

immediately and season it thoroughly with pepper and salt   Serve with the topping of parsley

Nutrition Info: Calories: 288 Carbohydrate: 10g Protein: 18g Fat: 10g Sugar: 4g Sodium: 482mg

Dover Sole

INGREDIENTS for Servings: 2

2 sole fillets Kosher salt as needed Freshly ground black pepper 1 garlic clove, minced 4 tablespoons unsalted butter	4 tablespoons dry white wine The zest of 1 lemon 2 tablespoons fresh lemon juice Fresh parsley for garnishing, chopped

DIRECTIONS and Cooking Time: 30 Minutes
Prepare your Sous-vide water bath to a temperature of 134-degrees Fahrenheit   Season the sole with some pepper and salt   Divide the soles into their own medium-sized zip bags and divide the butter, lemon zest, wine, garlic and lemon juice between the bags   Seal the bags using the immersion method and cook for 30 minutes   Once done, remove the bags from the water and arrange them on a serving plate   Spoon some of your cooking liquid over the fish and garnish with parsley. Serve!

Nutrition Info: Per serving:Calories: 595 ;Carbohydrate: 27g ;Protein: 53g ;Fat: 28g ;Sugar: 8g ;Sodium: 370mg

Buttery Cockles With Peppercorns

INGREDIENTS for Servings: 2

4 oz canned cockles ¼ cup dry white wine 1 diced celery stalk 1 diced parsnip 1 quartered shallot 1 bay leaf 1 tbsp black peppercorns 1 tbsp olive oil 8 tbsp butter, room temperature	1 tbsp minced fresh parsley 2 garlic cloves, minced Salt to taste 1 tsp freshly cracked black pepper ¼ cup panko breadcrumbs 1 baguette, sliced

DIRECTIONS and Cooking Time: 1 Hour 30 Minutes
Prepare a water bath and place the Sous Vide in it. Set to 154 F. Place the cockles, shallots, celery, parsnip, wine, peppercorns, olive oil and bay leaf in a vacuum-sealable bag. Release air by the water displacement method, seal and submerge the bag in the water bath. Cook for 60 minutes.   Using a blender, pour the butter, parsley, salt, garlic and ground pepper. Mix at medium speed until combined. Put the mixture into a plastic bag and roll it. Move into the fridge and allow chilling.   Once the timer has stopped, remove the snail and veggies. Discard the cooking juices. Heat a skillet over high heat. Top the cockles with butter,

sprinkle some breadcrumbs over and cook for 3 minutes until melted. Serve with warm baguette slices.

Amazing Lemon Salmon With Basil

INGREDIENTS for Servings: 4

2 pounds salmon	Juice of 1 lemon
2 tbsp olive oil	¼ tsp garlic powder
1 tbsp chopped basil	Sea salt and black
Zest of 1 lemon	pepper to taste

DIRECTIONS and Cooking Time: 35 Minutes
Prepare a water bath and place the Sous Vide in it. Set to 115 F. Place the salmon in a vacuum-sealable bag. Release air by the water displacement method, seal and submerge the bag in the water bath. Cook for 30 minutes. Meanwhile, in a bowl combine well the pepper, salt, basil, lemon juice, and garlic powder until emulsified. Once the timer has stopped, remove the salmon and transfer to a plate. Reserve the cooking juices. Heat olive oil in a pan over high heat and sauté the garlic slices. Set aside the garlic. Put the salmon in the pan and cook for 3 minutes until golden. Plate and top with the garlic slices.

Shrimp Cocktail

INGREDIENTS

For Shrimp:	2 small tomatoes
1 pound raw shrimp, peeled and deveined	1 chipotle pepper in adobo sauce
salt and freshly ground black pepper, to taste	3 cloves garlic
	¼ cup tomato paste
1 tablespoon butter	1 tablespoon honey
For Cocktail Sauce:	1 tablespoon lime
¼ cup fresh cilantro, plus more for garnishing	juice
	salt and freshly ground black pepper, to taste

DIRECTIONS and Cooking Time: 35 Mins Cooking Temperature: 132°f
Attach the sous vide immersion circulator using an adjustable clamp to a Cambro container or pot filled with water and preheat to 132°F. Season shrimp evenly with salt and black pepper. Into a cooking pouch, add shrimp and butter. Seal pouch tightly after squeezing out the excess air. Place pouch in sous vide bath and set the cooking time for 15-35 minutes. Remove pouch from sous vide bath and carefully open it. Remove shrimp from pouch. With paper towels, pat shrimp completely dry. Refrigerate until chilled. For cocktail sauce: in a food processor, add all ingredients and pulse until well-combined. Remove shrimp cocktail from refrigerator. Into a large serving bowl, place cocktail sauce and shrimp. Garnish with cilantro and serve.

Juicy Scallops With Chili Garlic Sauce

INGREDIENTS for Servings: 2

2 tbsp yellow curry powder	1 tbsp lemon juice
	6 scallops
1 tbsp tomato paste	Cooked brown rice,
½ cup coconut cream	for serving
1 tsp chili garlic sauce	Fresh cilantro, chopped

DIRECTIONS and Cooking Time: 75 Minutes
Prepare a water bath and place the Sous Vide in it. Set to 134 F. Combine the coconut cream, tomato paste, curry powder, lime juice, and chili-garlic sauce. Place the mixture with the scallops in a vacuum-sealable bag. Release air by the water displacement method, seal and submerge the bag in the water bath. Cook for 60 minutes. Once the timer has stopped, remove the bag and transfer to a plate. Serve the brown rice and top with the scallops. Garnish with cilantro.

Saffron Infused Halibut

INGREDIENTS

For Halibut:	For Tomato Compote:
4 x 5-ounce boneless fresh halibut fillets, cut into thick cubes	2 tablespoons water
	3 tablespoons fresh basil, chopped
kosher salt, to taste	1 tablespoon fresh orange zest, finely chopped
⅓ cup fish broth	
3 tablespoons butter	
1 tablespoon fresh orange zest, finely chopped	½ teaspoon freshly ground black pepper
	For Zucchini:
15 Spanish saffron threads	2 zucchinis
	1 tablespoon extra-virgin olive oil
2 tablespoons extra-virgin olive oil	1 tablespoon fresh parsley, chopped
2 tablespoons garlic, finely chopped	1 tablespoon fresh mint, chopped
2 tablespoons shallots, finely chopped	1 teaspoon fresh lemon zest, grated
½ cup cherry tomatoes, halved lengthwise	pinch of salt
	For Garnish:
	2 tablespoons fresh chives, minced

DIRECTIONS and Cooking Time: 25 Mins Cooking Temperature: 140°f
Attach the sous vide immersion circulator using an adjustable clamp to a Cambro container or pot filled with water and preheat to 140°F. For the halibut: season halibut cubes with a little kosher salt and keep aside. Into a pan over a low heat, add remaining ingredients and cook for 3 minutes, beating continuously. Remove from heat. Between 2 cooking pouches, divide halibut cubes and butter

mixture evenly. Seal pouches tightly after squeezing out the excess air and keep aside. For the tomato compote: in a pan, heat oil over medium heat and sauté garlic until golden. Add water and shallots and cook for 3-4 minutes. Stir in remaining ingredients and remove from heat. Keep aside to cool. Into a cooking pouch, add tomato mixture. Seal pouch tightly after squeezing out the excess air and keep aside. For zucchini in a bowl: add all ingredients and toss to coat well. Into a cooking pouch, add zucchini mixture. Seal pouch tightly after squeezing out the excess air. Place all pouches in sous vide bath and set the cooking time for 17 minutes, plus a separate timer for 12 minutes. After 12 minutes, remove pouches of tomato compote and zucchini. Carefully, open pouches. Remove zucchini from pouch, reserving cooking liquid into bowl. Transfer tomato compote into another bowl. With vegetable peeler, shape zucchini into ribbons. Transfer zucchini ribbons into the bowl of reserved cooking liquid and toss to coat. After the full 17 minutes, remove pouches of halibut from sous vide bath and carefully open them. Remove halibut cubes from pouches. Divide zucchini ribbons onto serving plates evenly. Place fish cubes over ribbons, followed by tomato compote evenly. Garnish with chives and serve.

Swordfish Steak

INGREDIENTS for Servings: 2

2 pieces /6 ounces swordfish steaks 2 tablespoons extra virgin olive oil 4 sprigs fresh thyme	Zest and juice of 2 lemons Kosher salt as needed Freshly ground black pepper

DIRECTIONS and Cooking Time: 30 Minutes
Prepare your Sous-Vide water bath using your immersion circulator and raise the temperature to 130-degrees Fahrenheit Season the sword fish with pepper and salt and add to a zip bag Add the olive oil, lemon juice, zest, thyme and seal using the immersion method Submerge underwater and cook for 30 minutes Remove the bag from the water and take out the sword fish Pat it dry using a kitchen towel Make sure to reserve the cooking liquid Heat up your grill to 600-700 degrees Fahrenheit and add the sword fish, sear 2 minutes per side Place the dish to your serving plate and allow it to rest for about 5 minutes Divide the Swordfish amongst two serving plates and drizzle the reserved cooking liquid. Serve!

Nutrition Info: Calories: 476 Carbohydrate: 11g Protein: 32g Fat: 33g Sugar: 2g Sodium: 136mg Special Tips If you want the fish to have a brighter, shiny texture, you may spritz it with some lime before serving!

Minty Sardines

INGREDIENTS for Servings: 3

2 pounds sardines 3 garlic cloves, crushed 1 large lemon, freshly juiced	¼ cup olive oil 2 sprigs fresh mint Salt and black pepper to taste

DIRECTIONS and Cooking Time: 1 Hour 20 Minutes
Wash and clean each fish but keep the skin. Pat dry using a kitchen paper. In a large bowl, combine olive oil with garlic, lemon juice, fresh mint, salt, and pepper. Place the sardines in a large vacuum-sealable bag along with the marinade. Cook in a water bath for one hour at 104 F. Remove from the bath and drain but reserve the sauce. Drizzle fish with sauce and steamed leek.

Perfect Scallops In Citrus Sauce

INGREDIENTS for Servings: 4

2lb. scallops, cleaned 2 lemons /1 quartered, 1 zested and juiced 2 tablespoons ghee 2 shallots, chopped	¼ cup pink grapefruit juice ¼ cup orange juice 2 tablespoons acacia honey Salt and pepper, to taste

DIRECTIONS and Cooking Time: 30 Minutes
Preheat Souse Vide cooker to 122F. Rinse scallops and drain. Season scallops with salt and pepper. Divide scallops between two Sous Vide bags. Place 2 quarters lemon in each bag and vacuum seal. Cook the scallops 30 minutes. Finishing steps: Make the sauce; heat ghee in a saucepan. Add the chopped shallots and cook until tender 4 minutes. Remove the scallops from the bag and sear on both sides in a lightly greased skillet. Remove the scallops from the skillet. Deglaze the pan with orange juice. Pour in pink grapefruit juice and lemon juice. Add shallots and lemon zest. Simmer until half reduces the sauce. Stir in honey and simmer until thickened. Serve scallops with sauce.

Nutrition Info: Calories 279 Total Fat 2g Total Carb 17g Dietary Fiber 1g Protein 37g

Crispy Frog Legs

INGREDIENTS for Servings: 2

1 lb. frog legs Kosher salt and pepper as needed 2 tablespoons unsalted butter 1 minced garlic clove	1 teaspoon red pepper flakes 3 tablespoons finely chopped fresh parsley 2 tablespoon lemon juice

DIRECTIONS and Cooking Time: 45 Minutes

Prepare your Sous-vide water bath to a temperature of 135-degrees Fahrenheit Season the legs with salt and pepper   Take a large-sized, heavy-duty resealable zip bag and add the frog legs. Seal the bag using the immersion method   Submerge the bag underwater and cook for 45 minutes   Once cooked, take the bag out from the water bath and pat the legs dry using the kitchen towel   Take a non-stick skillet, place it over medium-high heat and melt the butter The moment the butter starts to brown, add the frog legs along with the red pepper flakes, garlic and season with pepper and salt   Cook for about 2 minutes, flip it, and cook for another 2 minutes Remove them from the heat and serve with lemon juice and parsley

Nutrition Info: Calories: 300 Carbohydrate: 8g Protein: 20g Fat: 3g Sugar: 1g Sodium: 212mg

Sweet Chili Shrimp Stir-fry

INGREDIENTS for Servings: 6

1½ pound shrimp	1 tbsp soy sauce
3 dried red chilis	2 tsp sugar
1 tbsp grated ginger	½ tsp cornstarch
6 garlic cloves, smashed	3 green onions, chopped
2 tbsp champagne wine	

DIRECTIONS and Cooking Time: 40 Minutes
Prepare a water bath and place the Sous Vide in it. Set to 135 F.   Combine the ginger, garlic cloves, chilis, champagne wine, sugar, soy sauce, and cornstarch. Place the peeled shrimp with the mixture in a vacuum-sealable bag. Release air by the water displacement method, seal and submerge in the water bath. Cook for 30 minutes.   Place green onions in a skillet over medium heat. Add in oil and cook for 20 seconds. Once the timer has stopped, remove the cooked shrimp and transfer to a bowl. Garnish with onion. Serve with rice.

Party Shrimp Cocktail

INGREDIENTS for Servings: 2

1 pound shrimp, peeled and deveined	4 tbsp mayonnaise
Salt and black pepper to taste	2 tsp freshly squeezed lemon juice
4 tbsp fresh dill, chopped	2 tsp tomato puree
1 tbsp butter	1 tbsp tabasco sauce
2 tbsp green onions, minced	4 oblong dinner rolls
	8 leaves of lettuce
	½ lemon, sliced into wedges

DIRECTIONS and Cooking Time: 40 Minutes
Prepare a water bath and place the Sous Vide in it. Set to 149 F. For the seasoning, combine well the mayonnaise, green onions, lemon juice, tomato puree, and Tabasco sauce. Season with salt and pepper.

Place the shrimp and seasoning in a vacuum-sealable bag. Add 1 tbsp of dill and 1/2 tbsp of butter in each pack. Release air by the water displacement method, seal and submerge the bag in the water bath. Cook for 15 minutes.   Preheat the oven over 400 F. and cook the dinner rolls for 15 minutes. Once the timer has stopped, remove the bag and drain. Put the shrimp in a bowl with the dressing and mix well. Serve on top of the lettuce rolls with lemon.

Speedy North-style Salmon

INGREDIENTS for Servings: 4

1 tbsp olive oil	Zest and juice of 1 lemon
4 salmon fillets, skin-on	2 tbsp yellow mustard
Salt and black pepper to taste	2 tsp sesame oil

DIRECTIONS and Cooking Time: 30 Minutes
Prepare a water bath and place Sous Vide in it. Set to 114 F. Season salmon with salt and pepper. Combine lemon zest and juice, oil, and mustard. Place the salmon in 2 vacuum-sealable bags with the mustard mixture. Release air by the water displacement method, seal and submerge the bags in the bath. Cook for 20 minutes. Heat sesame oil in a skillet. Once the timer has stopped, remove the salmon and pat dry. Transfer the salmon into the skillet and sear for 30 seconds per side.

Lime-parsley Poached Haddock

INGREDIENTS for Servings: 4

4 haddock fillets, skin on	6 tbsp butter
½ tsp salt	2 tsp chopped fresh parsley
Zest and juice of 1 lime	1 lime, quartered

DIRECTIONS and Cooking Time: 75 Minutes
Prepare a water bath and place the Sous Vide in it. Set to 137 F.   Season the fillets with salt and place in 2 vacuum-sealable bags. Add butter, half the lime zest and lime juice, and 1 tbsp of parsley. Release air by the water displacement method. Transfer into the fridge and allow to chill for 30 minutes. Seal and submerge the bags in the water bath. Cook for 30 minutes. Once the timer has stopped, remove the fillets and pat dry with kitchen towel. Heat the remaining butter in a skillet over medium heat and sear the fillets for 45 seconds each side, spooning the melted butter over the top. Pat dry with kitchen towel and transfer to a plate. Garnish with lime quarters and serve.

Savory Creamy Cod With Parsley

INGREDIENTS for Servings: 6

For Cod	1 cup half-and-half
6 cod fillets	cream
Salt to taste	1 finely chopped
1 tbsp olive oil	white onion
3 sprigs fresh parsley	2 tbsp dill, chopped
For Sauce	2 tsp black
1 cup white wine	peppercorns

DIRECTIONS and Cooking Time: 40 Minutes

Prepare a water bath and place the Sous Vide in it. Set to 148 F. Place seasoned with salt cod fillets in vacuum-sealable bags. Add olive oil and parsley. Release air by the water displacement method, seal and submerge the bag in the water bath. Cook for 30 minutes. Heat a saucepan over medium heat, add in wine, onion, black peppercorns and cook until reduced. Stir in half-and-half cream until thickened. Once the timer has stopped, plate the fish and drizzle with sauce.

Swordfish With Mango Salsa

INGREDIENTS

For Salsa:	3 tablespoons sugar
5½ ounces fresh raspberries, washed	3 tablespoons fine sea salt
5½ ounces fresh mango, peeled, pitted and chopped	4-4½ cups cool water
	4 x 4-ounce swordfish fillets
1½ ounces red onion, minced	½ cup butter
⅓ cup fresh cilantro, chopped	3 tablespoons balsamic vinegar
1 small jalapeño pepper, minced	1¾ tablespoons honey
	1½ tablespoons Dijon mustard
2 tablespoons fresh lime juice	salt and freshly ground white pepper,
For Swordfish:	to taste

DIRECTIONS and Cooking Time: 35 Mins Cooking Temperature: 127°f

For the salsa: to a bowl, add all ingredients and mix. Refrigerate overnight, covered. For the swordfish: in a large bowl, dissolve sugar and salt in cool water. Place swordfish fillets and refrigerate for 3 hours. Attach the sous vide immersion circulator using an adjustable clamp to a Cambro container or pot filled with water and preheat to 127°F. Into a pan, add butter and cook until golden brown, swirling pan continuously. Remove from heat and add vinegar, honey, Dijon mustard, salt and white pepper, beating until well-combined. Remove fish fillet from bowl of cold water and lightly season with salt and white pepper. Between 4 cooking pouches, divide fish fillets. Add 2-3 tablespoons of brown butter to each pouch. Seal pouches tightly after squeezing out the excess air. Place pouches in sous vide bath and set the cooking time for 30 minutes. Remove pouches from sous vide bath and carefully open them. Remove

fish fillets from pouches. With paper towels, pat fillets completely dry. With a blow torch, toast each fillet until a slight crust is formed. Divide fillets onto serving plates and drizzle evenly with brown butter. Place salsa evenly alongside each fillet and serve.

Ahi Tuna

INGREDIENTS

⅓ cup honey	¼ cup ponzu sauce
1 tablespoon chili-garlic sauce	1 pound ahi tuna

DIRECTIONS and Cooking Time: 30 Mins Cooking Temperature: 120°f

Into a small bowl, add all ingredients except tuna, and beat until well-combined. Into a cooking pouch, add tuna and honey mixture. Seal pouch tightly after squeezing out the excess air and refrigerate for 1 hour. Attach the sous vide immersion circulator using an adjustable clamp to a Cambro container or pot filled with water and preheat to 120°F. Place pouch in sous vide bath and set the cooking time for 30 minutes. Remove pouch from sous vide bath and carefully open it. Remove tuna from pouch. Cut tuna into desired sized slices, and serve immediately.

Scallop Sashimi With Yuzu Vinaigrette

INGREDIENTS for Servings: 4

4-8 dry, large-sized sea scallops	1 head Belgian endive, base trimmed up and halved lengthwise.
2 tablespoons red grapefruit juice	The halves should then be cut lengthwise
1 tablespoon soy sauce	into ¼ inch wedges
1 teaspoon lime juice	1 avocado, pitted,
1 teaspoon finely minced, medium-hot red Chili	peeled, halved and cut lengthwise into ½ inch thick slices
1 teaspoon Japanese sweet cooking wine	1 red grapefruit
1 tablespoon extra-virgin olive oil	Sea salt as needed 2 shiso leaves for serving
8 mint leaves	

DIRECTIONS and Cooking Time: 30 Minutes

Prepare your Sous-vide water bath to a temperature of 122-degrees Fahrenheit Add the scallops in a large-sized, resealable bag and seal it using the immersion method and cook for 30 minutes. Let the bags chill for 20 minutes in an ice bath While they are chilling, take a bowl and mix together the grapefruit juice, Japanese cooking wine, soy sauce, lime juice, red chili and oil until they are finely blended Taste your vinaigrette to ensure it has a nice tangy, salty flavor, sweet and spicy Transfer your chilled scallops to a cutting board and discard any excess liquid   Slice the scallops horizontally into ¼ inch thick coins using a sharp knife.   Serve with 2 shiso leaves placed in the center of a chilled plate, and arrange your scallop coins alongside the Belgian endive wedges on top   Scatter some avocado slices and grapefruit around the scallops with a final drizzle of vinaigrette   Sprinkle some salt and serve!

Nutrition Info: Calories: 232 Carbohydrate: 34g Protein: 13g Fat: 10g Sugar: 8g Sodium: 559mg

Light Sea Bass With Dill

INGREDIENTS for Servings: 3

1 pound Chilean sea bass, skinless	Salt and black pepper to taste
1 tbsp olive oil	1 tbsp dill

DIRECTIONS and Cooking Time: 35 Minutes
Prepare a water bath and place the Sous Vide in it. Set to 134 F. Season the sea bass with salt and pepper and place in a vacuum-sealable bag. Add the dill and olive oil. Release air by the water displacement method, seal and submerge the bag in the water bath. Cook for 30 minutes. Once the timer has stopped, remove the bag and transfer the sea bass to a plate.

Basic Cooked Shrimp

INGREDIENTS for Servings: 4

1 tablespoon olive oil	1 1/2 pounds large shrimp /shelled, deveined
2 sprigs chervil, parsley or tarragon	
1/2 teaspoon Kosher salt	1/2 teaspoon baking soda

DIRECTIONS and Cooking Time: 45 Minutes
Preheat water to 135°F in a sous vide cooker or with an immersion circulator.   Vacuum-seal shrimp, olive oil, herbs, salt and baking soda in a sous vide bag, or use a plastic zip-top freezer bag /remove as much air as possible from the bag before sealing. Arrange shrimp in a single layer in bag, submerge bag in water and cook for 45 minutes.   Remove shrimp from cooking bag and blot dry with paper towels. Serve as desired and enjoy!

Nutrition Info: Calories: 232; Total Fat: 6g; Saturated Fat: 1g; Protein: 39g; Carbs: 3g; Fiber: 0g; Sugar: 0g

Mussels In Fresh Lime Juice

INGREDIENTS for Servings: 2

1 pound fresh mussels, debearded	½ cup freshly squeezed lime juice
1 medium-sized onion, peeled and finely chopped	¼ cup fresh parsley, finely chopped
Garlic cloves, crushed	1 tbsp rosemary,
	finely chopped
	2 tbsp olive oil

DIRECTIONS and Cooking Time: 40 Minutes
Place mussels along with lime juice, garlic, onion, parsley, rosemary, and olive oil in a large vacuum-sealable bag. Cook en Sous Vide for 30 minutes at 122 F. Serve with green salad.

Dijon Cream Sauce With Salmon

INGREDIENTS for Servings: 2

4 skinless salmon fillets	1 tablespoon lemon juice
1 bunch of spinach	Salt and pepper as needed
½ cup Dijon mustard	
1 cup heavy cream	

DIRECTIONS and Cooking Time: 45 Minutes
Prepare your Sous-vide water bath to a temperature of 115-degrees Fahrenheit   Season the salmon with salt   Transfer to a resealable bag and seal using the immersion method. Cook for 45 minutes   Take a pan and place it on a medium heat and add the spinach and cook until wilted   Add the lemon juice, pepper and salt, and keep cooking over a low heat   Take another saucepan and place it over medium heat   Add the heavy cream and Dijon mustard. Let it all boil a bit and then lower down the heat   Mix them well and season with salt and pepper   Take out the cooked salmon, drizzle the sauce on top, assemble the spinach on the side, and serve!

Nutrition Info: Per serving:Calories: 204 ;Carbohydrate: 7g ;Protein: 28g ;Fat: 8g ;Sugar: 3g ;Sodium: 489mg

Garlic & Herbs Cod

INGREDIENTS for Servings: 2

2 medium cod fillets	2 tbsp unsalted butter
2 garlic cloves, minced	1 tbsp olive oil
1 tbsp fresh rosemary, chopped	Juice of 1 lemon
1 tbsp fresh thyme, chopped	Salt and pepper to taste

DIRECTIONS and Cooking Time: 30 Minutes
Preheat the water bath to 135ºF.   Rub the cod fillets with salt and pepper, and put them into the vacuum bag adding rosemary, thyme, butter, minced garlic and lemon juice.   Seal the bag and set the timer for 30 minutes.   When the time is up, sear the fish in a cast iron skillet in 1 tbsp olive oil on both sides and serve over white rice.

Nutrition Info: Per serving:Calories 200, Carbohydrates 18 g, Fats 8 g, Protein 22 g

Herby Lemon Salmon

INGREDIENTS for Servings: 2

2 skinless salmon fillets	1 shallot, sliced into thin rings
Salt and black pepper to taste	1 tbsp basil leaves, lightly chopped
¾ cup extra virgin olive oil	3 oz mixed greens
1 tsp allspice	1 lemon

DIRECTIONS and Cooking Time: 45 Minutes

Prepare a water bath and place the Sous Vide in it. Set to 128 F.   Place the salmon and season with salt and pepper in a vacuum-sealable bag. Add in shallot rings, olive oil, allspice, and basil. Release air by the water displacement method, seal and submerge the bag in the water bath. Cook for 25 minutes.   Once the timer has stopped, remove the bag and transfer the salmon to a plate. Mix the cooking juices with some lemon juice and top salmon fillets. Serve.

Buttered Scallops

INGREDIENTS for Servings: 3

3 tsp butter (2 tsp for cooking + 1 tsp for searing)	½ lb scallops Salt and black pepper to taste

DIRECTIONS and Cooking Time: 55 Minutes

Make a water bath, place Sous Vide in it, and set to 140 F. Pat dry scallops using a paper towel. Place scallops, salt, 2 tablespoons of butter, and pepper in a vacuum-sealable bag. Release air by the water displacement method, seal and submerge the bag in the water bath and set the timer for 40 minutes.   Once the timer has stopped, remove and unseal the bag. Pat dry the scallops using a paper towel and set aside. Set a skillet over medium heat and the remaining butter. Once it has melted, sear the scallops on both sides until golden brown. Serve with a side of buttered mixed vegetables.

Salmon Rillettes

INGREDIENTS for Servings: 2

½ lb. salmon fillets, skin and pin bones removed	2 shallots, peeled and minced
1 teaspoon sea salt	1 garlic clove, peeled and minced
6 tablespoons unsalted butter	½ oz. lemon juice

DIRECTIONS and Cooking Time: 20 Minutes

Take a Sous Vide water bath and preheat it to a temperature of 130-degrees Fahrenheit using your immersion circulator   Add the salmon fillets, unsalted butter, sea salt, garlic cloves, shallots, and lemon juice in a heavy-duty, resealable bag and seal it

using the immersion method   Submerge underwater and cook for 20 minutes   Take the salmon out from the bag and break into small portions   Divide the salmon between 8 crocks and season each of them with lemon butter sauce from the bag   Put the crocks in the fridge and chill for 2 hours   Serve as a spread with some bread slices

Nutrition Info: Calories: 277 Carbohydrate: 0g Protein: 20g Fat: 21g Sugar: 0g Sodium: 411mg

Brown Butter Scallops

INGREDIENTS

1 x 4¼-ounce package scallops	salt and freshly ground black pepper, to taste
2 teaspoons brown butter, divided	

DIRECTIONS and Cooking Time: 40 Mins Cooking Temperature: 140°f

Attach the sous vide immersion circulator using an adjustable clamp to a Cambro container or pot filled with water and preheat to 140°F.   With paper towels, pat scallops.   Into a cooking pouch, add scallops, 1 teaspoon brown butter, salt and black pepper. Seal pouch tightly after squeezing out the excess air. Place pouch in sous vide bath and set the cooking time for 35-40 minutes.   Remove pouch from sous vide bath and carefully open it. Remove scallops from pouch. With paper towels, pat scallops completely dry.   In a pan, melt remaining brown butter over high heat, and sear scallops for 30 seconds per side.   Serve immediately.

Lobster Rolls

INGREDIENTS for Servings: 2

2 lobster tails	A pinch of black pepper
1 tablespoon butter	
2 green onions, chopped	2 teaspoons lemon juice
3 tablespoons mayonnaise	Buttered Buns for serving
A pinch of salt	

DIRECTIONS and Cooking Time: 25 Minutes

Prepare your Sous-vide water bath to a temperature of 140-degrees Fahrenheit   Pour the water into a small pot and bring to a boil   Cut the lobster tails down the center from the top of the shell   Once the water has reached boiling point, submerge the lobsters and cook for 90 seconds   Remove them and soak in cold water for 5 minutes   Crack the shells and remove the tails from the shell   Add the shells in a bag and add the butter. Seal the bag using the immersion method, and cook for 25 minutes   Remove the tails from the water bath and pat them dry. Place them in a small bowl and chill for 30 minutes   Chop up the tail and mix with the mayonnaise, green onions, salt, pepper, and lime juice. Serve with some toasted, buttered buns

Nutrition Info: Per serving:Calories: 556 ;Carbohydrate: 23g ;Protein: 79g ;Fat: 21g ;Sugar: 3g ;Sodium: 513mg

Garlic Shrimps

INGREDIENTS for Servings: 4

16 shrimps, peeled and deveined	1 shallot, minced
1 tbsp unsalted butter, melted	2 garlic cloves, minced

DIRECTIONS and Cooking Time: 25 Minutes
Preheat your cooking machine to 125ºF. Put all ingredients in the vacuum bag. Seal the bag, put it into the water bath and set the timer for 25 minutes. Serve immediately as an appetizer or tossed with penne pasta.

Nutrition Info: Per serving:Calories 153, Carbohydrates 9 g, Fats 1 g, Protein 27 g

Crab Mango Salad

INGREDIENTS for Servings: 2

2 blue swimmer crabs	2 tablespoons olive oil
1 large-sized mango	1 tablespoon lime juice
¼ cup halved cherry tomatoes	1 tablespoon freshly squeezed orange juice
1 cup rocket lettuce	
¼ julienned red onion	2 teaspoons honey
Salt and pepper as needed	

DIRECTIONS and Cooking Time: 45 Minutes
Prepare your Sous-vide water bath to a temperature of 154-degrees Fahrenheit Take a pot of water and let it boil Add the crabs in and let them boil for 60 seconds Chop the legs of the crabs, using pincers, and put them in a heavy-duty, resealable bag. Zip it up using the immersion method Submerge underwater and cook for 45 minutes Add the cooked crabs to an ice bath Add all the dressing ingredients in a bowl. Mix them well Take the crab meat out of the crab and transfer to your serving dish Add the dressing to the crab meat and toss well to coat them Serve!

Nutrition Info: Calories: 148 Carbohydrate: 7g Protein: 24g Fat: 2g Sugar: 3g Sodium: 518mg

Sesame Tuna With Ginger Sauce

INGREDIENTS for Servings: 6

Tuna:	1 inch ginger, grated
3 tuna steaks	2 shallots, minced
Salt and black pepper to taste	1 red chili, minced
	3 tbsp water
⅓ cup olive oil	2 ½ lime juice

2 tbsp canola oil	1 ½ tbsp rice vinegar
½ cup black sesame seeds	2 ½ tbsp soy sauce
	1 tbsp fish sauce
½ cup white sesame seeds	1 ½ tbsp sugar
	1 bunch green lettuce
Ginger Sauce:	leaves

DIRECTIONS and Cooking Time: 45 Minutes
Start with the sauce: place a small pan over low heat and add olive oil. Once it has heated, add ginger and chili. Cook for 3 minutes Add sugar and vinegar, stir and cook until sugar dissolves. Add water and bring to a boil. Add in soy sauce, fish sauce, and lime juice and cook for 2 minutes. Set aside to cool. Make a water bath, place Sous Vide in it, and set to 110 F. Season the tuna with salt and pepper and place in 3 separate vacuum-sealable bag. Add olive oil, release air from the bag by the water displacement method, seal and submerge the bag in the water bath. Set the timer for 30 minutes. Once the timer has stopped, remove and unseal the bag. Place tuna aside. Place a skillet over low heat and add canola oil. While heating, mix sesame seeds in a bowl. Pat dry tuna, coat them in sesame seeds and sear top and bottom in heated oil until seeds start to toast. Slice tuna into thin strips. Layer a serving platter with lettuce and arrange tuna on the bed of lettuce. Serve with ginger sauce as a starter.

Seafood Mix With Tomato, Wine And Parsley

INGREDIENTS for Servings: 4

2 pounds seafood mix, thawed	1 tsp dried oregano
	2 tbsp olive oil
1 cup tomatoes in own juice, diced	Salt and pepper to taste
½ cup dry white wine	Lemon juice for sprinkling
1 bay leaf	
2 garlic cloves, minced	Chopped parsley for sprinkling

DIRECTIONS and Cooking Time: 2 Hours
Preheat your cooking machine to 140ºF. Sprinkle the thawed seafood mix with salt and pepper and put it into the vacuum bag adding tomatoes, bay leaf, dried oregano, garlic, olive oil and white wine. Seal the bag, put it into the water bath and cook for 2 hours. Serve over rice sprinkled with freshly chopped parsley and lemon juice.

Nutrition Info: Per serving:Calories 369, Carbohydrates 18 g, Fats 25 g, Protein 18 g

Shrimp Cocktail Slider

INGREDIENTS for Servings: 2

Kosher salt and pepper as needed	10 small-sized shrimps, peeled and

4 tablespoons fresh dill, chopped	de-veined
	2 teaspoons ketchup
1 tablespoon unsalted butter	Tabasco sauce
	4 small-sized, oblong dinner rolls
4 tablespoons mayonnaise	8 small-sized leaves of butter lettuce
2 tablespoons red onions, minced	½ lemon, sliced into wedges
2 teaspoons freshly squeezed lemon juice	

DIRECTIONS and Cooking Time: 15 Minutes
Prepare your Sous-vide water bath to a temperature of 149-degrees Fahrenheit   Take a bowl and add the mayonnaise, red onion, lemon juice, ketchup and Tabasco sauce in it. Whisk them well to create the seasoning   Take the mixture and season it well with pepper and salt and divide the mixture and shrimps equally between two heavy-duty, resealable plastic bags   Add 1 tablespoon of dill and ½ tablespoon of butter to each of the bags   Seal the bags using the immersion method, submerge and cook for 15 minutes   Preheat your oven to 400-degrees Fahrenheit and warm the rolls for about 10 minutes   Remove them and slice in half lengthwise   Once done, remove the contents of the bag and strain over a medium bowl   Transfer the shrimps to the bowl with the dressing. Give it a nice toss   Take 2 lettuce leaves and place the shrimp mixture on top of the lettuce rolls   Serve with lemon

Nutrition Info: Per serving: Calories: 375 ; Carbohydrate: 15g ; Protein: 17g ; Fat: 28g ; Sugar: 8g ; Sodium: 443mg

Sweet Buttered Scallops With Pancetta

INGREDIENTS for Servings: 6

12 large scallops	4 pancetta slices
1 tbsp olive oil	2 tbsp honey
Salt and black pepper to taste	2 tbsp butter

DIRECTIONS and Cooking Time: 45 Minutes
Prepare a water bath and place the Sous Vide in it. Set to 126 F.   Preheat an oven to 390 F. Combine the scallops with olive oil, salt and pepper. Place in a vacuum-sealable bag. Release air by the water displacement method, seal and submerge the bag in the water bath. Cook for 30 minutes.   Transfer the pancetta to a baking tray, lined with aluminium foil, and brush both sides with honey and pepper. Bake for 20 minutes. Transfer to a plate. Reserve the pancetta fat.   Once the timer has stopped, remove the scallops and pat dry with kitchen towel. Melt butter and 1 tbsp of the pancetta fat in a skillet over medium heat. Put the scallops and cook for 1 minute per side until golden brown. Slice the pancetta into small pieces. Plate the scallops. Garnish with pancetta.

Dill Baby Octopus Bowl

INGREDIENTS for Servings: 4

1 pound baby octopus	Salt and black pepper to taste
1 tbsp olive oil	
1 tbsp freshly squeezed lemon juice	1 tbsp dill

DIRECTIONS and Cooking Time: 60 Minutes
Prepare a water bath and place the Sous Vide in it. Set to 134 F. Place the octopus in a vacuum-sealable bag. Release air by the water displacement method, seal and submerge the bag in the water bath. Cook for 50 minutes. Once the timer has stopped, remove the octopus and pat dry. Mix the octopus with some olive oil and lemon juice. Season with salt, pepper and dill.

Halibut With Sweet Sherry & Miso Glaze

INGREDIENTS for Servings: 4

1 tbsp olive oil	2½ tbsp soy sauce
2 tbsp butter	4 fillets halibut
⅓ cup sweet sherry	2 tbsp chopped scallions
⅓ cup red miso	
¼ cup mirin	2 tbsp chopped fresh parsley
3 tbsp brown sugar	

DIRECTIONS and Cooking Time: 50 Minutes
Prepare a water bath and place the Sous Vide in it. Set to 134 F. Heat the butter in a saucepan over medium-low heat. Stir in sweet sherry, miso, mirin, brown sugar, and soy sauce for 1 minute. Set aside. Allow to cool. Place the halibut in 2 vacuum-sealable bags. Release air by the water displacement method, seal and submerge the bags in the water bath. Cook for 30 minutes.   Once the timer has stopped, remove the halibut from the bags and pat dry with kitchen towel. Reserve cooking juices. Heat a saucepan over high heat and pour in cooking juices. Cook until reduced by half.   Heat olive oil in a skillet over medium heat and transfer the fillets. Sear for 30 seconds each side until crispy. Serve the fish and drizzle with Miso Glaze. Garnish with scallions and parsley.

Coconut Cod Stew

INGREDIENTS for Servings: 6

2 pounds fresh cod /cut into fillets	Salt and freshly ground black pepper, to taste
1 can /15 ounces coconut milk /divided	1 can /15 ounces crushed tomatoes
1 tablespoon olive oil	1 teaspoon fish sauce
1 sweet onion /julienned	1 teaspoon lime juice
1 red bell pepper	Sriracha hot sauce, to

/julienned 4 garlic cloves /minced	taste 2 tablespoon chopped fresh cilantro leaves

DIRECTIONS and Cooking Time: 30 Minutes

Preheat water to 130°F in a sous vide cooker or with an immersion circulator. Season cod fillets with salt and pepper and vacuum-seal with 1/4 cup coconut milk in a sous vide bag /or use a plastic zip-top freezer bag, removing as much air as possible from the bag before sealing. Submerge bag in water and cook for 30 minutes. Immediately begin preparing the sauce. Heat olive oil in a nonstick skillet over medium-high heat and sauté onion and bell pepper until softened, 3 to 4 minutes, stirring frequently. Add garlic and sauté about 1 minute more, stirring constantly. Add undrained tomatoes, fish sauce, lime juice, sriracha sauce and remaining coconut milk and stir until thoroughly combined. Season sauce to taste with salt and pepper, reduce heat to low and simmer until the end of the cooking time for the cod, stirring occasionally. Remove cod from cooking bag, add to sauce and turn gently to coat with sauce. Let stew stand for about 5 minutes. Garnish stew with cilantro leaves to serve. Enjoy!

Nutrition Info: Calories: 400; Total Fat: 18g; Saturated Fat: 13g; Protein: 40g; Carbs: 23g; Fiber: 5g; Sugar: 2g

Pan Tomate Espelette Shrimp

INGREDIENTS for Servings: 4

1 lb. shrimps, peeled, de-veined 1 tablespoon extra-virgin olive oil ¾ teaspoon Piment d'Espelette ½ high-quality loaf of bread cut up into 1½ inch slices	Kosher salt as needed 1 garlic clove, halved 2 beefsteak tomatoes, 1 sliced horizontally, the other sliced into wedges Flaky sea salt

DIRECTIONS and Cooking Time: 25 Minutes

Prepare your Sous-vide water bath to a temperature of 122ºF Take a large-sized bowl and put the shrimps in it along with the olive oil, a pinch of kosher salt and the Piment d'Espelette Whisk it well and transfer the mixture to a large-sized heavy-duty zip bag. Seal the bag using the immersion method Submerge the bag underwater and cook for 25 minutes Place a grill pan over a medium-high heat for 5 minutes before the shrimps are done Carefully arrange the bread slices in a single layer in your pan and toast them on both sides Once toasted, remove the bread and rub one side of the slices with the garlic clove Rub the tomato halves over your toast as well and divide them between your serving plates Once cooked, remove the bag and drain the liquid Return the grill pan to a medium-high heat and add the

shrimp a single layer Sear for 10 seconds and divide the shrimps among the tomato bread Drizzle the olive oil over your shrimps Sprinkle some salt over and serve with the tomato wedges! Nutrition Info: Per serving:Calories 238, Carbohydrates 25 g, Fats 6 g, Protein 21 g

Cilantro Trout

INGREDIENTS for Servings: 4

2 pounds trout, 4 pieces 5 garlic cloves 1 cup cilantro leaves, finely chopped	1 tbsp sea salt 4 tbsp olive oil 2 tbsp rosemary, finely chopped ¼ cup freshly squeezed lemon juice

DIRECTIONS and Cooking Time: 60 Minutes

Clean and rinse well the fish. Pat dry with a kitchen paper and rub with salt. Combine garlic with olive oil, cilantro, rosemary, and lemon juice. Use the mixture to fill each fish. Place in a separate vacuum-sealable bags and seal. Cook en Sous Vide for 45 minutes at 131 F.

Coriander-garlic Squids

INGREDIENTS for Servings: 4

4 4oz. squids, cleaned ¼ cup chopped coriander 4 cloves garlic, minced 2 chili pepper, chopped	¼ cup olive oil 2 teaspoons minced ginger ¼ cup vegetable oil 1 lemon, cut into wedges Salt and pepper, to taste

DIRECTIONS and Cooking Time: 2 Hours

Set the Sous vide cooker to 136F. Place the squids and 2 tablespoons olive oil in a Sous Vide bags. Season to taste and vacuum seal the bag. Submerge in water and cook 2 hours. Finishing steps: Heat remaining olive oil in a skillet. Add garlic, chili pepper, and ginger and cook 1 minute. Add half the coriander and stir well. Remove from the heat. Remove the squids from the bag. Heat vegetable oil in a skillet, until sizzling hot. Add the squid and cook 30 seconds per side. Transfer the squids onto a plate. Top with garlic-coriander mixture and sprinkle with the remaining coriander. Serve with lemon.

Nutrition Info: Calories 346 Total Fat 29g Total Carb 7g Dietary Fiber 7g Protein 12g

Salmon With Sweet Potato Puree

INGREDIENTS for Servings: 2

2 pieces skin-on salmon fillets	¼ cup coconut milk 1 bunch rainbow

Olive oil	chard
2 sprigs thyme	1 small-sized grated
4 garlic cloves	ginger
3 pieces sweet	Soy sauce
potatoes	1 bunch radish
	Sea salt

DIRECTIONS and Cooking Time: 60 Minutes
Prepare your Sous-vide water bath to a temperature of 122-degrees Fahrenheit   Take a resealable zipper bag and add in the salmon, 2 garlic cloves, thyme, and olive oil.   Seal the bag using the immersion method, submerge underwater and cook for 1 hour   Wrap the potatoes in foil and roast them in the oven for 45 minutes at 375-degrees Fahrenheit   Cut the potatoes in half and then, carefully scoop out the flesh and put it in a blender with the coconut milk and blend them together. Season with pepper and salt   Steam the chard for 3 minutes   Take another pan and add the olive oil, minced garlic, grated ginger together with the chard and soy sauce. Sauté for a while   Cut the radish in half and drizzle the olive oil on top   Roast for 30 minutes at 375-degrees Fahrenheit   Then, sear the salmon in a hot pan with a pinch of salt   Assemble on your serving platter by placing the potato, chard and finally the salmon on top of everything   Scatter some roasted radish over and serve!

Nutrition Info: Calories: 579 Carbohydrate: 3g Protein: 42g Fat: 33g Sugar: 1g Sodium: 493mg

Yummy Cheesy Lobster Risotto

INGREDIENTS for Servings: 4

1 tall lobster, shell removed	¾ cup Arborio rice
Salt and black pepper to taste	2 tbsp red wine
	¼ cup grated Grana Padano cheese
6 tbsp butter	2 minced chives
2½ cups chicken stock	

DIRECTIONS and Cooking Time: 55 Minutes
Prepare a water bath and place the Sous Vide in it. Set to 138 F. Season the lobster with salt and pepper and place in a vacuum-sealable bag with 3 tbsp of butter. Release air by the water displacement method, seal and submerge the bag in the water bath. Cook for 25 minutes.   Heat 3 tbsp of butter in a skillet over medium heat and cook the rice. Stir in 1/4 cup of chicken stock. Keep cooking until the stock evaporated. Add 1/4 cup of chicken stock more. Repeat the process for 15 minutes until the rice is creamy.   Once the timer has stopped, remove the lobster and chop in bites. Add the lobster to the rice. Stir the remaining chicken stock and red wine. Cook until liquid is absorbed. Top with Grana Padano cheese and season with salt and pepper. Garnish with chives and more cheese.

Sage Salmon With Coconut Potato Mash

INGREDIENTS for Servings: 2

2 salmon fillets, skin-on	4 garlic cloves
	¼ cup coconut milk
2 tbsp olive oil	1 bunch rainbow chard
2 sprigs sage	
3 potatoes, pelled and chopped	1 tbsp grated ginger
	1 tbsp soy sauce
	Sea salt to taste

DIRECTIONS and Cooking Time: 1 Hour 30 Minutes
Prepare a water bath and place the Sous Vide in it. Set to 122 F. Place salmon, sage, garlic, and olive oil in a vacuum-sealable bag. Release air by the water displacement method, seal and submerge the bag in the water bath. Cook for 1 hour.   Heat an oven to 375 F. Brush the potatoes with oil and bake for 45 minutes. Transfer potatoes to a blender and add in coconut milk. Season with salt and pepper. Blend for 3 minutes, until smooth.   Heat olive oil in a skillet over medium heat and sauté ginger, chard and soy sauce.   Once the timer has stopped, remove the salmon and transfer to a hot pan. Sear for 2 minutes. Transfer to a plate, add the potato mash, and top with char to serve.

APPETIZERS & SNACKS

Carrots & Nuts Stuffed Peppers

INGREDIENTS for Servings: 5

4 shallots, chopped	1 tbsp soy sauce
4 carrots, chopped	1 tbsp ground cumin
4 garlic cloves, minced	2 tsp paprika
1 cup raw cashews, soaked and drained	1 tsp garlic powder
1 cup pecans, soaked and drained	1 pinch cayenne pepper
1 tbsp balsamic vinegar	4 fresh thyme sprigs
	Zest of 1 lemon
	4 bell peppers, tops cut off and seeded

DIRECTIONS and Cooking Time: 2 Hours 35 Minutes
Prepare a water bath and place the Sous Vide in it. Set to 186 F.   Combine in a blender the carrots, garlic, shallots, cashews, pecans, balsamic vinegar, soy sauce, cumin, paprika, garlic powder, cayenne, thyme, and lemon zest. Mix until roughly.   Pour the mixture into the bell peppers shells and place in a vacuum-sealable bag. Release air by the water displacement method, seal and submerge the bag in the water bath. Cook for 1 hour and 15 minutes. Once the timer has stopped, remove the peppers and transfer to a plate.

Stuffed Collard Greens

INGREDIENTS for Servings: 3

1 pound collard greens, steamed	1 tbsp olive oil
1 pound lean ground beef	Salt and black pepper to taste
1 small onion, finely chopped	1 tsp fresh mint, finely chopped

DIRECTIONS and Cooking Time: 65 Minutes
Boil a large pot of water and add in greens. Briefly cook, for 2-3 minutes. Drain and gently squeeze the greens and set aside.   In a large bowl, combine ground beef, onion, oil, salt, pepper, and mint. Stir well until incorporated. Place leaves on your work surface, vein side up. Use one tablespoon of the meat mixture and place it in the bottom center of each leaf. Fold the sides over and roll up tightly. Tuck in the sides and gently transfer to a large vacuum-sealable bag. Seal the bag and cook in sous vide for 45 minutes at 167 F.

Luxury And Rich French Fondue

INGREDIENTS for Servings: 12

1 clove garlic, cut in half	3 tablespoons flour
1 cup dry white wine	3 tablespoons Kirsch
12 ounces Swiss	1/4 teaspoon freshly grated nutmeg
cheese, shredded	A pinch of paprika
12 ounces Cheddar cheese	Salt and ground black pepper, to taste

DIRECTIONS and Cooking Time: 40 Minutes
Preheat a sous vide water bath to 170 degrees F. Rub the inside of a pan with the garlic halves. In the pan, cook wine over a high heat; bring to a boil and turn the heat to medium-low.   In a mixing bowl, combine cheeses and flour; now, gradually stir this mixture into the wine.   Continue cooking until cheese is melted completely. Transfer this mixture to cooking pouches; add the remaining ingredients and seal tightly.   Submerge the cooking pouches in the water bath; cook for 35 minutes.   Pour your fondue into a warm serving bowl and serve immediately.

Nutrition Info: 191 Calories; 14g Fat; 3g Carbs; 16g Protein; 4g Sugars

Herby And Garlicky Corn On The Cob

INGREDIENTS for Servings: 6

2 sticks butter, melted	1 teaspoon shallot powder
1 tablespoon paprika	6 ears corn
1 tablespoon fresh chives, chopped	Flaked sea salt and white pepper, to taste
1 teaspoon granulated garlic	

DIRECTIONS and Cooking Time: 30 Minutes
Preheat a sous vide water bath to 183 degrees F. Toss corn on the cob with all ingredients.   Place the seasoned corn in cooking pouches; seal tightly. Submerge the cooking pouches in the water bath; cook for 25 minutes.   Taste, adjust the seasonings, and serve right away. Bon appétit!

Nutrition Info: 397 Calories; 37g Fat; 32g Carbs; 6g Protein; 2g Sugars

Citrus Chili Shrimp

INGREDIENTS for Servings: 4

2 pounds fresh shrimps, cleaned and deveined	¼ teaspoon black pepper, ground
1 large lemon, freshly juiced	½ teaspoon sea salt
tablespoons olive oil	¼ teaspoon chili pepper, ground
2 tablespoons fresh parsley, finely chopped	Serve with: Spring onions and lemon wedges

DIRECTIONS and Cooking Time: 45 Minutes;

Clean and devein the shrimps. Rinse under cold running water and pat dry with a kitchen paper. In a medium bowl, combine shrimps along with other ingredients and refrigerate to marinate for 20 minutes. Now, place the shrimps along with all juices in a large Ziploc bag. Seal the bag and cook en sous vide for 45 minutes at 131 degrees.

Nutrition Info: Calories: 395 Total Fat: 19g Saturated Fat: 2g; Trans Fat: 0g Protein: 59g; Net Carbs: 9g

Spicy Cauliflower Steaks

INGREDIENTS for Servings: 5

1 pound cauliflower, sliced	1 tsp sriracha
1 tbsp turmeric	1 tbsp chipotle
1 tsp chili powder	1 tbsp heavy
½ tsp garlic powder	2 tbsp butter

DIRECTIONS and Cooking Time: 35 Minutes
Prepare a water bath and place the Sous Vide in it. Set to 185 F. Whisk together all of the ingredients, except cauliflower. Brush the cauliflower steaks with the mixture. Place them in a vacumm-sealable bag. Release air by the water displacement method, seal and submerge the bag in water bath.Set the timer for 18 minutes. Once the timer has stopped, remove the bag and preheat your grill and cook the steaks for a minute per side.

Apple Cider Smelts

INGREDIENTS for Servings: 4

1 pound smelts, cleaned	½ cup extra-virgin olive oil
1 cup apple cider vinegar	1 teaspoon dried thyme
½ cup white wine	1 teaspoon sea salt
1 tablespoon fresh rosemary, finely chopped	Serve with: Steamed bell peppers

DIRECTIONS and Cooking Time: 45 Minutes;
In a large bowl, combine apple cider with wine, olive oil, rosemary, thyme, and sea salt. Submerge smelts in this mixture and refrigerate for one hour. Remove the fish from the marinade and drain but reserve the liquid. Place in a large Ziploc and cook en sous vide for 40 minutes at 122 degrees. Drizzle with some marinade before serving.

Nutrition Info: Calories: 397 Total Fat: 29g Saturated Fat: 3g; Trans Fat: 0g Protein: 27g; Net Carbs: 1g

Cheesy Taco Dip

INGREDIENTS for Servings: 10

1 pound pork, ground	3 garlic cloves, chopped
1/2 pound beef, ground	12 ounces cream of celery soup
1 teaspoon Taco seasoning	1 cup processed American cheese
1/2 cup medium-hot taco sauce	Sea salt and ground black pepper, to taste
1 cup shallots, chopped	

DIRECTIONS and Cooking Time: 2 Hours 5 Minutes
Preheat a sous vide water bath to 140 degrees F. Place all ingredients in cooking pouches; seal tightly. Submerge the cooking pouches in the water bath; cook for 2 hours. Season, adjust the seasonings and serve with veggie sticks or tortilla chips. Enjoy!

Nutrition Info:195 Calories; 12g Fat; 7g Carbs; 24g Protein; 2g Sugars

Traditional French Béarnaise Sauce

INGREDIENTS for Servings: 12

4 tablespoons Champagne vinegar	1/2 cup dry white wine
1 tablespoon fresh tarragon, finely chopped	5 egg yolks
3 tablespoons shallots, finely chopped	2 sticks butter, melted
	1 tablespoon fresh lemon juice

DIRECTIONS and Cooking Time: 45 Minutes
Preheat a sous vide water bath to 148 degrees F. In a pan, place the vinegar, wine, tarragon, and shallots; bring to a rolling boil. Turn down heat to simmer. Continue cooking for 12 minutes. Strain the mixture through a fine-mesh strainer into a food processor. Fold in the egg yolks and blitz mixture until uniform and smooth. Place the sauce in cooking pouches; seal tightly. Submerge the cooking pouches in the water bath; cook for 25 minutes. Add the contents from the cooking pouches to a mixing dish; add the butter and lemon juice; mix with an immersion blender until smooth. Serve with your favorite roasted vegetable bites. Bon appétit!

Nutrition Info:175 Calories; 12g Fat; 1g Carbs; 4g Protein; 3g Sugars

Nutty Baked Sweet Potatoes

INGREDIENTS for Servings: 2

1 pound sweet potatoes, sliced	¼ cup walnuts
Salt to taste	1 tbsp coconut oil

DIRECTIONS and Cooking Time: 3 Hours 45 Minutes
Prepare a water bath and place the Sous Vide in it. Set to 146 F. Place the potatoes and salt in a vacuum-sealable bag. Release air by the water displacement method, seal and submerge the bag in the water bath.

Cook for 3 hours. Heat a skillet over medium heat and toast the walnuts. Chop them. Preheat the over to 375 F and lined a baking tray with parchment foil. Once the timer has stopped, remove the potatoes and transfer to the baking tray. Sprinkle with coconut oil and bake for 20-30 minutes. Toss once. Serve topped with toasted walnuts.

Tarragon Asparagus Mix

INGREDIENTS for Servings: 3

1 ½ lb medium asparagus	1 tbsp parsley, chopped
5 tbsp butter	1 tbsp + 1 tbsp fresh dill, chopped
2 tbsp lemon juice	
½ tsp lemon zest	1 tbsp + 1 tbsp tarragon, chopped
1 tbsp chives, sliced	

DIRECTIONS and Cooking Time: 25 Minutes
Make a water bath, place the Sous Vide in it, and set to 183 F. Cut off and discard the tight bottoms of the asparagus. Place the asparagus in a vacuum-sealable bag. Release air by the water displacement method, seal and submerge in water bath and set timer for 10 minutes. Once the timer has stopped, remove the bag and unseal. Place a skillet over low heat, add in butter and steamed asparagus. Season with salt and pepper and toss continually. Add lemon juice and zest and cook for 2 minutes. Turn heat off and add parsley, 1 tablespoon of dill, and 1 tablespoon of tarragon. Toss evenly. Garnish with remaining dill and tarragon. Serve warm as a side dish.

Paprika & Rosemary Potatoes

INGREDIENTS for Servings: 4

8 oz fingerling potatoes	1 tbsp butter
Salt and black pepper to taste	1 sprig rosemary
	1 tsp paprika

DIRECTIONS and Cooking Time: 55 Minutes
Prepare a water bath and place the Sous Vide in it. Set to 178 F. Combine the potatoes with salt, paprika and pepper. Place them in a vacuum-sealable bag. Release air by the water displacement method, seal and submerge the bag in the water bath. Cook for 45 minutes. Once the timer has stopped, remove the potatoes and cut by the half. Heat the butter in a skillet over medium heat and stir in rosemary and potatoes. Cook for 3 minutes. Serve in a plate. Garnish with salt.

Salmon With Curried Tomatoes

INGREDIENTS for Servings: 4

2 pounds salmon fillets	3 tablespoons fresh basil, chopped
1 cup grape tomatoes,	½ teaspoon sea salt
diced	¼ teaspoon black pepper, ground
1 tablespoon red curry paste	Serve with:
tablespoons olive oil	Steamed asparagus

DIRECTIONS and Cooking Time: 40 Minutes;
Wash the grape tomatoes and finely dice. Set aside. Rinse the salmon fillets under cold running water and pat dry with a kitchen paper. Gently rub the fillets with salt and pepper and place in a large Ziploc bag along with olive oil, basil, curry, and diced tomatoes. Seal the bag and cook en sous vide for 40 minutes at 131 degrees.

Nutrition Info: Calories: 444 Total Fat: 22g Saturated Fat: 4g; Trans Fat: 0g Protein: 45g; Net Carbs: 2g

Beef Patties

INGREDIENTS for Servings: 4

1 pound lean ground beef	2 garlic cloves, crushed
1 egg	¼ cup olive oil
2 tbsp almonds, finely chopped	Salt and black pepper to taste
2 tbsp almond flour	¼ cup parsley leaves, finely chopped
1 cup onions, finely chopped	

DIRECTIONS and Cooking Time: 1 Hour 55 Minutes
In a bowl, combine ground beef with finely chopped onions, garlic, oil, salt, pepper, parsley, and almonds. Mix well with a fork and gradually add some almond flour. Whisk in one egg and refrigerate for 40 minutes. Remove the meat from the refrigerator and gently form into one-inch-thick patties, about 4-inches in diameter. Place in a two separate vacuum-sealable bags and cook in sous vide for one hour at 129 F.

Gingery Squash Veggies

INGREDIENTS for Servings: 8

14 ounces butternut squash	1 tsp lemon juice
1 tbsp grated ginger	Salt and black pepper to taste
1 tsp butter, melted	¼ tsp turmeric

DIRECTIONS and Cooking Time: 70 Minutes
Prepare a water bath and place the Sous Vide in it. Set to 185 F. Peel and slice the squash into wedges. Place all the ingredients in a vacuum-sealable bag. Shake to coat well. Release air by the water displacement method, seal and submerge the bag in water bath. Set the timer for 55 minutes. Once the timer has stopped, remove the bag. Serve warm.

Scallops With Bacon

INGREDIENTS for Servings: 6

10 ounces scallops	½ onion, grated
3 ounces bacon, sliced	½ tsp white pepper
	1 tbsp olive oil

DIRECTIONS and Cooking Time: 50 Minutes
Prepare a water bath and place the Sous Vide in it. Set to 140 F. Top the scallops with the grated onion and wrap with bacon slices. Sprinkle with white pepper and drizzle with oil. Place in a plastic bag. Release air by the water displacement method, seal and submerge the bag in water bath.Set the timer for 35 minutes. Once the timer has stopped, remove the bag. Serve.

Oven Baked Yam Chips

INGREDIENTS for Servings: 4

Coarse sea salt and freshly ground black pepper, to taste	1 pound yams, peeled and cubed
2 tablespoons extra-virgin olive oil	1/2 teaspoon Hungarian paprika
	1/3 teaspoon ancho chili powder

DIRECTIONS and Cooking Time: 1 Hour 30 Minutes
Preheat a sous vide water bath to 183 degrees F. Season the yams with salt and pepper. Add the yams to a cooking pouch; seal tightly. Submerge the cooking pouch in the water bath; cook for 60 minutes. Remove the yams from the cooking pouch and pat them dry. Preheat an oven to 350 degrees F. Arrange the yams on a parchment-lined baking sheet in a single layer. Drizzle olive oil over sous vide yams; sprinkle Hungarian paprika and ancho chili powder over them. Bake approximately 25 minutes. Bon appétit!

Nutrition Info:193 Calories; 9g Fat; 36g Carbs; 8g Protein; 6g Sugars

Cherry Chicken Bites

INGREDIENTS for Servings: 3

1 pound chicken breast, boneless and skinless, cut into bite-sized pieces	1 cup cherry tomatoes, whole
1 cup red bell pepper, chopped into chunks	1 cup olive oil
	1 tsp Italian seasoning mix
1 cup green bell pepper, chopped into chunks	1 tsp cayenne pepper
	½ tsp dried oregano
	Salt and black pepper to taste

DIRECTIONS and Cooking Time: 1 Hour And 40 Minutes
Rinse the meat under cold running water and pat dry with a kitchen paper. Cut into bite-sized pieces and set aside. Wash the bell peppers and cut them into chunks. Wash the cherry tomatoes and remove the green stems. Set aside. In a bowl, combine olive oil with Italian seasoning, cayenne, salt, and pepper. Stir until well incorporated. Add the meat and coat well with the marinade. Set aside for 30 minutes to allow flavors to meld and penetrate into the meat. Place the meat along with vegetables in a large vacuum-sealable bag. Add three tablespoons of the marinade and seal the bag. Cook in sous vide for 1 hour at 149 F.

Winter Lamb Stew

INGREDIENTS for Servings: 3

1 pound lamb neck fillets	2 tablespoons extra-virgin olive oil
1 cup green beans, chopped	¼ cup of lemon juice, freshly juiced
1 small red bell pepper, chopped	½ teaspoon salt
1 garlic clove, crushed	¼ teaspoon black pepper, ground
1 small carrot, chopped	Serve with:
	Cabbage salad

DIRECTIONS and Cooking Time: 1 Hour
Wash the meat under cold running water and pat dry with a kitchen paper. Cut into bite-sized pieces and rub with salt, pepper, garlic. Drizzle with lemon juice and set aside. Wash the green beans and carrot. Cut into small pieces and set aside. Wash the bell pepper and cut in half. Remove the seeds and chop into small pieces. Set aside. Place the meat along with vegetables and olive oil in a large Ziploc bag. Seal the bag and cook en sous vide for 1 hour at 154 degrees.

Nutrition Info: Calories: 399 Total Fat: 27g Saturated Fat: 5g; Trans Fat: 0g Protein: 49g; Net Carbs: 8g

Buttery Yams

INGREDIENTS for Servings: 4

1 pound yams, sliced	½ cup heavy cream
8 tbsp butter	Salt to taste

DIRECTIONS and Cooking Time: 1 Hour 10 Minutes
Prepare a water bath and place the Sous Vide in it. Set to 186 F. Combine the heavy cream, yams, kosher salt, and butter. Place in a vacuum-sealable bag. Release air by the water displacement method, seal and submerge the bag in the water bath. Cook for 60 minutes. Once the timer has stopped, remove the bag and pour the contents into a bowl. Using a Food processor mix well and serve.

Mustard Drumsticks

INGREDIENTS for Servings: 5

2 pounds chicken drumsticks	2 tbsp coconut aminos
	1 tsp pink Himalayan

¼ cup Dijon mustard 2 garlic cloves, crushed	salt ½ tsp black pepper

DIRECTIONS and Cooking Time: 1 Hour

Rinse drumsticks under cold running water. Drain in a large colander and set aside. In a small bowl, combine Dijon with crushed garlic, coconut aminos, salt, and pepper. Spread the mixture over the meat with a kitchen brush and place in a large vacuum-sealable bag. Seal the bag and cook in sous vide for 45 minutes at 167 F.

Cod Bite Balls

INGREDIENTS for Servings: 5

12 ounces minced cod 2 ounces bread 1 tbsp butter ¼ cup flour 1 tbsp semolina	2 tbsp water 1 tbsp minced garlic Salt and black pepper to taste ¼ tsp paprika

DIRECTIONS and Cooking Time: 105 Minutes

Prepare a water bath and place the Sous Vide in it. Set to 125 F.   Combine the bread and water and mash the mixture. Add in the remaining ingredients and mix well to combine. Make balls out of the mixture. Spray a skillet with cooking spray and cook the bite balls over medium heat about 15 seconds per side, until lightly toasted. Place the cod bites in a vacuum-sealable bag. Release air by the water displacement method, seal and submerge the bag in water bath. Set the timer for 1 hour and 30 minutes. Once the timer has stopped, remove the bag and plate the cod bites. Serve.

Party-friendly Mini Sliders

INGREDIENTS for Servings: 8

1/2 pound ground sirloin Sea salt and freshly ground black pepper, to taste 1 /25-ounce envelope onion soup mix 4 tablespoons mayonnaise	1/2 pound ground pork 1 tablespoon Dijon mustard 1 banana shallot, chopped 3/4 pound Gorgonzola cheese, crumbled 16 miniature burger buns

DIRECTIONS and Cooking Time: 3 Hours 15 Minutes

Preheat a sous vide water bath to 145 degrees F. Thoroughly combine ground meat, salt, pepper, and envelope onion soup mix in a mixing dish. Shape the mixture into 16 meatballs with your hands. Flatten each portion into a small patty, about 1/2-inches-thick.   Transfer the prepared patties to cooking pouches; seal tightly.   Submerge the cooking pouches in the water bath; cook for 3 hours.   Heat a

grill pan over medium-high flame. Grill burgers for 1 to 2 minutes on each side, working in batches. Divide the mayonnaise, mustard and shallot among the bottom buns. Now, top each with a slider, and finish with Gorgonzola cheese. Cover with the top of the bun and serve immediately.

Nutrition Info: 314 Calories; 24g Fat; 18g Carbs; 26g Protein; 5g Sugars

Spinach & Mushroom Quiche

INGREDIENTS for Servings: 2

1 cup of fresh Cremini mushrooms, sliced 1 cup of fresh spinach, chopped 2 large eggs, beaten 2 tbsp whole milk	1 garlic clove, minced ¼ cup Parmesan cheese, grated 1 tbsp butter ½ tsp salt

DIRECTIONS and Cooking Time: 20 Minutes

Wash the mushrooms under cold running water and thinly slice them. Set aside. Wash the spinach thoroughly and roughly chop it. In a large vacuum-sealable bag, place mushrooms, spinach, milk, garlic, and salt. Seal the bag and cook in sous vide for 10 minutes at 180 F. Meanwhile, melt the butter in a large saucepan over a medium heat. Remove the vegetable mixture from the bag and add to a saucepan. Cook for 1 minute, and then add beaten eggs. Stir well until incorporated and cook until eggs are set. Sprinkle with grated cheese and remove from heat to serve.

Beef Pepper Meat

INGREDIENTS for Servings: 2

pound beef tenderloin, cut into bite-sized pieces 1 large onion finely chopped 1 tablespoon butter, melted 1 tablespoon fresh parsley, finely chopped 1 teaspoon dried thyme, ground	1 tablespoon lemon juice, freshly squeezed 1 tablespoon tomato paste ½ teaspoon sea salt ½ teaspoon black pepper, freshly ground Serve with: Cooked carrots

DIRECTIONS and Cooking Time: 6 Hours

Combine the ingredients in a large Ziploc bag. Seal the bag and cook en sous vide for 6 hours at 158 degrees. Remove from the water bath and open the bag. Serve immediately.

Nutrition Info: Calories: 560 Total Fat: 27g Saturated Fat: 16g; Trans Fat: 0g Protein: 61g; Net Carbs: 1g

Spicy Pickled Beets

INGREDIENTS for Servings: 4

12 oz beets, sliced	2/3 cup white vinegar
½ jalapeno pepper	2/3 cup water
1 diced garlic clove	2 tbsp pickling spice

DIRECTIONS and Cooking Time: 50 Minutes
Prepare a water bath and place the Sous Vide in it. Set to 192 F. In 5 mason jars, combine jalapeño pepper, beets and garlic cloves. Heat a saucepan and boil the pickling spice, water and white vinegar. Drain and pour over the beets mixture inside the jars. Seal and submerge the jars in the water bath. Cook for 40 minutes. Once the timer has stopped, remove the jars and allow cooling. Serve.

Glazed Baby Carrots

INGREDIENTS for Servings: 4

1 cup baby carrots	Salt and black pepper
4 tbsp brown sugar	to taste
1 cup chopped shallot	1 tbsp dill
1 tbsp butter	

DIRECTIONS and Cooking Time: 3 Hours 10 Minutes
Prepare a water bath and place Sous Vide in it. Set to 165 F. Place all the ingredients in a vacuum-sealable bag. Shake to coat. Release air by the water displacement method, seal and submerge in water bath.Set the timer for 3 hours. Once the timer has stopped, remove the bag. Serve warm.

Kaffir Lime Drumsticks

INGREDIENTS for Servings: 7

16 ounces chicken drumsticks	Salt and white pepper to taste
2 tbsp cilantro leaves	1 tbsp olive oil
1 tsp dried mint	1 tbsp chopped Kaffir lime leaves
1 tsp thyme	

DIRECTIONS and Cooking Time: 80 Minutes
Prepare a water bath and place the Sous Vide in it. Set to 153 F. Place all the ingredients in a vacuum-sealable bag. Massage to coat the chicken well. Release air by the water displacement method, seal and submerge the bag in water bath. Set the timer for 70 minutes. Once done, remove the bag. Serve warm.

Classic Ragout

INGREDIENTS for Servings: 3

1 pound lamb chops, cut into 1-inch thick pieces	1 medium-sized tomato, chopped
2 small carrots, finely chopped	½ teaspoon salt
	½ tablespoon Cayenne pepper,
½ cup of green peas tablespoons extra-virgin olive oil	ground
	¼ teaspoon black pepper, ground
	Serve with:
	Fresh lettuce salad

DIRECTIONS and Cooking Time: 1 Hour 20 Minutes;
Wash the lamb chops under cold running water and pat dry with a kitchen paper. Rub the lamb chops with salt, Cayenne pepper, and black pepper. Set aside. Wash the carrots and tomato. Peel and chop into small pieces. Set aside. Place the meat along with olive oil and green peas in a large Ziploc bag. Seal the bag and cook for 1 hour at 158 degrees. Remove the bag from the water bath and set aside to cool for a while. Transfer all to a heavy-bottomed pot and add carrots and tomato. Add one cup of water and bring it to a boil. Reduce the heat to low and cover with a lid. Cook for 20 minutes and remove from the heat.

Nutrition Info: Calories: 492 Total Fat: 24g Saturated Fat: 6g; Trans Fat: 0g Protein: 46g; Net Carbs: 19g

Italian Chicken Fingers

INGREDIENTS for Servings: 3

1 pound chicken breast, boneless and skinless	½ tsp cayenne pepper
	2 tsps mixed Italian herbs
1 cup almond flour	¼ tsp black pepper
1 tsp minced garlic	2 eggs, beaten
1 tsp salt	¼ cup olive oil

DIRECTIONS and Cooking Time: 2 Hours 20 Minutes
Rinse the meat under cold running water and pat dry with a kitchen paper. Season with mixed Italian herbs and place in a large vacuum-sealable. Seal the bag and cook in sous vide for 2 hours at 167 F. Remove from the water bath and set aside. Now combine together flour, salt, cayenne, Italian herbs, and pepper in a bowl and set aside. In a separate bowl, beat the eggs and set aside. Heat up olive oil in a large skillet, over medium heat. Dip the chicken into the beaten egg and coat with the flour mixture. Fry for 5 minutes on each side, or until golden brown.

Mushroom Beef Tips

INGREDIENTS for Servings: 3

1 pound beef stew meat, cubed	1 cup beef stock
	½ teaspoon salt
1 cup button mushrooms, chopped	¼ teaspoon black pepper, ground
1 small onion, chopped	2 tablespoons olive oil
	Serve with:
1 garlic clove, crushed	Fresh tomato salad

DIRECTIONS and Cooking Time: 8 Hours 15 Minutes;
In a medium bowl, combine meat, garlic, onion, olive oil, salt, and pepper. Mix well and place all in a large

Ziploc bag. Seal the bag and cook for 8 hours at 185 degrees.   Remove the meat from the water bath and set aside to cool for a while. Transfer all to a heavy-bottomed pot and add beef stock and mushrooms. Stir well and bring it to a boil. Reduce the heat to low and cover with a lid. Add some water if needed and cook for 10 more minutes.

Nutrition Info: Calories: 383 Total Fat: 19g Saturated Fat: 5g; Trans Fat: 0g Protein: 48g; Net Carbs: 6g

Cheesy And Crispy Polenta Squares

INGREDIENTS for Servings: 6

1/2 pound polenta	2 cups water
2 cups broth, preferably homemade	1 stick butter, diced
1/2 cup Monterey-Jack cheese, freshly grated	Salt and pepper, to taste
	1 teaspoon paprika

DIRECTIONS and Cooking Time: 2 Hours 20 Minutes
Preheat a sous vide water bath to 185 degrees F. Add the polenta, water, broth and butter to cooking pouches; seal tightly.   Submerge the cooking pouches in the water bath; cook for 2 hours 10 minutes.   Place sous vide polenta in a mixing bowl. Add shredded cheese, salt, pepper, and paprika; stir to combine well. Spoon the polenta into a baking pan; cover and chill overnight.   Cut polenta into squares and spritz with a nonstick cooking spray.   Place under a preheated broiler for 6 to 7 minutes, flipping halfway through. You can top polenta squares with some extra cheese if desired. Bon appétit!

Nutrition Info: 225 Calories; 12g Fat; 1g Carbs; 1g Protein; 3g Sugars

Kielbasa Bites In Beer And Apple Jelly Sauce

INGREDIENTS for Servings: 12

2 ½ pounds kielbasa, cut into 1/2-inch thick slices	2 bay leaves
4 ounces lager beer	1 /18-ounce jar apple jelly
1 teaspoon mixed whole peppercorns	2 tablespoons spicy brown mustard

DIRECTIONS and Cooking Time: 2 Hours 5 Minutes
Preheat a sous vide water bath to 150 degrees F. Place kielbasa, beer, bay leaves, and peppercorns in cooking pouches; add apple jelly and mustard; seal tightly.   Submerge the cooking pouches in the water bath; cook for 2 hours. Serve with cocktail sticks.

Nutrition Info: 241 Calories; 12g Fat; 5g Carbs; 11g Protein; 7g Sugars

Lobster Tails

INGREDIENTS for Servings: 6

1 pound lobster tails, pelled	¼ tsp onion powder
½ lemon	1 tbsp rosemary
½ tsp garlic powder	1 tsp olive oil

DIRECTIONS and Cooking Time: 50 Minutes
Prepare a water bath and place the Sous Vide in it. Set to 140 F.   Season lobster with garlic and onion powder. Place in a vacuum-sealable bag. Add the rest of the ingredients and shake to coat. Release air by the water displacement method, seal and submerge the bag in water bath.Set the timer for 40 minutes. Once the timer has stopped, remove the bag. Serve warm.

Pickled Pineapple Salsa

INGREDIENTS for Servings: 4

1/2 pineapple, peeled, cored and chopped	1 red onion, sliced
1 jalapeno pepper, stemmed, seeded and finely chopped	1/2 teaspoon whole allspice
	2 whole cloves
1/3 cup white distilled vinegar	1/2 teaspoon ground ginger
1/2 teaspoon coriander seeds	1 bay leaf, crumbled
	1 cinnamon stick
1/2 teaspoon mustard seed	Kosher salt and freshly ground black pepper, to taste

DIRECTIONS and Cooking Time: 40 Minutes
Preheat a sous vide water bath to 145 degrees F. Divide all ingredients among cooking pouches and seal tightly.   Submerge the cooking pouches in the water bath; cook for 35 minutes.   Remove the contents of the cooking pouches to a bowl and let it cool down fully. Store in a clean glass jar for up to a week. Enjoy!

Nutrition Info: 58 Calories; 2g Fat; 13g Carbs; 7g Protein; 14g Sugars

Creamy Artichoke Dip

INGREDIENTS for Servings: 6

2 tbsp butter	18 oz frozen spinach, thawed
2 onions, quartered	
3 cloves garlic, minced	5 oz green chilies
15 oz artichoke hearts, chopped	3 tbsp mayonnaise
	3 tbsp whipped cream cheese

DIRECTIONS and Cooking Time: 1 Hour 45 Minutes
Make a water bath, place Sous Vide in it, and to 181 F. Divide onions, garlic, artichoke hearts, spinach, and green chilies into 2 vacuum-sealable bags. Release air by the water displacement method, seal and submerge the bags in the water bath. Set the timer for

30 minutes to cook. Once the timer has stopped, remove and unseal the bags. Puree the ingredients using a blender. Place a pan over medium heat and add in butter. Put in vegetable puree, lemon juice, mayonnaise, and cream cheese. Season with salt and pepper. Stir and cook for 3 minutes. Serve warm with vegetable strips.

Vanilla Apricots With Whiskey

INGREDIENTS for Servings: 4

2 apricots, pitted and quartered	½ cup ultrafine sugar
	1 tsp vanilla extract
½ cup rye whiskey	Salt to taste

DIRECTIONS and Cooking Time: 45 Minutes
Prepare a water bath and place Sous Vide in it. Set to 182 F. Place all ingredients in a vacuum-sealable bag. Release air by the water displacement method, seal and submerge in water bath. Cook for 30 minutes. Once the timer has stopped, remove the bag and transfer into an ice bath.

Dijon Chicken Filets

INGREDIENTS for Servings: 4

1 pound chicken filets	1 tbsp lemon zest
3 tbsp Dijon mustard	1 tsp thyme
2 onions, grated	1 tsp oregano
2 tbsp cornstarch	Garlic salt and black
½ cup milk	pepper to taste
	1 tbsp olive oil

DIRECTIONS and Cooking Time: 65 Minutes
Prepare a water bath and place the Sous Vide in it. Set to 146 F. Whisk together all the ingredients and place in a vacuum-sealable bag. Release air by the water displacement method, seal and submerge the bag in water bath.Set the timer for 45 minutes. Once the timer has stopped, remove the bag and transfer to a saucepan and cook over medium heat for 10 minutes.

Broccoli & Blue Cheese Mash

INGREDIENTS for Servings: 6

1 head broccoli, cut into florets	3 tbsp butter
	1 tbsp parsley
Salt and black pepper to taste	5 oz blue cheese, crumbled

DIRECTIONS and Cooking Time: 1 Hour 40 Minutes
Prepare a water bath and place the Sous Vide in it. Set to 186 F. Place broccoli, butter, salt, parsley, and black pepper in a vacuum-sealable bag. Release air by the water displacement method, seal and submerge the bag in the water bath. Cook for 1 hour and 30 minutes. Once the timer has stopped, remove the bag and transfer into a blender. Put the cheese inside

and mix on high speed for 3-4 minutes until smooth. Serve.

Orange Duck With Paprika & Thyme

INGREDIENTS for Servings: 4

16 ounces duck legs	1 tbsp orange juice
1 tsp orange zest	2 tsp sesame oil
2 tbsp Kaffir leaves	½ tsp paprika
1 tsp salt	½ tsp thyme
1 tsp sugar	

DIRECTIONS and Cooking Time: 15 Hours 10 Minutes
Prepare a water bath and place the Sous Vide in it. Set to 160 F. Dump all the ingredients in a vacuum-sealable bag. Massage to combine well. Release air by the water displacement method, seal and submerge the bag in water bath.Set the timer for 15 hours. Once the timer has stopped, remove the bag. Serve warm.

Jarred Pumpkin Bread

INGREDIENTS for Servings: 4

1 egg, beaten	1 tsp cinnamon
6 tbsp canned pumpkin puree	¼ tsp nutmeg
	1 tbsp sugar
6 ounces flour	¼ tsp salt
1 tsp baking powder	

DIRECTIONS and Cooking Time: 3 Hours 40 Minutes
Prepare a water bath and place the Sous Vide in it. Set to 195 F. Sift the flour along with the baking powder, salt, cinnamon, and nutmeg in a bowl. Stir in beaten egg, sugar and pumpkin puree. Mix to form a dough. Divide the dough between two mason jars and seal. Place in water bath and cook for 3 hours and 30 minutes. Once the time passed, remove the jars and let it cool before serving.

Aromatic Lamb With Dill

INGREDIENTS for Servings: 4

2 pounds lamb, tender cuts	3 tablespoons fresh dill, finely chopped
1 tablespoon sea salt	2 basil leaves, whole
½ cup vegetable oil	Serve with:
1 teaspoon freshly ground red pepper	Sour cream

DIRECTIONS and Cooking Time: 6 Hours 15 Minutes; Rinse well the meat and place on a clean working surface. Using a sharp paring knife, cut into 3-inches long and 2-inces thick pieces. Place in a Ziploc along with other ingredients. Cook en sous vide for 6 hours at 140 degrees. Remove from the water bath and set aside.   Preheat the oven to 400 degrees. Line some baking paper over a baking sheet and place lamb cuts along with sauce.   Bake for 15 minutes, or until lightly charred on top.   Serve with sour cream.

Nutrition Info: Calories: 670 Total Fat: 41g Saturated Fat: 13g; Trans Fat: 0g Protein: 62g; Net Carbs: 6g

Ahi Tuna Steak

INGREDIENTS for Servings: 4

2 pounds Ahi tuna steaks	¼ cup fresh coriander, finely chopped
3 garlic cloves, minced	½ teaspoon cumin, ground
2 tablespoons lemon juice, freshly juiced	½ teaspoon salt
4 tablespoons olive oil	¼ teaspoon black pepper, ground
½ teaspoon smoked paprika	Serve with: Steamed bell peppers

DIRECTIONS and Cooking Time: 45 Minutes;
Rinse the steaks under cold running water and pat dry with a kitchen paper. Set aside.   In a large bowl, combine olive oil, lemon juice, garlic, paprika, cumin, salt, and pepper. Mix well and add the meat. Coat the steaks and refrigerate for 30 minutes in this marinade. Now, place all in a large Ziploc bag. Seal the bag and cook en sous vide for 45 minutes at 131 degrees. Remove the steaks from the bag and sprinkle with fresh coriander.

Nutrition Info: Calories: 545 Total Fat: 24g Saturated Fat: 7g; Trans Fat: 0g Protein: 62g; Net Carbs: 3g

Turkey Salad With Cucumber

INGREDIENTS for Servings: 3

pound turkey breasts, skinless and boneless, cut into bite-sized pieces	1 medium-sized tomato, chopped
½ cup chicken broth	1 large red bell pepper, chopped
garlic cloves, minced	1 medium-sized cucumber
tablespoons olive oil	½ teaspoon Italian seasoning
1 teaspoon salt	Serve with:
¼ teaspoon Cayenne pepper	Greek Yogurt
2 bay leaves	

DIRECTIONS and Cooking Time: 2 Hours
Using a sharp paring knife, gently remove the skin from the breast. Cut the meat into half-inch thick slices and then into bite-sized pieces. Rinse well and season with salt, and cayenne pepper. Place in a large Ziploc along with chicken broth, garlic, and bay leaves. Seal the bag and cook en sous vide for 2 hours at 167 degrees. Remove from the water bath and set aside. Wash and prepare the vegetables. Place in a large bowl. Add turkey breast and season with Italian

seasoning mix and olive oil. Toss well to combine and serve immediately.

Nutrition Info: Calories: 415 Total Fat: 23g Saturated Fat: 6g; Trans Fat: 0g Protein: 41g; Net Carbs: 6g

Chicken Liver Spread

INGREDIENTS for Servings: 8

1pound chicken liver	2 tbsp soy sauce
6 eggs	3 tbsp vinegar
8 ounces bacon, minced	Salt and black pepper to taste
3 ounces shallot, chopped	4 tbsp butter
	½ tsp paprika

DIRECTIONS and Cooking Time: 5 Hours 15 Minutes
Prepare a water bath and place the Sous Vide in it. Set to 156 F.   Cook the bacon in a skillet over medium heat, add shallots and cook for 3 minutes. Stir in the soy sauce and vinegar. Transfer to a blender along with the remaining ingredients. Blend until smooth. Place all the ingredients in a mason jar and seal. Cook for 5 hours. Once the timer has stopped, remove the jar and serve.

Ginger Balls

INGREDIENTS for Servings: 3

1 pound ground beef	¼ cup fresh mint, finely chopped
1 cup onions, finely chopped	2 tsp ginger paste
3 tbsp olive oil	1 tsp cayenne pepper
¼ cup fresh cilantro, finely chopped	2 tsps salt

DIRECTIONS and Cooking Time: 1 Hour 30 Minutes
In a large bowl, combine ground beef, onions, olive oil, cilantro, mint, cilantro, ginger paste, cayenne pepper, and salt. Mold patties and refrigerate for 15 minutes. Remove from the refrigerator and transfer to separate vacuum-sealable bags. Cook in Sous Vide for 1 hour at 154 F.

Cheesy Pears With Walnuts

INGREDIENTS for Servings: 2

1 pear, sliced	2 cups rocket leaves
1 pound honey	Salt and black pepper to taste
½ cup walnuts	2 tbsp lemon juice
4 tbsp shaved Grana Padano cheese	2 tbsp olive oil

DIRECTIONS and Cooking Time: 55 Minutes
Prepare a water bath and place the Sous Vide in it. Set to 158 F. Combine the honey and pears. Place in a vacuum-sealable bag. Release air by the water displacement method, seal and submerge the bag in the water bath. Cook for 45 minutes. Once the timer

has stopped, remove the bag and transfer into a bowl. Top with the dressing.

White Wine Mussels

INGREDIENTS for Servings: 3

3 tbsp extra virgin olive oil 1 cup onions, finely chopped ¼ cup fresh parsley, finely chopped	1 pound fresh mussels 3 tbsp fresh thyme, chopped 1 tbsp lemon zest 1 cup dry white wine

DIRECTIONS and Cooking Time: 1 Hour 20 Minutes
In a medium-sized skillet, Heat the oil. Add onions and stir-fry until translucent. Add lemon zest, parsley, and thyme. Give it a good stir and transfer to a vacuum-sealable bag. Add mussels and one cup of dry white wine. Seal the bag and cook in Sous Vide for 40 minutes at 104 F.

Chicken & Mushrooms In Marsala Sauce

INGREDIENTS for Servings: 2

2 chicken breasts, boneless and skinless 1 cup Marsala wine 1 cup chicken broth 14 ounces mushrooms, sliced ½ tbsp flour	1 tbsp butter Salt and black pepper to taste 2 garlic cloves, minced 1 shallot, minced

DIRECTIONS and Cooking Time: 2 Hours 25 Minutes
Prepare a water bath and place the Sous Vide in it. Set to 140 F. Season the chicken with salt and pepper and place in a vacuum-sealable bag along with the mushrooms. Release air by the water displacement method, seal and submerge in water bath. Cook for 2 hours. Once the timer has stopped, remove the bag. Melt the butter in a pan over medium heat, whisk in the flour and the remaining ingredients. Cook until the sauce thickens. Add chicken and cook for 1 minute.

Milky Mashed Potatoes With Rosemary

INGREDIENTS for Servings: 4

2 pounds red potatoes 5 garlic cloves 8 oz butter 1 cup whole milk	3 sprigs rosemary Salt and white pepper to taste

DIRECTIONS and Cooking Time: 1 Hour 45 Minutes
Prepare a water bath and place the Sous Vide in it. Set to 193 F. Wash the potatoes and peel them and slice. Take the garlic, peel and mash them. Combine the potatoes, garlic, butter, 2tbsp of salt, and rosemary. Place in a vacuum-sealable bag. Release air by the water displacement method, seal and submerge the bag in the water bath. Cook for 1 hour and 30 minutes. Once the timer has stopped, remove the bag and transfer into a bowl and mash them. Stir the blended butter and milk. Season with salt and pepper. Top with rosemary and serve.

Spinach And Mushroom Quiche

INGREDIENTS for Servings: 2

1 cup of fresh Cremini mushrooms, sliced 1 cup of fresh spinach, chopped 2 large eggs, beaten 2 tablespoons whole milk	1 garlic clove, minced ¼ cup Parmesan cheese, grated 1 tablespoon butter ½ teaspoon salt Serve with: Greek yogurt

DIRECTIONS and Cooking Time: 5 Minutes;
Wash the mushrooms under cold running water and thinly slice them. Set aside. Wash the spinach thoroughly and roughly chop it. In a large Ziploc bag, place mushrooms, spinach, milk, garlic, and salt. Seal the bag and cook en sous vide for 10 minutes at 180 degrees. Meanwhile, melt the butter in a large saucepan over a medium-high heat. Remove the vegetable mixture from the bag and add it to a saucepan. Cook for 1 minute, and then add beaten eggs. Stir well until incorporated and cook until eggs are set. Just before removing from the heat, sprinkle with grated cheese. Serve warm.

Nutrition Info: Calories: 283 Total Fat: 19gSaturated Fat: 13g; Trans Fat: 0g Protein: 24g; Net Carbs: 5g

Tamari Corn On The Cob

INGREDIENTS for Servings: 8

1 pound corn on cob 1 tbsp butter ¼ cup tamari sauce	2 tbsp miso paste 1 tsp salt

DIRECTIONS and Cooking Time: 3 Hours 15 Minutes
Prepare a water bath and place the Sous Vide in it. Set to 185 F. Whisk together the tamari, butter, miso, and salt. Place the corn in a plastic bag and pour the mixture over. Shake to coat. Release air by the water displacement method, seal and submerge the bag in water bath.Set the timer for 3 hours. Once the timer has stopped, remove the bag. Serve warm.

Bacon-wrapped Turkey Leg

INGREDIENTS for Servings: 5

14 ounces turkey leg 5 ounces bacon, sliced	1 tbsp sour cream ½ tsp oregano

½ tsp chili flakes	½ tsp paprika
2 tsp olive oil	¼ lemon, sliced

DIRECTIONS and Cooking Time: 6 Hours 15 Minutes
Prepare a water bath and place the Sous Vide in it. Set to 160 F. Combine in a bowl the herbs and spices with the sour cream and brush over the turkey. Wrap in bacon and drizzle with olive oil. Place in a vacuum-sealable bag along with lemon. Release air by the water displacement method, seal and submerge the bag in water bath. Set timer for 6 hours. Once the timer has stopped, remove the bag and slice. Serve warm.

Cinnamon Persimmon Toast

INGREDIENTS for Servings: 6

4 Bread Slices, toasted	½ tsp Cinnamon
4 Persimmons, chopped	2 tbsp Orange Juice
3 tbsp Sugar	½ tsp Vanilla Extract

DIRECTIONS and Cooking Time: 4 Hours 10 Minutes
Prepare a water bath and place the Sous Vide in it. Set to 155 F. Place persimmons in a vacuum-sealable bag. Add in orange juice, vanilla extract, sugar, and cinnamon. Close the bag and shake well to coat the persimmon pieces. Release air by the water displacement method, seal and submerge the bag in water bath. Set the timer for 4 hours. Once the timer has stopped, remove the bag and transfer the persimmons to a food processor. Blend until smooth. Spread the persimmon mixture over toasted bread.

Radish Cheese Dip

INGREDIENTS for Servings: 4

30 small radishes, green leaves removed	1 cup water for steaming
1 tbsp Chardonnay vinegar	1 tbsp grapeseed oil
Sugar to taste	12 oz cream cheese

DIRECTIONS and Cooking Time: 1 Hour 15 Minutes
Make a water bath, place Sous Vide in it, and set to 183 F. Put the radishes, salt, pepper, water, sugar, and vinegar in a vacuum-sealable bag. Release air from the bag, seal and submerge in the water bath. Cook for 1 hour. Once the timer has stopped, remove the bag, unseal and transfer the radishes with a little of the steaming water into a blender. Add cream cheese and puree to get a smooth paste. Serve.

Chicken Wings With Ginger

INGREDIENTS for Servings: 4

2 pounds chicken wings	1 tsp cayenne pepper
	1 tbsp fresh thyme,

¼ cup extra virgin olive oil	finely chopped
4 garlic cloves	1 tbsp fresh ginger, grated
1 tbsp rosemary leaves, finely chopped	¼ cup lime juice
1 tsp white pepper	½ cup apple cider vinegar

DIRECTIONS and Cooking Time: 2 Hours 25 Minutes
Rinse the chicken wings under cold running water and drain in a large colander. In a large bowl, combine olive oil with garlic, rosemary, white pepper, cayenne pepper, thyme, ginger, lime juice, and apple cider vinegar. Submerge wings in this mixture and cover. Refrigerate for one hour. Transfer the wings along with the marinade in a large vacuum-sealable bag. Seal the bag and cook in sous vide for 1 hour and 15 minutes at 149 F. Remove from the vacuum-sealable bag and brown before serving. Serve and enjoy!

Sous Vide Pickled Rhubarb

INGREDIENTS for Servings: 8

2 pounds rhubarb, sliced	1 tbsp brown sugar
	¼ celery stalk, minced
7 tbsp apple cider vinegar	¼ tsp salt

DIRECTIONS and Cooking Time: 40 Minutes
Prepare a water bath and place the Sous Vide in it. Set to 180 F. Place all the ingredients in a vacuum-sealable bag. Shake to coat well. Release air by the water displacement method, seal and submerge the bag in water bath. Cook for 25 minutes. Once the timer has stopped, remove the bag. Serve warm.

Sweet Thighs With Sun-dried Tomatoes

INGREDIENTS for Servings: 7

2 pounds chicken thighs	1 yellow onions, chopped
3 ounces sun dried tomatoes, chopped	1 tbsp sugar
	2 tbsp olive oil
1 tsp rosemary	1 egg, beaten

DIRECTIONS and Cooking Time: 75 Minutes
Prepare a water bath and place the Sous Vide in it. Set to 149 F. Combine all the ingredients in a vacuum-sealable bag and shake to coat well. Release air by the water displacement method, seal and submerge the bag in water bath. Set the timer for 63 minutes. Once the timer has stopped, remove the bag and serve as desired.

Hot Chicken Wings

INGREDIENTS for Servings: 4

| 2 pound chicken wings | ¼ cup hot red sauce |
| ½ butter stick, melted | ½ tsp salt |

DIRECTIONS and Cooking Time: 4 Hours 15 Minutes
Prepare a water bath and place Sous Vide in it. Set to 170 F. Season chicken with salt and place in 2 vacuum-sealable bags. Release air by the water displacement method, seal and submerge in bath. Cook for 4 hours. Once done, remove the bags. Whisk the sauce and butter. Toss the wings with the mixture.

Sweet Tofu Kebabs With Veggies

INGREDIENTS for Servings: 8

1 zucchini, sliced	1 eggplant, sliced
1 yellow bell pepper, chopped	16 ounces tofu cheese
	¼ cup olive oil
1 red bell pepper, chopped	1 tsp honey
	Salt and black pepper to taste
1 green bell pepper, chopped	

DIRECTIONS and Cooking Time: 65 Minutes
Prepare a water bath and place the Sous Vide in it. Set to 186 F. Place the zucchini and eggplant in a vacuum-sealable bag. Place the bell pepper chunks in a vacuum-sealable bag. Release air by the water displacement method, seal and submerge the bags in the water bath. Cook for 45 minutes. After 10 minutes, heat a skillet over medium heat. Strain the tofu and pat dry. Chop into cubes. Brush with olive oil and transfer to the skillet and sear until golden brown each side. Transfer into a bowl, pour in honey and cover. Allow to chill. Once the timer has stopped, remove the bags and transfer all the contents into a bowl. Season with salt and pepper. Discard cooking juices. Place the veggies and tofu, alternating, into the kebabs.

Turkey Meatballs

INGREDIENTS for Servings: 4

12 ounces ground turkey	1 tbsp butter
	Salt and black pepper to taste
2 tsp tomato sauce	
1 egg	1 tbsp breadcrumbs
1 tsp cilantro	½ tsp thyme

DIRECTIONS and Cooking Time: 2 Hours 10 Minutes
Prepare a water bath and place the Sous Vide in it. Set to 142 F. Combine all the ingredients in a bowl. Shape the mixture into meatballs. Place in a vacuum-sealable bag. Release air by the water displacement method, seal and submerge the bag in water bath.Set the timer for 2 hours. Once the timer has stopped, remove the bag. Serve warm.

Curried Zucchinis

INGREDIENTS for Servings: 3

3 small zucchinis, diced	Salt and black pepper to taste
2 tsp curry powder	¼ cup cilantro
1 tbsp olive oil	

DIRECTIONS and Cooking Time: 40 Minutes
Make a water bath, place Sous Vide in it, and set to 185 F. Place zucchinis in a vacuum-sealable bag. Release air by the water displacement method, seal and submerge the bag in the water bath. Cook for 20 minutes. Once the timer has stopped, remove and unseal the bag. Place a skillet over medium, add olive oil. Once it has heated, add the zucchinis and the remaining listed ingredients. Season with salt and stir-fry for 5 minutes. Serve as a side dish.

Buttery & Sweet Duck

INGREDIENTS for Servings: 7

2 pounds duck wings	1 tsp black pepper
2 tbsp sugar	1 tsp salt
3 tbsp butter	1 tbsp tomato paste
1 tbsp maple syrup	

DIRECTIONS and Cooking Time: 7 Hours 10 Minutes
Prepare a water bath and place the Sous Vide in it. Set to 175 F. Whisk together the ingredients in a bowl and brush the wings with the mixture. Place the wings in a vacuum-sealable bag and pour over the remaining mixture. Release air by the water displacement method, seal and submerge the bag in water bath.Set the timer for 7 hours. Once the timer has stopped, remove the bag and slice. Serve warm.

Rich And Easy Pizza Dip

INGREDIENTS for Servings: 12

10 ounces Cottage cheese, at room temperature	1/2 teaspoon dried basil
	1/2 pound ground pork
2 cups Colby cheese, freshly grated	1 ounce pepperoni, sliced
1 cup Romano cheese, shredded	2 tablespoons green pepper, chopped
3/4 cup pasta sauce	1/4 cup black olives, sliced
1/2 teaspoon dried parsley	

DIRECTIONS and Cooking Time: 3 Hours 20 Minutes
Preheat a sous vide water bath to 145 degrees F. Divide all ingredients among cooking pouches, except for Colby cheese; seal tightly. Submerge the cooking pouches in the water bath; cook for 3 hours. Preheat your oven to 380 degrees F. Spritz a pie dish with a nonstick cooking spray. Transfer the contents of cooking pouches to the prepared pie dish. Top with

a freshly grated Colby cheese. Bake for 15 minutes or until it is done to your liking. Bon appétit!

Nutrition Info:230 Calories; 17g Fat; 4g Carbs; 14g Protein; 8g Sugars

Cayenne Potato Strips With Mayo Dressing

INGREDIENTS for Servings: 6

2 large gold potatoes, cut into strips	1 tsp paprika
Salt and black pepper to taste	½ tsp cayenne pepper
	1 egg yolk
1½ tbsp olive oil	2 tbsp cider vinegar
1 tsp thyme	¾ cup vegetable oil
	Salt and black pepper to taste

DIRECTIONS and Cooking Time: 1 Hour 50 Minutes
Prepare a water bath and place the Sous Vide in it. Set to 186 F. Place the potatoes with a pinch of salt in a vacuum-sealable bag. Release air by the water displacement method, seal and submerge in water bath. Cook for 1 hour and 30 minutes.   Once the timer has stopped, remove the potatoes and pat dry with kitchen towel. Discard cooking juices. Heat oil in a pan over medium heat. Add in fries and sprinkle with paprika, cayenne, thyme, black pepper, and the remaining salt. Stir for 7 minutes until the potatoes turn golden brown on all sides.   To make the mayo: mix well egg yolk and half of vinegar. Slowly, pour in veggie oil, while stirring, until smooth. Add the remaining vinegar. Season with salt and pepper and mix well. Serve with fries.

Bbq Tofu

INGREDIENTS for Servings: 8

15 ounces tofu	1 tsp onion powder
3 tbsp barbecue sauce	1 tsp salt
2 tbsp tamari sauce	

DIRECTIONS and Cooking Time: 2 Hours 15 Minutes
Prepare a water bath and place the Sous Vide in it. Set to 180 F.   Cut the tofu into cubes. Place it in a plastic bag. Release air by the water displacement method, seal and submerge the bag in water bath.Set the timer for 2 hours.   Once the timer has stopped, remove the bag and transfer to a bowl. Add the remaining ingredients and toss to combine.

Italian-style Tomato Dipping Sauce

INGREDIENTS for Servings: 10

2 pounds very ripe tomatoes, chopped with juices	Sea salt and ground black pepper, to taste
	1 teaspoon red pepper

1 cup scallions, chopped	flakes
3 cloves roasted garlic, pressed	1 teaspoon sugar
	2 tablespoons extra-virgin olive oil
2 teaspoons dried Italian herb seasoning	1 cup Parmigiano-Reggiano cheese, preferably freshly grated
2 heaping tablespoons fresh cilantro, roughly chopped	

DIRECTIONS and Cooking Time: 45 Minutes
Preheat a sous vide water bath to 180 degrees F. Add all ingredients, minus cheese, to cooking pouches; seal tightly. Submerge the cooking pouches in the water bath; cook for 40 minutes.   Place the prepared sous vide sauce in a serving bowl; top with grated Parmigiano-Reggiano cheese and serve with breadsticks. Bon appétit!

Nutrition Info:71 Calories; 3g Fat; 6g Carbs; 3g Protein; 4g Sugars

Delicious Artichokes With Simple Dip

INGREDIENTS for Servings: 6

6 artichokes, trimmed and cut into halves	6 cloves garlic, peeled
1 ½ sticks butter, room temperature	2 teaspoons lemon zest
	1/2 cup sour cream
Sea salt and freshly ground black pepper, to taste	1/2 cup mayonnaise

DIRECTIONS and Cooking Time: 1 Hour
Preheat a sous vide water bath to 183 degrees F. Place trimmed artichokes along with butter, garlic, lemon zest, salt and black pepper in cooking pouches; seal tightly. Submerge the cooking pouches in the water bath; cook for 50 minutes. Remove artichokes from the water bath and pat them dry. Then, blow torch artichokes to get the char marks.   Place artichokes on a serving platter.   In a bowl, mix the sour cream and mayonnaise. Serve artichokes with sour cream-mayo dip on the side. Bon appétit!

Nutrition Info:314 Calories; 21g Fat; 21g Carbs; 3g Protein; 9g Sugars

Tilapia In Soy Sauce

INGREDIENTS for Servings: 2

pound tilapia fillets	½ teaspoon sea salt
1 medium-sized carrot, sliced	¼ teaspoon black pepper, ground
1 medium-sized red pepper, finely chopped	1 tablespoon fresh parsley, finely chopped
tablespoons soy sauce	Serve with:
tablespoons olive oil	Lamb's lettuce

DIRECTIONS and Cooking Time: 1 Hour And 15 Minutes;

Rub each fillet with soy sauce and sprinkle with salt, pepper, and parsley. Place in a large Ziploc along with sliced carrot and finely chopped red bell pepper. Seal the bag and cook en sous vide for 1 hour and ten minutes at 131 degrees. Remove from the water bath and set aside. Heat up the olive oil in a large skillet, over medium-high heat. Add fillets and briefly cook for 2 minutes on each side, until nice golden brown color. Remove from the heat and serve.

Nutrition Info: Calories: 344 Total Fat: 12g Saturated Fat: 9g; Trans Fat: 0g Protein: 46g; Net Carbs: 7g

Shrimp Appetizer

INGREDIENTS for Servings: 8

1 pound shrimps	½ cup parsley
3 tbsp sesame oil	Salt and white pepper
3 tbsp lemon juice	to taste

DIRECTIONS and Cooking Time: 75 Minutes
Prepare a water bath and place the Sous Vide in it. Set to 140 F. Place all ingredients in a vacuum-sealable bag. Shake to coat the shrimp well. Release air by the water displacement method, seal and submerge the bag in water bath. Set the timer for 1 hour. Once the timer has stopped, remove the bag. Serve warm.

Spicy Butter Corn

INGREDIENTS for Servings: 5

5 ears yellow corn, husked	5 tbsp butter
1 tablespoon fresh parsley	½ tsp Cayenne pepper
	Salt to taste

DIRECTIONS and Cooking Time: 35 Minutes
Prepare a water bath and place the Sous Vide in it. Set to 186 F. Place 3 ears of corn in each vacuum-sealable bag. Release air by the water displacement method, seal and submerge the bags in the water bath. Cook for 30 minutes. Once the timer has stopped, remove the corn from the bags and transfer into a plate. Garnish with cayenne pepper and parsley.

Baby Carrots With Creamy Sesame Dressing

INGREDIENTS for Servings: 6

1 ½ pounds baby carrots	1 tablespoon lemon juice
Sea salt and white pepper, to taste	1 teaspoon maple syrup
2 teaspoons olive oil	1/3 cup sesame seeds, toasted
1 tablespoon fresh	
parsley, minced	1 tablespoon fresh dill leaves, chopped
1 tablespoon mint, minced	1/2 teaspoon mustard powder
Dressing:	
1/3 cup sour cream	

DIRECTIONS and Cooking Time: 1 Hour
Preheat a sous vide water bath to 183 degrees F. Add baby carrots, salt, white pepper, olive oil, parsley, and mint to cooking pouches; seal tightly. Submerge the cooking pouches in the water bath; cook for 55 minutes. Now, make the dressing by mixing all ingredients. Dress sous vide baby carrots and serve at room temperature. Enjoy!

Nutrition Info: 129 Calories; 1g Fat; 18g Carbs; 1g Protein; 6g Sugars

Asparagus With Garlic Dipping Sauce

INGREDIENTS for Servings: 8

1 ½ pounds asparagus spears, halved lengthwise	4 garlic cloves, minced
1/2 stick butter, melted	1/4 cup sour cream
	1/4 cup mayonnaise
Sea salt and black pepper, to taste	10 garlic cloves, smashed
1/2 cup plain yogurt	Salt and pepper, to taste

DIRECTIONS and Cooking Time: 40 Minutes
Preheat a sous vide water bath to 183 degrees F. Place asparagus spears, butter, salt, black pepper, and 4 garlic cloves in a large-sized cooking pouch; seal tightly. Submerge the cooking pouch in the water bath; cook for 30 minutes. In a bowl, mix the remaining ingredients to prepare a dipping sauce. Serve asparagus with garlic dipping sauce and enjoy!

Nutrition Info: 232 Calories; 15g Fat; 9g Carbs; 2g Protein; 7g Sugars

Kale Two-cheese Dip

INGREDIENTS for Servings: 10

1/2 pound Cottage cheese	2 garlic cloves, smashed
4 ounces Colby cheese, shredded	1 sun-dried Thai chili, finely chopped
1 cup ale	1 teaspoon mustard powder
1/4 cup Thai fish sauce	Sea salt and ground black pepper, to taste
1 cup kale leaves, chopped	

DIRECTIONS and Cooking Time: 50 Minutes
Preheat a sous vide water bath to 183 degrees F. Place all ingredients in cooking pouches; seal tightly. Submerge the cooking pouches in the water bath;

cook for 45 minutes.   Serve with tortilla chips, breadsticks or veggie chips. Enjoy!

Nutrition Info: 79 Calories; 6g Fat; 8g Carbs; 7g Protein; 1g Sugars

Chili Hummus

INGREDIENTS for Servings: 9

16 ounces chickpeas, soaked overnight and drained	¼ tsp chili powder
	½ tsp chili flakes
	½ cup olive oil
2 garlic cloves, minced	1 tbsp salt
1 tsp sriracha	6 cups water

DIRECTIONS and Cooking Time: 4 Hours 15 Minutes
Prepare a water bath and place the Sous Vide in it. Set to 195 F. Place the chickpeas and water in a plastic bag. Release air by the water displacement method, seal and submerge the bag in water bath.Set the timer for 4 hours.   Once the timer has stopped, remove the bag, drain the water and transfer the chickpeas to a food processor. Add in the remaining ingredients. Blend until smooth.

Onion & Bacon Muffins

INGREDIENTS for Servings: 5

1 onion, chopped	1 egg
6 ounces bacon, chopped	1 tsp baking soda
	1 tbsp vinegar
1 cup flour	¼ tsp salt
4 tbsp butter, melted	

DIRECTIONS and Cooking Time: 3 Hours 45 Minutes
Prepare a water bath and place the Sous Vide in it. Set to 196 F.   Meanwhile, in a skillet over medium heat, cook the bacon until crispy. Transfer to a bowl and add in onion to the bacon grease and cook for a few minutes, until soft.   Transfer to a bowl and stir in the remaining ingredients. Divide the muffin batter into 5 small jars. Make sure not to fill more than halfway. Place the jars into a water bath and set the timer for 3 hours and 30 minutes. Once the timer stopped, remove the jars and serve.

Leek & Garlic Eggs

INGREDIENTS for Servings: 2

2 cups fresh leek, chopped into bite-sized pieces	1 tbsp butter
	2 tbsp extra virgin olive oil
5 garlic cloves, whole	4 large eggs
	1 tsp salt

DIRECTIONS and Cooking Time: 35 Minutes
Whisk together eggs, butter, and salt. Transfer to a vacuum-sealable bag and cook in Sous Vide for ten minutes at 165 F. Gently transfer to a plate. Heat the

oil in a large skillet over medium heat. Add garlic and chopped leek. Stir-fry for ten minutes. Remove from the heat and use to top eggs.

Panko Yolk Croquettes

INGREDIENTS for Servings: 5

2 eggs plus 5 yolks	¼ tsp italian seasoning
1 cup panko breadcrumbs	
	½ tsp salt
3 tbsp olive oil	¼ tsp paprika
5 tbsp flour	

DIRECTIONS and Cooking Time: 60 Minutes
Prepare a water bath and place the Sous Vide in it. Set to 150 F. Place the yolk inside the water (without a bag or glass) and cook for 45 minutes, turning over halfway through. Let cool slightly. Beat the eggs along with the other ingredients, except the oil. Dip the yolks in the egg and panko mixture.   Heat the oil in a skillet. Fry the yolks for a few minutes per side, until golden.

Herrings With Kale

INGREDIENTS for Servings: 3

1 pound herrings, cleaned	1 tablespoon fresh basil, finely chopped
4 tablespoons extra virgin olive oil	1 teaspoon dried thyme, ground
2 tablespoons lime juice, freshly squeezed	2 garlic cloves, crushed
1 teaspoon sea salt	¾ cup fresh kale
¼ teaspoon red pepper flakes	1 teaspoon butter
	Serve with: Greek yogurt

DIRECTIONS and Cooking Time: 45 Minutes;
Wash the fish under cold running water and place in a large bowl. Add oil, lime juice, salt, pepper, basil, thyme, and garlic. Rub each fish with this mixture and refrigerate for one hour.   Transfer to a large Ziploc bag along with the marinade and cook en sous vide for 40 minutes at 122 degrees.   Meanwhile, melt the butter in a medium-sized saucepan over a medium-high heat. Add kale and cook for five minutes, until tender. Remove from the heat and serve with fish.

Nutrition Info: Calories: 487 Total Fat: 38g Saturated Fat: 7g; Trans Fat: 0g Protein: 49g; Net Carbs: 3g

Turkey In Orange Sauce

INGREDIENTS for Servings: 2

1 pound turkey breasts, skinless and boneless	1 teaspoon Cayenne pepper, ground
	½ teaspoon salt
1 tablespoon butter	¼ teaspoon black pepper, ground
3 tablespoons fresh	

orange juice	Serve with:
½ cup chicken stock	Grilled eggplants

DIRECTIONS and Cooking Time: 42 Minutes;
Rinse the turkey breasts under cold running water and pat dry. Set aside. In a medium bowl, combine orange juice, chicken stock, Cayenne pepper, salt, and pepper. Mix well and place the meat into this marinade. Refrigerate for 20 minutes. Now, place the meat along with marinade into a large Ziploc bag and cook en sous vide for 40 minutes at 122 degrees. In a medium nonstick saucepan, melt the butter over a medium-high temperature. Remove the meat from the bag and add it to the saucepan. Fry for about 2 minutes and remove from the heat.

Nutrition Info: Calories: 303 Total Fat: 9g Saturated Fat: 5g; Trans Fat: 0g Protein: 32g; Net Carbs: 13g

Portuguese Chicken In Tomato Sauce

INGREDIENTS for Servings: 3

1 ½ cup chicken fillets	2 tablespoons olive oil
4 garlic cloves, crushed	1 teaspoon dried basil
1 large onion, peeled and finely chopped	1 teaspoon salt
1 large tomato, finely chopped	½ teaspoon freshly ground black pepper
2 teaspoons fresh rosemary, finely chopped	¼ cup white wine
	Serve with:
	Steamed spinach

DIRECTIONS and Cooking Time: 1 Hour 15 Minutes;
Heat up the olive oil in a large skillet. Add onion and garlic. Stir-fry for 3-4 minutes, stirring constantly. Now add tomato, basil, rosemary, and wine. Continue to cook until tomato softens, for ten minutes. Remove from the heat and set aside. Rinse well the chicken and cut into bite-sized pieces. Place in a Ziploc along with tomato sauce and seal the bag. Cook en sous vide for one hour at 14

Nutrition Info: Calories: 352 Total Fat: 11g Saturated Fat: 7g; Trans Fat: 0g Protein: 32g; Net Carbs: 3g

"eat-me" Fruity Chorizo

INGREDIENTS for Servings: 4

2½ cups seedless white grapes, stems removed	4 chorizo sausages
	2 tbsp balsamic vinegar
1 tbsp fresh rosemary, chopped	Salt and black pepper to taste
2 tbsp butter	

DIRECTIONS and Cooking Time: 75 Minutes
Prepare a water bath and place the Sous Vide in it. Set to 165 F. Place the butter, white grapes, rosemary and chorizo in a vacuum-sealable bag. Shake well. Release air by the water displacement method, seal and submerge the bag in the water bath. Cook for 60 minutes. Once the timer has stopped, transfer the chorizo mix to a plate. In a hot saucepan pour the cooking liquids along with grapes and balsamic vinegar. Stir for 3 minutes. Top chorizo with grape sauce.

Skinny Sweet Potato Fries

INGREDIENTS for Servings: 4

1 ½ pounds sweet potatoes, peeled and cut into sticks	1/4 teaspoon ground allspice
1 cup water	2 tablespoons canola oil
1 tablespoon sea salt	

DIRECTIONS and Cooking Time: 1 Hour 15 Minutes
Preheat a sous vide water bath to 183 degrees F. Add sweet potatoes, water, salt, and allspice to cooking pouches; seal tightly. Submerge the cooking pouches in the water bath; cook for 60 minutes. Pat dry sweet potatoes. In a bowl, toss sweet potatoes with canola oil. Arrange sweet potatoes on a parchment-lined baking sheet. Preheat an oven to 400 degrees F. Bake for 10 minutes or until nice and crisp. Serve with your favorite sauce for dipping. Enjoy!

Nutrition Info:134 Calories; 8g Fat; 11g Carbs; 2g Protein; 0g Sugars

Green Pea Dip

INGREDIENTS for Servings: 8

2 cups green peas	1 tsp olive oil
3 tbsp heavy cream	Salt and black pepper to taste
1 tbsp tarragon	
1 garlic clove	¼ cup diced apple

DIRECTIONS and Cooking Time: 45 Minutes
Prepare a water bath and place the Sous Vide in it. Set to 185 F. Place all the ingredients in a vacuum-sealable bag. Release air by the water displacement method, seal and submerge the bag in water bath.Set the timer for 32 minutes. Once the timer has stopped, remove the bag and blend with a hand blender until smooth.

Eggplant Kebab

INGREDIENTS for Servings: 3

1 large eggplant, sliced into 1-inch thick slices	1 medium-sized tomato, finely chopped
1 small zucchini, sliced into 1-inch thick slices	1 teaspoon red pepper flakes
	3 tablespoons olive oil
1 large green bell	1 teaspoon salt

pepper, seeds removed and sliced 2 garlic cloves, crushed	Serve with: Sour cream or yogurt

DIRECTIONS and Cooking Time: 1 Hour

Wash the eggplant and zucchini. Slice into 1-inch thick pieces and set aside. Wash the bell pepper and cut in half. Remove the seeds and slice. Set aside. Wash the tomato and finely chop it. Set aside. Now, place all vegetables along with garlic, red pepper, olive oil, and salt in a large Ziploc bag. Seal the bag and cook en sous vide for 1 hour at 185 degrees.

Nutrition Info: Calories: 189 Total Fat: 16g Saturated Fat: 2g; Trans Fat: 0g Protein: 9g; Net Carbs: 9g

Creamy And Cheesy Seafood Dip

INGREDIENTS for Servings: 12

6 ounces scallops, chopped 6 ounces shrimp, chopped 2 cups broth, preferably homemade 1 ½ cups Colby cheese, shredded	1 ½ cups Gruyere cheese, shredded 1/2 teaspoon smoked paprika 1/2 teaspoons ground black pepper 1/2 teaspoon dried oregano

DIRECTIONS and Cooking Time: 40 Minutes

Preheat a sous vide water bath to 132 degrees F. Simply put all ingredients into cooking pouches; seal tightly. Submerge the cooking pouches in the water bath; cook for 35 minutes. Transfer the sous vide

dipping sauce to a nice serving bowl; serve with dippers of choice. Bon appétit!

Nutrition Info:206 Calories; 12g Fat; 2g Carbs; 25g Protein; 2g Sugars

Beef Steak With Shallots And Parsley

INGREDIENTS for Servings: 4

1 large beef steak, about 2 pounds 2 tablespoons Dijon mustard 1 tablespoon fresh parsley leaves, finely chopped 1 teaspoon fresh rosemary, finely chopped	3 tablespoons olive oil 1 tablespoon shallot, finely chopped ½ teaspoon dried thyme 1 garlic clove, crushed Serve with: Red cabbage salad

DIRECTIONS and Cooking Time: 1 Hour

Clean the beef steak and cut into 1-inch thick slices. Set aside. In a small bowl, combine Dijon mustard with olive oil. Add parsley, rosemary, shallot, thyme, and garlic. Rub the meat with this mixture and place in a Ziploc. Cook en sous vide for one hour at 136 degrees for medium, or at 154 for well done. Serve with red cabbage salad.

Nutrition Info: Calories: 521 Total Fat: 25g Saturated Fat: 9g; Trans Fat: 0g Protein: 63g; Net Carbs: 4g

DESSERTS RECIPES

Homemade Vanilla Bourbon

INGREDIENTS for Servings: 6

1 cup granulated sugar	6 split vanilla beans
½ cup water	Soda for serving
½ cup bourbon	Lemon wedges for serving

DIRECTIONS and Cooking Time: 2 Hours 10 Minutes
Prepare a water bath and place the Sous Vide in it. Set to 135 F. Combine the sugar, vanilla beans, water and bourbon and place in a vacuum-sealable bag. Release air by the water displacement method, seal and submerge the bag in the water bath. Cook for 2 hours. Once the timer has stopped, remove the bag and strain the mixture. Allow chilling all night. Serve with one-part syrup, two parts soda with ice. Garnish with a lemon wedge.

Vanilla Ice Cream

INGREDIENTS for Servings: 4

2 cups half-and-half	6 egg yolks
½ cup sugar	1 teaspoon vanilla

DIRECTIONS and Cooking Time: 1 Hour Plus Freezing
Preheat the water bath to 180°F. Whisk together all ingredients. Pour into bag and seal. Place in water bath and cook 1 hour. After 1 hour, pass ice cream base through a strainer to remove any clumps. Transfer to refrigerator and cool completely. Churn in an ice cream machine according to machine instructions. Freeze.

Nutrition Info: Calories 291 Total Fat 268g Total Carb 1.72g Dietary Fiber 0g Protein 63g

Sous Vide Chocolate Cupcakes

INGREDIENTS for Servings: 6

5 tbsp butter, melted	1 tsp baking soda
1 egg	1 tsp vanilla extract
3 tbsp cocoa powder	1 tsp apple cider vinegar
1 cup flour	
4 tbsp sugar	Pinch of sea salt
½ cup heavy cream	

DIRECTIONS and Cooking Time: 3 Hours 15 Minutes
Prepare a water bath and place the Sous Vide in it. Set to 194 F. Whisk together the wet ingredients in one bowl. Combine the dry ingredients in another bowl. Combine the two mixtures gently and divide the batter between 6 small jars. Seal the jars and submerge the bag in water bath. Set the timer for 3

hours Once the timer has stopped, remove the bag. Serve chilled.

Gingery Gin Tonic With Lemons

INGREDIENTS for Servings: 4

1 cup gin	1 ¼ cups tonic water
1 cup ice	1 lemon, cut into wedges
1 inch ginger piece, peeled	

DIRECTIONS and Cooking Time: 2 Hours 15 Minutes
Prepare a water bath and place the Sous Vide in it. Set to 125 F. Place the gin, ginger and half of the lemon wedges in a vacuum-sealable bag. Release air by the water displacement method, seal and submerge the bag in water bath. Set the timer for 2 hours. Once the timer has stopped, remove the bag. Let cool completely. Serve with ice and remaining lemon wedges.

Asian-style Rice Pudding With Almonds

INGREDIENTS for Servings: 5

5 tbsp basmati rice	3 tbsp sugar
2 (14-oz) cans coconut milk	3 tbsp cashews, chopped
5 cardamom pods, crushed	Slivered almonds for garnish

DIRECTIONS and Cooking Time: 7 Hours 30 Minutes
Prepare a water bath and place the Sous Vide in it. Set to 182 F. In a bowl, combine the coconut milk, sugar, and 1 cup water. Pour the rice and mix well. Divide the mixture between the jars. Add a cardamom pod to each pot. Seal and submerge in the bath. Cook for 3 hours. Once the timer has stopped, remove the jars. Allow cooling for 4 hours. Serve and top with cashews and almonds.

Cinnamon & Citrus Yogurt

INGREDIENTS for Servings: 4

½ cup yogurt	4 cups full cream milk
½ tbsp orange zest	1 tsp cinnamon
½ tbsp lemon zest	
½ tbsp lime zest	

DIRECTIONS and Cooking Time: 3 Hours 15 Minutes
Prepare a water bath and place the Sous Vide in it. Set to 113 F. Warm the milk in a pot until 182 F. Transfer to an ice bath and allow cooling until reached 110 F. Pour in yogurt and cinnamon. Add the citrus zest. Put the mixture into 4 canning jars and seal.

Immerse the jars in the water bath. Cook for 3 hours. Once the timer has stopped, remove the jars and serve.

Poached Pears

INGREDIENTS

brandy *	vanilla extract, as required
white wine *	
water *	
sugar *	4 pears, peeled and cored
2 strips orange peel	
cinnamon stick *	whipped cream, as required
star anise *	

DIRECTIONS and Cooking Time: 1 Hour 10 Mins Cooking Temperature: 176°f
Attach the sous vide immersion circulator using an adjustable clamp to a Cambro container or pot filled with water and preheat to 176°F. In a pan, mix brandy, wine, water, sugar, orange peel strips, cinnamon stick and star anise over a low heat and cook until heated sugar is dissolved. Stir in vanilla extract and remove from heat. Keep aside to cool. Into a cooking pouch, add pears and cooled syrup. Seal pouch tightly after squeezing out the excess air. Place pouch in sous vide bath and set the cooking time for 1 hour. Remove pouches from sous vide bath and immediately plunge into a large bowl of ice water to cool. Place pears onto a plate, transferring cooking liquid into a pan. Place pan over stove and cook until a syrupy consistency is reached. Pour syrup over pears and serve with a dollop of whipped cream.

Summer Mint & Rhubarb Mojito

INGREDIENTS for Servings: 12

2 cups diced rhubarb	1 cup water
1 cup sugar	5 sprigs mint

DIRECTIONS and Cooking Time: 1 Hour 45 Minutes
Prepare a water bath and place the Sous Vide in it. Set to 182 F. Combine all the ingredients and place in a vacuum-sealable bag. Release air by the water displacement method, seal and submerge the bag in the water bath. Cook for 1 hour 30 minutes. Once the timer has stopped, remove the bag and drain the contents. Reserve the fruit. Allow chilling.

Creamy Chocolate Infused With Blood Orange

INGREDIENTS

For Pots de Crème	¼ cup milk
1 cup heavy whipping cream	3 large egg yolks
	2 dashes Angostura bitters
juice of one blood orange	For Whipped Cream:

2 tablespoons plus 2 teaspoons granulated sugar	½ cup chilled heavy whipping cream
⅛ teaspoon kosher salt	1 tablespoon maple syrup
3½ ounces bittersweet chocolate, chopped	1 tablespoon bourbon
	¼ teaspoon vanilla bean paste

DIRECTIONS and Cooking Time: 40 Mins Cooking Temperature: 180°f
Attach the sous vide immersion circulator using an adjustable clamp to a Cambro container or pot filled with water and preheat to 180°F. Into a small pan add whipping cream, orange juice, milk, granulated sugar and salt, and beat over medium heat until well-combined. Bring to a gentle boil, stirring continuously. Remove from heat and immediately add chocolate, beating continuously until smooth and completely melted. Keep aside to cool for 2 minutes, stirring occasionally. Add egg yolks, one at a time then, beating until well-combined. Add Angostura bitters and beat to combine. Through a fine mesh strainer, strain the mixture. Divide mixture into 4 canning jars evenly and close the lids tightly. Place jars in sous vide bath and set the cooking time for 35 minutes. Remove the jars from sous vide bath and place onto a wire rack to cool completely. After cooling, transfer the jars into refrigerator for at least 2 hours (or until set). Meanwhile, for the whipped cream: pre-chill the bowl of a stand mixer for at least 10 minutes. In the chilled bowl, add all ingredients and, with whisk attachment, mix on medium speed until soft peaks form. Place whipped cream over pots de crème and serve.

Blueberry Clafoutis

INGREDIENTS for Servings: 4

1 piece of whole egg	¼ teaspoon of vanilla extract
¼ cup of heavy cream	
¼ cup of almond flour	Just a pinch of salt
1 tablespoon of granulated sugar	½ a cup of fresh blueberries
2 teaspoon of coconut flour	4 pieces of 4 ounce screw top – hinge closure canning jar
¼ teaspoon of baking powder	

DIRECTIONS and Cooking Time: 60 Minutes
Set your water bath to 185° Fahrenheit Tale a small bowl and add all of the ingredients except blueberries Set up your jars on your work surface and grease with some cooking spray Divide the prepared batter evenly among the 4 jars Top it up with 2 tablespoon of blueberries Attach the lids with fingertip lightness /to ensure that the air is able to escape once submerged under water Put them in your water bat and cook for 1 hour Remove the jar from the bath

and open it up   Enjoy warm with a sprinkle of sugar or crème anglaise

Nutrition Info: Calories: 228, Fat 3g, Protein 5g, Dietary Fiber 2g

Warm Vanilla Quince

INGREDIENTS for Servings: 2

2 peeled quince	½ tsp salt
1 vanilla bean	1 tbsp butter
2 tbsp dark brown sugar	Vanilla ice cream

DIRECTIONS and Cooking Time: 50 Minutes
Prepare a water bath and place the Sous Vide in it. Set to 175 F. Slice the quince by the half. Remove the core. Combine the vanilla bean with brown sugar and salt. Soak vanilla seeds with the mixture.   Place the quinces and the mixture in a vacuum-sealable bag. Release air by water displacement method, seal and submerge in the water bath. Cook for 45 minutes. Once the timer has stopped, remove the quinces and transfer to a bowls. Sprinkle the quinces with the butter sauce. Serve with vanilla ice cream.

Lemon Curd

INGREDIENTS for Servings: 8

1 cup butter	12 egg yolks
1 cup sugar	5 lemons

DIRECTIONS and Cooking Time: 75 Minutes
Prepare a water bath and place the Sous Vide in it. Set to 168 F.   Grate the zest from lemons and place in a bowl. Squeeze the juice and add to the bowl as well. Whisk on the yolks and sugar and transfer to a vacumm-sealable bag. Release air by the water displacement method, seal and submerge the bag in water bath.Set the timer for 1 hour.   Once the timer has stopped, remove the bag and transfer the cooked lemon curd to a bowl and place in an ice bath. Let chill completely.

Apple & Cardamom Gin

INGREDIENTS for Servings: 4

1 pink lady apple cored, sliced into rings	1 cup Gin
	1 green cardamom pod

DIRECTIONS and Cooking Time: 120 Minutes
Prepare your Sous Vide water bath using your immersion circulator and raise the temperature to 134-degrees Fahrenheit.   Add all the above ingredients to a resealable zip bag.   Seal using the immersion method. Cook for 2 hours.   Once done, take the bag out from the water bath and transfer to

an ice bath.   Strain into a large bowl and transfer to a container   Serve chilled!

Nutrition Info: Calories: 152 Carbohydrate: 22g Protein: 0g Fat: 0g Sugar: 19g Sodium: 7mg

Salted Caramel Ice Cream

INGREDIENTS for Servings: 6

1 ½ cup sugar	1 teaspoon vanilla bean paste
1 ¾ cups heavy cream	
1 teaspoon sea salt	Pinch of kosher salt
1 cup whole milk	Tools Required
5 egg yolks	Ice Cream Maker

DIRECTIONS and Cooking Time: 30 Minutes
Set up your Sous Vide immersion circulator to a temperature of 180-degrees Fahrenheit and prepare your water bath.   Heat up 1 cup of sugar in a large-sized nonstick saucepan, making sure to keep stirring it until it begins to melt.   Swirl until the sugar has melted and is slightly browned.   Whisk in 1 cup of heavy cream and cook until the mixture is smooth. Stir in salt and remove the heat and allow the mixture to cool down.   Take a food processor and add the egg yolks, vanilla, 3/4 cup of cream, ½ cup of sugar, milk and purée for 30 seconds.   Transfer the mixture to a resealable zip bag and seal using the immersion method.   Cook for 30 minutes underwater.   Stir caramel* into the bag and allow it to chill overnight. Allow the mixture to cool. Churn the mixture in ice cream maker   Freeze and serve!

Nutrition Info: Per serving:Calories: 1013 ;Carbohydrate: 94g ;Protein: 12g ;Fat: 68g ;Sugar: 94g ;Sodium: 526mg

Mexican Chocolate Pots

INGREDIENTS

1 x 3½-ounce bar Mexican chocolate, chopped	3 egg yolks
	2 teaspoons cocoa powder
1 tablespoon sugar	¼ teaspoon vanilla extract
⅓ cup whole milk	
1 cup heavy whipping cream pus more for topping	⅛ teaspoon sea salt chocolate shavings, for serving

DIRECTIONS and Cooking Time: 30 Mins Cooking Temperature: 180°f
Attach the sous vide immersion circulator using an adjustable clamp to a Cambro container or pot filled with water and preheat to 180°F.   In a heatproof bowl, mix together chocolate and sugar. Keep aside. Into a pan, add milk and cream and cook until heated completely.   Remove from heat and pour mixture over chocolate and sugar. Keep aside for 5 minutes. Meanwhile, in another small bowl, add egg yolks, vanilla extract, cocoa powder and salt, and beat until well-combined.   After 5 minutes, stir the chocolate

mixture until well-combined and smooth. Add egg mixture and beat until well-combined. Fill the ramekins evenly with chocolate mixture. Arrange ramekins on a rack in the sous vide bath. (Water level should be halfway up the sides of ramekins). Using plastic wrap, cover the ramekins. Set the cooking time for 30 minutes. Remove from sous vide bath and keep aside for 20 minutes to cool. Refrigerate for at least 2 hours before serving. Top with chocolate shavings and a dollop of whipped cream, and serve.

Flan Custard
INGREDIENTS

¾ cup granulated sugar	1 x 12-fluid-ounce can evaporated milk
1 x 14-ounce can condensed milk	1 teaspoon pure vanilla extract
12 large egg yolks	

DIRECTIONS and Cooking Time: 2 Hours Cooking Temperature: 180°f
Attach the sous vide immersion circulator using an adjustable clamp to a Cambro container or pot filled with water and preheat to 180°F. Into a pan, add sugar and heat until liquefied completely. Pour liquefied sugar evenly into 4 x ½-pint jars and keep aside to cool. Into a bowl, add condensed milk, evaporated milk, egg yolks and vanilla extract, and gently stir to combine. Through a cheesecloth, strain mixture. Pour strained mixture over liquefied sugar in each jar, leaving just enough room for the lid to close tightly. Carefully arrange ramekins over the rack in sous vide bath. Set the cooking time for 2 hours. Carefully, remove ramekins from sous vide bath. Place ramekins onto wire rack to cool completely. After cooling, refrigerate to chill before serving.

Gingered Peaches With Cardamom
INGREDIENTS for Servings: 4

1 pound peaches, halved	1 tbsp butter
1 tsp cardamom seeds, freshly ground	½ tsp ground ginger
	½ tsp salt
	Fresh basil, chopped

DIRECTIONS and Cooking Time: 1 Hour 15 Minutes
Prepare a water bath and place the Sous Vide in it. Set to 182 F. Combine the butter, peaches, ginger, cardamom, and salt. Place in a vacuum-sealable bag. Release air by the water displacement method, seal and submerge the bag in the water bath. Cook for 60 minutes. Once the timer has stopped, remove the bag and transfer into a bowl. Garnished with basil and serve.

Creamy Blueberry Mousse
INGREDIENTS for Servings: 8

1 pound blueberries	¼ tsp ground cinnamon
¼ cup sugar	1 cup heavy cream
3 tbsp lemon juice	1 tsp vanilla extract

DIRECTIONS and Cooking Time: 60 Minutes
Prepare a water bath and place the Sous Vide in it. Set to 182 F. Combine blueberries, sugar, lemon juice, and cinnamon and place in a vacuum-sealable bag. Release air by the water displacement method, seal and submerge the bag in the water bath. Cook for 30 minutes. Once ready, remove the bag and transfer the contents to a blender. Stir until smooth. Whisk the cream and vanilla. Pour in the blueberries mix and combine well. Transfer into 8 serving bowls. Allow chilling.

Bacon Infused Bourbon
INGREDIENTS for Servings: 8

2 cups bourbon	8 oz. smoked bacon, cooked until crisp
3 tablespoon bacon fat reserved from cooking	3 tablespoons light brown sugar

DIRECTIONS and Cooking Time: 60 Minutes
Prepare your Sous Vide water bath using your immersion circulator and raise the temperature to 150-degrees Fahrenheit. Add all the listed ingredients to a resealable zip bag. Seal using the immersion method. Cook for 1 hour. Once done, take the bag out from the water bath and strain the contents through a fine-mesh strainer into a large bowl Transfer the bourbon to the refrigerator and chill until the pork fat solidifies on top. Skim off the fat Then, strain the bourbon a second time through a cheesecloth-lined strainer. Pass it to a storage container and store in the refrigerator.

Nutrition Info: Calories: 274 Carbohydrate: 14g Protein: 6g Fat: 19g Sugar: 13g Sodium: 316mg

Chocolate Chip Cookies
INGREDIENTS for Servings: 12 Cookies

½ cup flour	1/3 cup granulated sugar
½ teaspoon baking powder	1 small egg
1 pinch salt	½ cup mini chocolate chips
3 tablespoons unsalted softened butter	1 teaspoon vanilla paste

DIRECTIONS and Cooking Time: 30 Minutes
Set the cooker to 195F. In a small bowl, combine flour, baking powder, and salt. In a separate large bowl, cream butter and sugar until fluffy. Fold in the

egg and vanilla paste, and stir until smooth. Mix in the flour mixture and stir until just combined. Fold in the chocolate chips. Roll the dough between two pieces of baking paper and cut out the cookies using a cookie cutter. Divide the cookies between two Sous Vide cooking bags. Vacuum seal the cookies and submerge in a water bath. Cook 30 minutes. Finishing steps: Remove the bag from the water bath. Cool completely before opening. Remove the cookies from the bag and serve.

Nutrition Info: Calories 44 Total Fat 4g Total Carb 7g Dietary Fiber 1g Protein 9g

Cinnamon Poached Pears With Ice Cream

INGREDIENTS for Servings: 4

3 peeled pears	Zest of 1 lemon
3 cups hard apple cider	1 vanilla bean, split
1 cup sugar	1 cinnamon stick
	Ice cream for serving

DIRECTIONS and Cooking Time: 1 Hour 15 Minutes
Prepare a water bath and place the Sous Vide in it. Set to 194 F. Place all the ingredients in a vacuum-sealable bag. Release air by the water displacement method, seal and submerge the bag in the water bath. Cook for 60 minutes. Once the timer has stopped, remove the pears and set aside. Drain the juices into a hot pot. Cook for 10 minutes. Cut the pears by the half and remove the seeds. Serve ice cream and top with the pears.

Cheesecake

INGREDIENTS for Servings: 6

12 oz. cream cheese at room temperature	2 eggs
½ cup sugar	Zest of 1 lemon
¼ cup creole cream cheese	½ tablespoon vanilla extract

DIRECTIONS and Cooking Time: 90 Minutes
Set up your Sous Vide immersion circulator to a temperature of 176-degrees Fahrenheit and prepare your water bath. Take a bowl and add both cream cheeses, and sugar and whisk them well Gradually add the eggs one by one and keep beating until well combined. Add the zest and vanilla and mix well. Pour the cheesecake mixture into 6 different jars of 6 ounces and distribute evenly Seal the jars with a lid. Place the jars underwater and let them cook for 90 minutes. Once done, remove from the water bath and chill until they are cooled Serve chilled with a topping of fresh fruit compote.

Nutrition Info: Per serving:Calories: 615 ;Carbohydrate: 56g ;Protein: 8g ;Fat: 41g ;Sugar: 40g ;Sodium: 418mg

Sugar-free Chocolate Chip Cookies

INGREDIENTS for Servings: 6

1/3 cup chocolate chips	½ tsp baking soda
	4 tbsp butter, melted
7 tbsp heavy cream	¼ tsp salt
2 eggs	1 tbsp lemon juice
½ cup flour	

DIRECTIONS and Cooking Time: 3 Hours 45 Minutes
Prepare a water bath and place the Sous Vide in it. Set to 194 F. Beat the eggs along with the cream, lemon juice, salt, and baking soda. Stir in flour and butter. Fold in the chocolate chips. Divide the dough between 6 ramekins. Wrap them well with plastic foil and place the ramekins in the water bath. Cook for 3 hours and 30 minutes. Once the timer has stopped, remove the ramekins.

Sensuous White Chocolate Cheese Cake

INGREDIENTS for Servings: 8

16 ounce of cream cheese	1 teaspoon of cake flour
¼ cup of sour cream	1 teaspoon of vanilla extract
2 tablespoon of granulated sugar	10 ounce of white chocolate
1 large sized eggs	

DIRECTIONS and Cooking Time: 120 Minutes
Carefully prepare your sous vide water bath to a temperature of 176° Fahrenheit using the immersion cooker Take a medium sized bowl and mix your cream cheese, sugar, sour cream and mix everything on medium setting until combined well With the mixer running, add your eggs one at a time, making sure to combine the previous one before adding another Add cake flour, vanilla extract and mix everything for 3 seconds Keep it on the side Take a small microwave safe bowl and add white chocolate Place your bowl in the microwave and heat it up on high settings in 30 second intervals until the whole chocolate has melted Add your melted chocolate to the cheesecake batter and combine well Divide the batter amongst eight 470nk glass canning jars and seal them up loosely 1 Place your jars in your water bath and let it cook for 2h ours 1 Remove the water bath 1 Place your jars in the fridge and let it chill for 4 hours 1 Serve with some toppings of seasonal fruit

Nutrition Info: Calories: 130, Protein 8g, Dietary Fiber: 4g

Grand Marnier

INGREDIENTS for Servings: 12

Zest of 8 large orange	2 cups brandy
	½ cup ultrafine sugar

DIRECTIONS and Cooking Time: 90 Minutes
Prepare your Sous Vide water bath using your immersion circulator and raise the temperature to 180-degrees Fahrenheit. Add all the listed ingredients to a resealable zip bag. Seal using the immersion method. Cook for 90 minutes. Strain and discard the orange zest. Allow it to chill and serve when needed!

Nutrition Info: Calories: 191 Carbohydrate: 39g Protein: 4g Fat: 2g Sugar: 31g Sodium: 31mg

Mulled Wine

INGREDIENTS for Servings: 2

½ bottle red wine	1 vanilla pod, sliced in
Juice of 2 oranges, peel of 1	half lengthways
1 cinnamon stick	1-star anise
1 bay leaf	2 oz. caster sugar

DIRECTIONS and Cooking Time: 60 Minutes
Prepare your Sous Vide water bath using your immersion circulator and raise the temperature to 140-degrees Fahrenheit. Add all the listed ingredients to a large bowl. Divide the mixture across two resealable zip bags and seal using the immersion method. Cook for 1 hour. Serve chilled!

Nutrition Info: Calories: 206 Carbohydrate: 17g Protein: 1g Fat: 0g Sugar: 11g Sodium: 0mg

Swedish Rosemary Snaps

INGREDIENTS for Servings: 10

3 sprigs fresh rosemary + plus extra for storage	1 bottle vodka
	4 strips of fresh orange peel

DIRECTIONS and Cooking Time: 120 Minutes
Prepare your Sous Vide water bath using your immersion circulator and raise the temperature to 135-degrees Fahrenheit. Add the vodka, 3 sprigs rosemary, and 3 strips of orange peel to a resealable zip bag. Seal using the immersion method. Cook for 2 hours. Once done, take the bag out from the water bath and pass through metal mesh strainer into bowl. Put one fresh sprig of rosemary and one strip of orange peel into bottle. Pour the prepared snaps into bottle. Chill and serve!

Nutrition Info: Calories: 236 Carbohydrate: 14g Protein: 0g Fat: 0g Sugar: 11g Sodium: 4mg

Brioche Bread Pudding

INGREDIENTS for Servings: 4

1 cup whole milk	¼ cup maple syrup
1 cup heavy cream	1 teaspoon vanilla bean paste
½ cup granulated sugar	½ teaspoon kosher salt
2 tablespoons orange juice	4 cups brioche, cut up into 1 inch cubes
1 tablespoon orange zest	

DIRECTIONS and Cooking Time: 120 Minutes
Set up your Sous Vide immersion circulator to a temperature of 170-degrees Fahrenheit and prepare your water bath. Take a large bowl and add the milk, heavy cream, sugar, maple syrup, orange zest, juice, vanilla bean paste, and salt. Mix well and add the brioche. Toss well Divide the mixture among 4 mason jars of 4-ounces size and gently seal them using the finger-tip method Cook for 2 hours underwater. Heat up your broiler and place the jars in the broiler. Brown for 2-3 minutes (with lids removed) and serve.

Nutrition Info: Per serving:Calories: 246 ;Carbohydrate: 19g ;Protein: 7g ;Fat: 16g ;Sugar: 3g ;Sodium: 164mg

Spiced Rum

INGREDIENTS for Servings: 10

1 bottle rum	2 whole black peppercorns
1 vanilla bean, split lengthwise	½ piece star anise
2 whole cloves	2 pieces of 3-inch fresh orange zest
½ cinnamon stick	

DIRECTIONS and Cooking Time: 120 Minutes
Prepare your Sous Vide water bath using your immersion circulator and raise the temperature to 153-degrees Fahrenheit. Add all the listed ingredients to a resealable zipper bag. Seal using the immersion method and cook for 2 hours. Once cooked, transfer it to an ice bath and chill. Strain to bottle and serve the drink!

Nutrition Info: Calories: 416 Carbohydrate: 1g Protein: 0g Fat: 0g Sugar: 0g Sodium: 3mg

Rice Pudding With Rum & Cranberries

INGREDIENTS for Servings: 6

½ cup dried cranberries soaked in ½ cup of rum overnight and drained	2 cups rice
	3 cups milk
	1 tsp cinnamon
	½ cup brown sugar

DIRECTIONS and Cooking Time: 2 Hours 15 Minutes

Prepare a water bath and place the Sous Vide in it. Set to 140 F. Combine all the ingredients in a bowl and transfer to 6 small jars. Seal them and submerge in water bath.Set the timer for 2 hours. Once the timer has stopped, remove the jars. Serve warm or chilled.

Mind Boggling Peach Cobbler

INGREDIENTS for Servings: 6

1 cup of self-rising flour	1 cup of whole milk
1 cup of granulated sugar	8 tablespoons of unsalted melted butter
1 teaspoon of vanilla extract	2 cups of roughly chopped peaches

DIRECTIONS and Cooking Time: 3 Hours
Set up your Sous Vide immersion circulator to a temperature of 195 ºF and prepare your water bath Prepare 6 half pint canning jars with butter Whisk flour, sugar in a large bowl, whisk in milk and vanilla and mix Stir in butter and peaches Divide the batter between jars and wipe sides, seal gently Cook for 3 hours Remove the jars and place on cooling rack, rest for 10 minutes and enjoy!

Nutrition Info: Per serving:Calories 329, Carbohydrates 7 g, Fats 25 g, Protein 19 g

Raspberry Ice Cream

INGREDIENTS for Servings: 6

2 cups raspberries	½ cup granulated sugar
½ cup fine sugar	
1 cup heavy cream	1 teaspoon vanilla paste
1 cup milk	
5 egg yolks	

DIRECTIONS and Cooking Time: 1 Hour 30 Minutes
Set the cooker to 180F. Combine the raspberries and fine sugar in Sous Vide bag. Seal the bag using water immersion technique. Cook the raspberries 30 minutes in a water bath. Remove the bag from the water. Finishing steps: Remove the bag from the cooker and strain the raspberries through the fine mesh sieve, pressing to remove pulp. Discard the seeds. Combine heavy cream, milk, egg yolks, granulated sugar, and vanilla paste in a food blender. Blend until smooth. Stir in the raspberry mixture and transfer all into a large bag. Seal the bag using water immersion technique and cook in Sous Vide cooker for 1 hour. When the timer goes off, remove the bag from the cooker and lace into ice-cold water bath 30 minutes. Churn the mixture in an ice cream machine until set. Serve.

Nutrition Info: Calories 218 Total Fat 13g Total Carb 26g Dietary Fiber 7g Protein 5g

Amaretto Crème Brulée

INGREDIENTS for Servings: 12

12 egg yolks	2 ounces Amaretto
¾ cup sugar	1-quart heavy cream
½ teaspoon salt	

DIRECTIONS and Cooking Time: 60 Minutes
Set up your Sous Vide immersion circulator to a temperature of 181-degrees Fahrenheit and prepare your water bath. Add the salt, and egg yolks to a bowl and mix them well. Add the Amaretto liqueur to egg mixture and combine them well. Add in the heavy cream and whisk. Then, strain the whole mixture into a bowl through a metal mesh strainer. Allow the mixture to rest. Then fill up the 4-ounce mason jars, making sure that there is ½ inch space at the top Gently tighten the lid and submerge underwater. Cook for 1 hour. Chill in your fridge for 2 hours and sprinkle sugar on top. Broil or caramelize the sugar using a blowtorch and serve!

Nutrition Info: Per serving:Calories: 457 ;Carbohydrate: 35g ;Protein: 6g ;Fat: 31g ;Sugar: 33g ;Sodium: 41mg

Rice & Cardamom Pudding

INGREDIENTS for Servings: 8

½ cup raisins	1 cup heavy cream
½ cup dark rum	3 strips lemon peel
5 tablespoons unsalted butter	3 crushed cardamom pods, crushed and wrapped in cheese cloth
1/3 cup light brown sugar	
4 cups cooked wild rice blend	1 teaspoon vanilla extract
1 cup whole milk	Cinnamon

DIRECTIONS and Cooking Time: 120 Minutes
Set up your Sous Vide immersion circulator to a temperature of 181-degrees Fahrenheit and prepare your water bath. Put the raisins and rum into a small microwave bowl and heat for 1 minute. Allow it to cool and remove the raisins using slotted spoon. Take a medium non-stick skillet and place it over medium-high heat. Add the butter and then brown sugar and heat it up. Stir until it has melted and simmer for 5 minutes. Add the cooked rice, milk, cream, lemon peel, cardamom and vanilla to butter mixture and bring the mixture to a boil. Lower down the heat to low and simmer for about 2 minutes. Remove from the heat and stir in raisins, spoon the mixture into resealable zip bag and seal using the immersion method. Cook for 2 hours underwater. Once cooked, take the bag out from the water bath and pour the mixture into a large bowl. Stir well and discard cardamom pod bundle alongside the lemon peels. Sprinkle cinnamon and serve!

Nutrition Info:Per serving:Calories: 362 ;Carbohydrate: 50g ;Protein: 12g ;Fat: 13g ;Sugar: 38g ;Sodium: 132mg

Cinnamon Pineapple With Cheese Yogurt

INGREDIENTS for Servings: 8

1 whole pineapple	1 cup white wine
1 tsp Chinese five-spice	For Whipping Cheese Yogurt
2 tsp orange zest	1 ½ tbsp vanilla yogurt
1 tsp crushed pink peppercorns	Grated star anise
¼ tsp nutmeg	9 oz whipping cheese
¼ tsp cinnamon	3 ½ oz natural yogurt
1 tsp allspice	3 ½ oz crushed ginger nut biscuits
3 ½ oz dark brown sugar	

DIRECTIONS and Cooking Time: 12 Hours 10 Minutes
Prepare a water bath and place the Sous Vide in it. Set to 186 F. Combine all the ingredients and place in a vacuum-sealable bag. Release air by the water displacement method, seal and submerge the bag in the water bath. Cook for 12 hours. Blend all the ingredients for the cheese yogurt cream and allow chilling in the fridge. Once the timer has stopped, remove the pineapple and transfer to plates. Serve topped with the cheese yogurt cream.

Orange Pots Du Créme With Chocolate

INGREDIENTS for Servings: 6

⅔ cup chopped chocolate	Zest of 1 large orange
6 egg yolks	⅛ tsp orange extract
1⅓ cups fine white sugar	2 tbsp orange juice
3 cups half and half	2 tbsp chocolate-flavored liqueur
1 tsp vanilla extract	

DIRECTIONS and Cooking Time: 65 Minutes + 5 Hours
Prepare a water bath and place the Sous Vide in it. Set to 196 F. With an electric mixer, combine the egg yolks and sugar. Mix for 1-2 minutes until creamy. Heat the cream in a saucepan over medium heat and add in vanilla, orange zest and extract. Cook on Low heat for 3-4 minutes. Set aside and allow to cool for 2-3 minutes. Melt the chocolate in the microwave. Once the mixture has cooled, pour the cream mixture into the egg mixture and stir. Add the melted chocolate and stir until combined. Add in orange juice and chocolate liqueur. Pour the chocolate mixture into mason jars. Seal with a lid and submerge the jars in the

water bath, Cook for 45 minutes. Once the timer has stopped, remove the jars and allow to cool for 5 minutes.

Apple Sauce

INGREDIENTS for Servings: 8

4 pounds apples /peeled, cored, sliced	1 lemon /juiced
1/4 cup brown sugar	1/2 teaspoon cinnamon
	1/4 teaspoon nutmeg

DIRECTIONS and Cooking Time: 45 Minutes
Preheat water to 180°F in a sous vide cooker or with an immersion circulator. Vacuum-seal apples, brown sugar, lemon juice, cinnamon and nutmeg in a sous vide bag or use a plastic zip-top freezer bag /remove as much air as possible from the bag before sealing. Submerge bag in water and cook for 45 minutes. Remove bag from cooking water and mash apples in pouch to desired consistency. For a smoother sauce, empty cooking bag into a food processor and puree to desired consistency. Serve applesauce immediately or refrigerate for later use. Enjoy!

Nutrition Info:Calories: 77; Total Fat: 0g; Saturated Fat: 0g; Protein: 0g; Carbs: 20g; Fiber: 3g; Sugar: 17g

Peach And Almond Yogurt

INGREDIENTS for Servings: 4

2 cup whole milk	¼ cup mashed peeled peaches
4 ounces ground almonds	¼ tsp vanilla sugar
2 tbsp yogurt	1 tbsp honey

DIRECTIONS and Cooking Time: 11 Hour 20 Minutes
Prepare a water bath and place the Sous Vide in it. Set to 110 F. Heat the milk in a saucepan until the temperature reaches 142 F. Let cook at 110 F. Stir yogurt, honey, peaches and sugar. Divide the mixture between 4 jars. Seal the jars and immerse in water bath. Cook for 11 hour. Once timer has stopped, remove the jars. Stir in almonds and serve.

Tomato Shrub

INGREDIENTS for Servings: 12

2 cups diced tomatoes	2 cups red wine vinegar
2 cups granulated sugar	1 cup water

DIRECTIONS and Cooking Time: 1 Hour 30 Minutes
Prepare your Sous Vide water bath using your immersion circulator and raise the temperature to 180-degrees Fahrenheit. Add all the listed ingredients to a resealable zip bag and seal using the immersion method. Cook for 1 ½ hour. Once done,

remove and strain the contents into a bowl. Discard any solids and transfer to storing jar. Serve as needed!

Nutrition Info: Calories: 126 Carbohydrate: 30g Protein: 1g Fat: 0g Sugar: 28g Sodium: 80mg

Orange Cheesy Mousse

INGREDIENTS for Servings: 8

2 cups milk	¼ cup powdered
6 tbsp white wine	sugar
vinegar	Grand Marnier liquor
4 oz chocolate chips	1 tbsp orange zest
	2 oz goat cheese

DIRECTIONS and Cooking Time: 1 Hour 25 Minutes
Prepare a water bath and place the Sous Vide in it. Set to 172 F. Place the milk and vinegar in a vacuum-sealable bag. Release air by the water displacement method, seal and submerge the bag in the water bath. Cook for 60 minutes. Once the timer has stopped, remove the bag and reserve the curds. Discard the remaining liquid. Strain the curds for 10 minutes. Allow chilling for 1 hour. Prepare a water bath to medium heat and add the chocolate chips. Cook until melted. Transfer to a blender and stir the sugar, orange zest, grand Marnier, goat cheese. Mix until smooth. Serve into individual bowls.

Chocolate & Ricotta Mousse

INGREDIENTS for Servings: 8

2 quarts' whole milk	¼ cup powdered
6 tablespoons white	sugar
wine vinegar	Grand Marnier liquor
4 oz. semisweet	1 tablespoon orange
chocolate chips	zest
	2 oz. ricotta

DIRECTIONS and Cooking Time: 60 Minutes
Set up your Sous Vide immersion circulator to a temperature of 172-degrees Fahrenheit and prepare your water bath. Put the milk and vinegar to a resealable zip bag. Seal using the immersion method and cook for 1 hour. Once done, remove the bag and skim the curds from top and transfer to a strainer lined with cheesecloth. Discard any remaining liquid. Let it sit and drain the curd for about 10 minutes. Then chill for 1 hour. Prepare your double broiler by setting a bowl over a small saucepan filled with 1 inch of water Bring the water to a low simmer over medium heat. Add the chocolate chips to a bowl of the double boiler and cook until it has melted. Transfer to a food processor. Add the sugar, orange zest, grand mariner, ricotta, and then process until smooth Transfer to individual bowls and serve!

Nutrition Info: Per serving:Calories: 472 ;Carbohydrate: 37g ;Protein: 6g ;Fat: 35g ;Sugar: 34g ;Sodium: 103mg

Maple Potato Flan

INGREDIENTS for Servings: 6

1 cup milk	½ cup sweet potatoes
1 cup heavy whipping	puree
cream	¼ cup maple syrup
3 whole eggs	½ tsp pumpkin spice
3 egg yolks	Sugar for garnish

DIRECTIONS and Cooking Time: 1 Hour 10 Minutes
Prepare a water bath and place Sous Vide in it. Set to 168 F Combine the milk, heavy cream, whole eggs, egg yolks, sweet potatoes puree, maple syrup, and pumpkin spice. Mix until smooth. Pour into mason jars. Seal and submerge in the water bath. Cook for 1 hour. Once ready, remove the jars and allow chilling. Sprinkle with sugar, place under broiler until the sugar is caramelized, and serve.

Banana Buckwheat Porridge

INGREDIENTS for Servings: 4

2 cups buckwheat	1 tsp vanilla extract
1 banana, mashed	1 ½ cup water
½ cup condensed milk	¼ tsp salt
1 tbsp butter	

DIRECTIONS and Cooking Time: 12 Hours 15 Minutes
Prepare a water bath and place the Sous Vide in it. Set to 180 F. Place the buckwheat in a vacumm-sealable bag. Whisk the remaining ingredients in a bowl. Pour this mixture over the buckwheat. Release air by the water displacement method, seal and submerge the bag in water bath.Set the timer for 12 hours. Once the timer has stopped, remove the bag. Serve warm.

Chocolate Pots De Crème

INGREDIENTS for Servings: 12

1 cup fruit-forward	12 oz. semisweet
red wine	chocolate chips
½ cup granulated	1 cup whole milk
sugar	½ cup heavy cream
8 ounces	8 large egg yolks
unsweetened dark	A pinch of kosher salt
chocolate, finely	
chopped up	

DIRECTIONS and Cooking Time: 45 Minutes
Set up your Sous Vide immersion circulator to a temperature of 180-degrees Fahrenheit and prepare your water bath. Take a medium-sized saucepan and place it over medium-high heat. Add the wine and sugar and bring the mixture to a boil, reduce heat

to medium-low and simmer for 20 minutes. Remove and allow it to cool for 10 minutes. Transfer to a food processor and add the chocolate chips, unsweetened dark chocolate, milk, cream, salt, and egg yolks. Blend well until smooth. Then, transfer the mixture to a resealable bag and seal using the immersion method, cook for 45 minutes. Once cooked, remove the bag and transfer the contents to a food processor. Blend for 2 minutes. Divide the mixture among 12 ramekins and cover them with plastic wrap. Chill for 4 hours and serve!

Nutrition Info:Per serving:Calories: 793 ;Carbohydrate: 56g ;Protein: 13g ;Fat: 62g ;Sugar: 51g ;Sodium: 494mg

Doce De Banana

INGREDIENTS for Servings: 4

5 small ripe bananas, firm but ripe, peeled and cut up into chunks	6 whole cloves
1 cup brown sugar	Whipped cream for serving
2 cinnamon sticks	Vanilla ice-cream for serving

DIRECTIONS and Cooking Time: 40 Minutes
Set up your Sous Vide immersion circulator to a temperature of 176-degrees Fahrenheit and prepare your water bath. Put the bananas, brown sugar, cinnamon sticks, and cloves to a resealable bag. Seal using the immersion method and cook for 30-40 minutes. Remove the bag and allow the contents to cool. Open the bag and remove the cinnamon sticks and cloves. Serve warm in a bowl with a topping of whipped cream and vanilla ice cream.

Nutrition Info:Per serving:Calories: 310 ;Carbohydrate: 80g ;Protein: 1g ;Fat: 0g ;Sugar: 65g ;Sodium: 9mg

Almond Nectarine Pie

INGREDIENTS for Servings: 6

3 cups nectarines, peeled and diced	1 tsp vanilla extract
	1 tsp almond extract
8 tbsp butter	1 cup milk
1 cup sugar	1 cup flour

DIRECTIONS and Cooking Time: 3 Hours 20 Minutes
Prepare a water bath and place the Sous Vide in it. Set to 194 F. Grease small jars with cooking spray. Gather the nectarines amongst the jars. In a bowl, mix sugar and butter. Add the almond extract, whole milk and vanilla extract, mix well. Stir the self-rising flour and blend until solid. Place the batter into the jars. Seal and submerge the jars in the water bath. Cook for 180 minutes. Once the timer has stopped, remove the jars. Serve.

Lemon And Crème Brulee

INGREDIENTS for Servings: 4

6 large egg yolks	4 tablespoon, freshly squeezed lemon juice
1 and 1/3 cup, superfine sugar	1 teaspoon, vanilla extract
3 cups of heavy whip cream	1 cup, fresh blueberries
2 lemon zest	

DIRECTIONS and Cooking Time: 1 Hour 10 Minutes
Set up your Sous Vide immersion circulator to a temperature of 195ºF and prepare your water bath Take an electric mixer and whisk in egg yolks, sugar until you have a creamy mixture, keep it on the side Take a medium saucepan and place it over medium heat, add cream and heat it up Add lemon zest, lemon juice, vanilla and stir simmer for 4-5 minute over low heat Remove the cream mixture from heat and allow it to cool, once cooled transfer a small amount into egg mix and whisk well Add remaining cream mixture into the egg and stir Divide the blueberries among six pieces of mini mason jars and pour the egg cream mix over the blueberries divide the mixture amongst the jars Tightly seal the lid and submerge, cook for 45 minutes Remove the jars from water bath and chill for 5 hours Caramelize a layer of sugar on top using a blowtorch and serve!

Nutrition Info:Per serving:Calories 154, Carbohydrates 5 g, Fats 10 g, Protein 11 g

Greek Yogurt

INGREDIENTS for Servings: 4

3 tablespoons plain yogurt with live active cultures /or yogurt starter	4 cups whole milk

DIRECTIONS and Cooking Time: 24 Hours
In a large saucepan over low heat, warm milk to 185°F, stirring occasionally to prevent scalding. Remove milk from heat and let cool to 100°F to 110°F /use a cold-water or ice-water bath to speed milk cooling if desired, but watch milk temperature closely. Meanwhile, preheat water to 115°F in a sous vide cooker or with an immersion circulator. Whisk plain yogurt into milk , pour into a large canning jar and screw on lid. Submerge jar in water bath and incubate for 24 hours. Line a strainer with a double layer of cheesecloth. Pour yogurt into strainer and let stand until whey is drained and yogurt is thickened, about 4 hours. Spoon yogurt into 4 small canning jars and refrigerate until chilled through before serving. Stored in the covered jars, yogurt will keep in the refrigerator for up to one month. Enjoy!

Nutrition Info:Calories: 160; Total Fat: 3g; Saturated Fat: 2g; Protein: 23g; Carbs: 9g; Fiber: 0g; Sugar: 7g

Banana Cream

INGREDIENTS for Servings: 4

5 bananas, chopped	6 whole cloves
1 cup brown sugar	Whipped cream for serving
2 cinnamon sticks	Vanilla ice-cream for serving
5 drops vanilla extract	

DIRECTIONS and Cooking Time: 60 Minutes
Prepare a water bath and place the Sous Vide in it. Set to 182 F. Place banana, brown sugar, vanilla, cinnamon sticks, and cloves in a vacuum-sealable bag. Release air by the water displacement method, seal and submerge the bag in the water bath. Cook for 40 minutes. Once the timer has stopped, remove the bag and allow cooling. Discard the cinnamon sticks and cloves. Serve warm whipped with cream.

Mocha Mini Brownies In A Jar

INGREDIENTS for Servings: 10

⅔ cup white chocolate, chopped	1 tbsp coconut extract
8 tbsp butter	1 tbsp coffee liqueur
⅔ cup superfine sugar	½ cup all-purpose flour
2 egg yolks	Ice cream, for serving
1 egg	
2 tbsp instant coffee powder	

DIRECTIONS and Cooking Time: 3 Hours 17 Minutes
Prepare a water bath and place Sous Vide in it. Set to 196 F. Heat the chocolate and butter in a pot or in the microwave. Fold sugar into the chocolate-butter mixture until dissolved. Pour the egg yolks one by one and stir well. Add in whole egg and continue mixing. Pour in coffee powder, coconut extract and coffee liqueur. Add in flour and stir until combined well. Pour the chocolate mixture into 10 mini mason jars. Seal with a lid and submerge the jars in the water bath, Cook for 3 hours. Once the timer has stopped, remove the jars and allow to cool for 1 minute.

Cookie Dough

INGREDIENTS for Servings: 6

½ cup softened butter	1 ¼ cups almond flour
¾ cup brown sugar	½ cup salted caramel chips
1 teaspoon molasses	
1 medium egg	

DIRECTIONS and Cooking Time: 10 Minutes
Preheat your cooker to 171F. Cream the butter with sugar in a large bowl. Fold in molasses and egg. Stir until smooth. Fold in the almond flour and mix until just combined. Add caramel chips and mix until incorporated. Refrigerate 1 hour. Remove the dough from the fridge and shape into 12 balls. Place the balls into Sous Vide bag and press each to ½-inch thick. Vacuum seal the bag and submerge in water. Cook the dough 10 minutes. Finishing steps: Remove the bag from the water bath and chill in a fridge 10 minutes. Open the bag carefully and serve the cookie dough.

Nutrition Info: Calories 253 Total Fat 19g Total Carb 19g Dietary Fiber 6g Protein 4g

Homemade Compote Of Strawberries

INGREDIENTS for Servings: 8

½ cup sugar	1 tbsp lemon zest
1 tbsp freshly squeezed lemon juice	1 tbsp cornstarch
	1 pound strawberries

DIRECTIONS and Cooking Time: 75 Minutes
Prepare a water bath and place the Sous Vide in it. Set to 18F. Combine well the sugar, lemon juice, lemon zest and cornstarch. Add strawberries and mix well. Place it in a vacuum-sealable bag. Release air by the water displacement method, seal and submerge the bag in the water bath. Cook for 60 minutes. Once the timer has stopped, remove the bag and transfer to a serving plate. Serve warm.

Kiwi & Vanilla Fresh Mint

INGREDIENTS for Servings: 2

2 peeled and sliced kiwis	2 generous tablespoons yogurt/ vanilla ice cream
2 tablespoons granulated sugar	Fresh mint leaves for garnishing
1 tablespoon freshly squeezed lemon juice	

DIRECTIONS and Cooking Time: 20 Minutes
Set up your Sous Vide immersion circulator to a temperature of 176-degrees Fahrenheit and prepare your water bath. Take a medium bowl and add the kiwi slices, sugar, lemon juice and stir. Transfer the mixture to a resealable zipper bag and seal using the immersion method. Cook for 20 minutes and remove the bag from the water bath. Divide the mixture between 2 serving plates. Scoop yogurt/ vanilla ice cream onto the plate next to your kiwi and garnish with some mint leaves. Serve!

Nutrition Info: Per serving:Calories: 148 ;Carbohydrate: 21g ;Protein: 5g ;Fat: 5g ;Sugar: 15g ;Sodium: 106mg

Basic Oatmeal From Scratch

INGREDIENTS for Servings: 4

1 cup oats	½ tsp vanilla extract
3 cups water	Pinch of sea salt

DIRECTIONS and Cooking Time: 8 Hours 10 Minutes
Prepare a water bath and place the Sous Vide in it. Set to 155 F. Combine all the ingredients in a vacumm-sealable bag. Release air by the water displacement method, seal and submerge the bag in water bath.Set the timer for 8 hours.   Once the timer has stopped, remove the bag. Serve warm.

Wine & Maple Poached Pears
INGREDIENTS

2 cups white wine	1¼ cups sugar
2 cups water	4 pears
1 cup maple syrup	

DIRECTIONS and Cooking Time: 1 Hour 5 Mins
Cooking Temperature: 176°f
Attach the sous vide immersion circulator using an adjustable clamp to a Cambro container or pot filled with water and preheat to 176°F.   Into a pan, add all ingredients except pears and simmer until sauce reduces a little.   Remove from heat and keep aside to cool.   Into a cooking pouch, add pears and syrup. Seal pouch tightly after squeezing out the excess air. Place pouch in sous vide bath and set the cooking time for 1 hour.   Remove pouch from sous vide bath and carefully open it.   Transfer pears onto a plate, drizzle with sauce, and serve.

Pumpkin Bread
INGREDIENTS

1 cup all-purpose flour	pinch of ground cloves
1 teaspoon baking powder	⅓ cup granulated sugar
¼ teaspoon baking soda	¼ cup dark brown sugar
2 teaspoons ground cinnamon	¾ cup canned pumpkin puree
½ teaspoon ground nutmeg	½ teaspoon salt
½ cup vegetable oil	2 large eggs

DIRECTIONS and Cooking Time: 3 Hours Cooking Temperature: 195°f
Attach the sous vide immersion circulator using an adjustable clamp to a Cambro container or pot filled with water and preheat to 195°F.   Generously grease 4 half-pint canning jars.   In a bowl, mix together flour, baking powder, baking soda and spices.   In another bowl, add oil, both sugars, pumpkin puree and salt.and beat until well-combined.   Add eggs, one at a time, beating until well-combined.   Add flour mixture into pumpkin mixture, and mix until just combined. Divide mixture evenly into prepared jars. (Each jar should be not full more than two-thirds full).   With a damp towel, wipe off sides and tops of jars. Tap the

jars onto a counter firmly to remove air bubbles. Close each jar. (Do not over-tighten jars because air will need to escape).   Place jars in sous vide bath and set the cooking time for 3 hours.   Remove the jars from sous vide bath and carefully remove the lids. Place jars onto a wire rack to cool completely. Carefully run a knife around the inside edges of the jars to loosen the bread from the walls.   Cut into slices and serve.

Pumpkin Pie Jars
INGREDIENTS for Servings: 6

1 large can pumpkin pie filling	2 tablespoons flour
1 egg + 3 egg yolks	1 can evaporated milk
½ teaspoon kosher salt	½ cup white sugar
1 tablespoon pumpkin pie spice	½ cup brown sugar
	Whipped cream and candied nuts for garnishing

DIRECTIONS and Cooking Time: 60 Minutes
Set up your Sous Vide immersion circulator to a temperature of 175-degrees Fahrenheit and prepare your water bath.   Add 1 large can of pumpkin pie filling, 2 tablespoons of flour, ½ teaspoon of kosher salt, 1 tablespoon of pumpkin pie spice, 1 egg and 3 egg yolks alongside 1 can of evaporated milk.   Whisk them well.   Pour the mixture into 6.4-ounce jars and seal them tightly.   Submerge underwater and cook for 1 hour.   Once done, remove the jars and chill for 8 hours.   Garnish with whipped cream and candied nuts.   Serve!

Nutrition Info: Per serving:Calories: 269 ;Carbohydrate: 24g ;Protein: 5g ;Fat: 17g ;Sugar: 3g ;Sodium: 145mg

Incredible Coffee Dessert
INGREDIENTS for Servings: 8

1/3 cup espresso	1/3 cup sugar
¾ cup milk	½ tsp salt
1 cup heavy cream	Whipped cream
6 oz white chopped chocolate	4 large egg yolks

DIRECTIONS and Cooking Time: 3 Hours 10 Minutes
Prepare a water bath and place the Sous Vide in it. Set to 182 F.   Heat a saucepan over medium heat and stir the heavy cream, espresso and milk. Remove from the heat and add the chocolate. Cook for 15 minutes. Combine egg yolks, salt, and sugar in a bowl. Mix in the chocolate mixture. Allow cooling. Place the mixture in a vacuum-sealable bag. Release air by water displacement method, seal and submerge in the bath. Cook for 30 minutes. Once done, transfer contents to small ramekins. Chill for 2 hours.

French Vanilla Custard Dessert

INGREDIENTS for Servings: 6

½ cup granulated sugar	8 large egg yolks
1 tsp vanilla bean paste	½ cup milk
	1 cup whipping cream

DIRECTIONS and Cooking Time: 5 Hours 25 Minutes
Prepare water bath and place Sous Vide in it. Set to 182 F. Whisk egg yolks, sugar, and vanilla paste. Heat whipping cream and milk in a pot over high heat. Mix in the egg mixture and allow cooling for 20 minutes. Put the mixture in 6 glass jars. Seal and submerge in the water bath. Cook for 45 minutes. Once the timer has stopped, remove the jars and allow cooling for 10 minutes. Transfer into an ice-water bath and allow chilling for 4 hours.

Coffee Buttery Bread

INGREDIENTS for Servings: 4

6 ounces white bread	½ tsp cinnamon
¾ cup butter	1 tsp brown sugar
6 tbsp coffee	

DIRECTIONS and Cooking Time: 3 Hours 15 Minutes
Prepare a water bath and place the Sous Vide in it. Set to 195 F. Slice the bread into strips and place in a vacumm-sealable bag. Whisk the other ingredients in a bowl and pour the mixture over the bread. Release air by the water displacement method, seal and submerge the bag in water bath.Set the timer for 3 hours. Once the timer has stopped, remove the bag. Serve warm.

Wine And Cinnamon Poached Pears

INGREDIENTS for Servings: 4

4 pears, peeled	1/3 cup sugar
2 cinnamon sticks	3 star anise
2 cups red wine	

DIRECTIONS and Cooking Time: 80 Minutes
Prepare a water bath and place the Sous Vide in it. Set to 175 F. Combine the wine, anise, sugar, and cinnamon in a large vacumm-sealable bag. Place the pears inside. Release air by the water displacement method, seal and submerge the bag in water bath.Set the timer for 1 hour. Once the timer has stopped, remove the bag. Serve the pears drizzle with the wine sauce.

Coconut Banana Oatrolls With Walnuts

INGREDIENTS for Servings: 4

2 cups rolled oats	1 tsp vanilla extract
3 cups coconut milk	1 cup of walnuts, chopped
3 cups skimmed milk	
3 mashed bananas	

DIRECTIONS and Cooking Time: 6-10 Hours 5 Minutes
Prepare a water bath and place the Sous Vide in it. Set to 182 F. Combine all the ingredients and place in a vacuum-sealable bag. Release air by the water displacement method, seal and submerge the bag in the water bath. Cook for 6-10 hours. Once the timer has stopped, remove the bags and transfer the oats into serving bowls. Top with walnuts.

Limoncello Vodka Cocktail

INGREDIENTS for Servings: 5

1 bottle vodka	1 cup granulated sugar
Grated zest/peel of 10-15 thoroughly washed lemons	1 cup water

DIRECTIONS and Cooking Time: 180 Minutes
Prepare your Sous Vide water bath using your immersion circulator and raise the temperature to 135-degrees Fahrenheit. Add the vodka and lemon zest to a large zip bag and seal using the immersion method. Cook for 2-3 hours. Take a saucepan and put it over medium-high heat Add the sugar and water and stir until the sugar dissolves to prepare the syrup Once done, take the bag out from the water bath and strain through metal mesh into a bowl. Stir in syrup. Pour Limoncello into bottles and serve!

Nutrition Info: Calories: 430 Carbohydrate: 61g Protein: 1g Fat: 0g Sugar: 53g Sodium: 8mg

Chocolate Pudding

INGREDIENTS for Servings: 4

½ cup milk	½ cup heavy cream
1 cup chocolate chips	4 tbsp cocoa powder
3 egg yolks	3 tbsp sugar

DIRECTIONS and Cooking Time: 55 Minutes
Prepare a water bath and place the Sous Vide in it. Set to 185 F. Whisk the yolks along with sugar, milk, and heavy cream. Stir in cocoa powder and chocolate chips. Divide the mixture between 4 jars. Seal and immerse the jars in the water bath. Set the timer for 40 minutes. Once the timer has stopped, remove the jars. Let cool before serving.

Peach With Lavender

INGREDIENTS

2 peaches, halved and pitted	¼ cup water
¼ cup honey	1 tablespoon dried lavender buds

DIRECTIONS and Cooking Time: 20 Mins Cooking Temperature: 185°f
Attach the sous vide immersion circulator using an adjustable clamp to a Cambro container or pot filled with water and preheat to 185°F. Into a cooking pouch, add all ingredients. Seal pouch tightly after squeezing out the excess air. Place pouch in sous vide bath and set the cooking time for 20 minutes. Remove pouch from sous vide bath and immediately plunge into a large bowl of ice water for 15-20 minutes. Open the pouch and transfer peaches into a bowl. Through a fine-mesh sieve, strain the poaching liquid into a bowl. Discard the lavender buds. Serve chilled peach halves chilled, along with pouching liquid.

Coconut And Almond Oatmeal

INGREDIENTS for Servings: 4

2 cups oatmeal	3 tbsp stevia extract
2 cups almond milk	1 tbsp butter
3 tbsp shredded coconut	¼ tsp ground anise
3 tbsp flaked almonds	Pinch of sea salt

DIRECTIONS and Cooking Time: 12 Hours 10 Minutes
Prepare a water bath and place the Sous Vide in it. Set to 180 F. Combine all the ingredients in a vacumm-sealable bag. Release air by the water displacement method, seal and submerge the bag in water bath.Set the timer for 12 hours. Once the timer has stopped, remove the bag and divide into 4 serving bowls.

Rhubarb & Blueberry Shrub Cocktail

INGREDIENTS for Servings: 12

2 cups sugar	1 cup diced blueberries
2 cups balsamic vinegar	1 cup water
1 cup diced rhubarb	

DIRECTIONS and Cooking Time: 1 Hour 45 Minutes
Prepare a water bath and place Sous Vide in it. Set to 182 F. Combine all the ingredients and place in vacuum-sealable bag. Release air by water displacement method, seal and submerge in the bath. Cook for 90 minutes. Once done, remove the bag and drain the contents. Reserve the fruit. Allow chilling.

Baked Ricotta

INGREDIENTS for Servings: 6

2 quarts whole milk	1 ½ teaspoon smoked salt
6 tablespoons white wine vinegar	1 teaspoon fresh ground smoked black pepper
2 large eggs	
2 tablespoons extra virgin olive oil	

DIRECTIONS and Cooking Time: 60 Minutes
Set up your Sous Vide immersion circulator to a temperature of 172-degrees Fahrenheit and prepare your water bath. Add the milk and vinegar to a resealable zip bag. Seal using the immersion method and cook for 1 hour. Preheat your oven to 350-degrees Fahrenheit. Remove the bag and skim the curd off the top. Then, pass the mixture through a strainer lined with a cheesecloth and discard any remaining liquid. Drain the curd for 10 minutes. Transfer drained curds to food processor alongside the eggs, salt, olive oil, and pepper. Process for 20 seconds. Divide the ricotta mixture between 6 oven proof ramekins and bake for 30 minutes until golden brown. Serve!

Nutrition Info: Per serving:Calories: 145 ;Carbohydrate: 3g ;Protein: 10g ;Fat: 10g ;Sugar: 0g ;Sodium: 342mg

Champagne Zabaglione

INGREDIENTS for Servings: 6

1 cup heavy cream	1 teaspoon vanilla extract
½ cup champagne	A pinch of kosher salt
½ cup ultrafine sugar	
4 large egg yolks	

DIRECTIONS and Cooking Time: 45 Minutes
Set up your Sous Vide immersion circulator to a temperature of 180-degrees Fahrenheit and prepare your water bath. Add all the listed ingredients to a blender and purée for 30 seconds. Transfer to a resealable zip bag and seal using the immersion method. Cook for 45 minutes and once done, transfer the bag to an ice bath. Serve immediately!

Nutrition Info: Per serving:Calories: 375 ;Carbohydrate: 28g ;Protein: 4g ;Fat: 27g ;Sugar: 27g ;Sodium: 62mg

Sous Vide Crème Brulee

INGREDIENTS for Servings: 4

¼ cup sugar	3 large egg yolks
1 pinch salt	Brown sugar, to sprinkle
1 cup heavy cream	

DIRECTIONS and Cooking Time: 1 Hour
Preheat Sous Vide cooker to 181F. Combine all ingredients in a food blender. Blend until smooth.

Transfer the content into Sous Vide bag. Fold the edges, and remove as much as air possible. Clip the bag to the side of your pot. Submerge the bag into a water bath and cook 60 minutes. Make sure you remove the bag after 30 minutes and shake gently. Finishing steps: Remove the bag from the cooker. Divide the bag content between four ramekins. Sprinkle the egg custard with brown sugar. Caramelize the sugar with a torch. Serve.

Nutrition Info:Calories 191 Total Fat 15g Total Carb 18g Dietary Fiber 0g Protein 6g

Cinnamon Spiced Apples

INGREDIENTS for Servings: 4

4 tart peeled apples	2 tablespoons raisins
1 lemon juice	¼ teaspoon fine sea
3 tablespoons	salt
unsalted butter	¼ teaspoon grated
2 tablespoons light	nutmeg
brown sugar	1/9 teaspoon vanilla
2 whole fresh dates	extract
pitted	Freshly whipped ice
1 tablespoon ground	cream
cinnamon	

DIRECTIONS and Cooking Time: 120 Minutes
Set up your Sous Vide immersion circulator to a temperature of 183-degrees Fahrenheit and prepare your water bath. Core the apples and toss the apples with lemon juice. Take a medium bowl and add the butter, brown sugar, dates, raisins, cinnamon, salt, vanilla, and nutmeg. Take a fork and mash the mixture into a chunky paste. Divide the mixture and fill the apple cores. Transfer the apple to a resealable zipper bag and seal using the immersion method. Cook for 2 hours. Remove the bags from the water bath. Take the apples out from the bag and place them on serving plates. Serve apples with whipped cream/ice cream.

Nutrition Info:Per serving:Calories: 259 ;Carbohydrate: 30g ;Protein: 0g ;Fat: 0g ;Sugar: 24g ;Sodium: 11mg

Sweet Candied Potatoes

INGREDIENTS for Servings: 8

2 lbs. sweet potatoes,	¼ cup maple syrup
peeled up and cut into	1 teaspoon kosher salt
¼ slices	1 cup chopped
½ cup unsalted butter	walnuts
2 oranges, juice and	1 cinnamon stick
zest	¼ cup brown sugar

DIRECTIONS and Cooking Time: 120 Minutes
Set up your Sous Vide immersion circulator to a temperature of 155-degrees Fahrenheit and prepare your water bath. Take a resealable bag and add the sweet potatoes and ¼ cup of butter. Seal using the

immersion method and cook for 2 hours. Preheat your oven to 350-degrees Fahrenheit. Remove the potatoes from the bag and pat dry. Arrange the potatoes evenly in a baking dish. Take a medium saucepan and bring ¼ cup of butter, brown sugar, maple syrup, orange zest, juice, walnuts, salt, and cinnamon stick to a boil. Remove from heat and pour over sweet potatoes, discard the cinnamon stick Bake for 30 minutes and serve warm!

Nutrition Info:Per serving:Calories: 320 ;Carbohydrate: 67g ;Protein: 3g ;Fat: 5g ;Sugar: 34g ;Sodium: 215mg

Dark Chocolate Mousse

INGREDIENTS for Servings: 4

2/3 cup dark	½ cup double cream
chocolate, chopped	½ tsp gelatin powder
½ cup milk	2 tbsp cold water

DIRECTIONS and Cooking Time: 24 Hours + 7 Hours
Preheat your Sous Vide machine to 194ºF. Place the chopped dark chocolate in the vacuum bag. Seal the bag, put it into the water bath and set the timer for 6 hours. When the time is up, pour the chocolate into a bowl and stir with a spoon. Pour the milk into a pan and warm it over medium heat. Soak the gelatin powder in 2 tbsp cold water and dissolve it in the warm milk. Carefully stir the milk-gelatin mixture into the chocolate paste until even and refrigerate for 25 minutes. Remove from the fridge, stir again and refrigerate for another 25 minutes. Beat the cream to peaks and combine with white chocolate mixture. Pour into single serve cups and refrigerate for 24 hours before serving.

Nutrition Info:Per serving:Calories 227, Carbohydrates 19 g, Fats 15 g, Protein 4 g

Chocolate Chili Cake

INGREDIENTS for Servings: 6

4 large eggs	½ lb. chocolate chips
4oz. unsalted butter	½ teaspoon chili
2 tablespoons cocoa	powder
powder	¼ cup brown sugar

DIRECTIONS and Cooking Time: 1 Hour 15 Minutes
Preheat the Sous Vide cooker to 115F. Place the chocolate chips, and butter into Sous Vide bag. Submerge in water and cook 15 minutes. Remove the bag and set the cooker to 170F. Prepare 6 4oz. Mason jars by coating with cooking spray. Beat the eggs with brown sugar until fluffy. Stir in the chocolate, cocoa powder, and chili powder. Divide the mixture between prepared mason jars and apply the lid on finger tight only. Submerge the jars in a water bath for 1 hour. Finishing steps: Remove the jars and place onto wire rack to cool completely.

Invert the cake onto a plate. Serve with raspberry ice cream

Nutrition Info: Calories 413 Total Fat 31g Total Carb 28g Dietary Fiber 9g Protein 6g

Lemony Muffins

INGREDIENTS for Servings: 6

2 eggs	1/3 cup heavy cream
1 cup flour	2 eggs
4 tbsp sugar	1 tsp baking soda
1 tbsp lemon juice	½ cup butter
1 tbsp lemon zest	

DIRECTIONS and Cooking Time: 3 Hours 45 Minutes
Prepare a water bath and place the Sous Vide in it. Set to 190 F. Beat the eggs and sugar until creamy. Gradually beat in the remaining ingredients. Divide the batter between 6 mason jars. Seal the jars and submerge the bag in water bath.Set the timer for 3 hours and 30 minutes. Once the timer has stopped, remove the jars. Let cool before serving.

Lemon & Berry Mousse

INGREDIENTS for Servings: 8

1 pound raspberries, halved	½ tsp salt
¼ cup light brown sugar	¼ tsp ground cinnamon
3 tbsp freshly squeezed lemon juice	1 cup heavy cream
	1 tsp vanilla extract
	1 cup crème fraiche

DIRECTIONS and Cooking Time: 65 Minutes
Prepare a water bath and place the Sous Vide in it. Set to 182 F. Place the raspberries, brown sugar, lemon juice, salt, and cinnamon in a vacuum-sealable bag. Release air by water displacement method, seal and submerge the bag in the water bath. Cook for 45 minutes. Once the timer has stopped, remove the bag and transfer the contents to a blender. Stir until smooth. Whisk the heavy cream and vanilla. Pour in the raspberries mix with the créme fraiche and combine well. Transfer into 8 serving bowls. Allow chilling.

Vanilla Cheesecake

INGREDIENTS for Servings: 6

12 oz cream cheese, at room temperature	2 eggs
½ cup sugar	Zest of 1 lemon
¼ cup mascarpone, at room temperature	½ tbsp vanilla extract

DIRECTIONS and Cooking Time: 1 Hour 45 Minutes
Prepare a water bath and place the Sous Vide in it. Set to 175 F. Combine cream cheese, mascarpone and sugar. Mix well. Stir in the eggs. Add in lemon zest and vanilla extract. Mix well. Pour the mixture in 6 mason jars. Seal and submerge in the water bath. Cook for 90 minutes. Once the timer has stopped, remove the jars and allow chilling. Top with fruit compote.

Pumpkin Crème Brulée

INGREDIENTS for Servings: 5

1 cup milk	¼ cup maple syrup
1 cup heavy whipping cream	½ teaspoon pumpkin spice
3 whole eggs	A pinch of kosher salt
3 egg yolks	Granulated sugar
½ cup pumpkin puree	

DIRECTIONS and Cooking Time: 60 Minutes
Set up your Sous Vide immersion circulator to a temperature of 167-degrees Fahrenheit and prepare your water bath. Take a large bowl and add the milk, heavy cream, 3 whole eggs, 3 egg yolks, ½ cup of pumpkin puree, ¼ cup of maple syrup, ½ teaspoon of pumpkin spice and a pinch of kosher salt. Whisk them well and keep whisking until it is combined and smooth. Pour the mixture into 6.4-ounce mason jars. Place the lid loosely and cook for 1 hour underwater. Allow them to chill. Spread a thin layer of sugar on top of the custard and caramelize with a blowtorch. Serve!

Nutrition Info: Per serving:Calories: 148 ;Carbohydrate: 21g ;Protein: 5g ;Fat: 5g ;Sugar: 15g ;Sodium: 106mg

APPENDIX : RECIPES INDEX

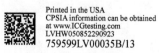
Printed in the USA
CPSIA information can be obtained
at www.ICGtesting.com
LVHW050852290923
759599LV00035B/13